Fraser's Horse Book

Alistair Fraser was born into a 'veterinary family' in 1903. He studied Veterinary Science at Liverpool and at the Pasteur Institute in Paris, taking a PhD at Cambridge University, and later held a commission in the Royal Army Veterinary Corps. He has spent over twenty years in practice in Berkshire, one of Britain's major horse training areas. He has hunted with hounds and played polo, and from 1963 to 1974 was Veterinary Surgeon to Her Majesty the Queen. He acted as Assistant Editor (1963–76) on the *Equine Veterinary Journal.* Dr Fraser now lives in Wiltshire.

Frank Manolson, DVM, was a member of the Royal College of Veterinary Surgeons. He practised in the United States, Canada, England and Central America. He died shortly before the publication of this book.

Tina Wommelsdorf has added notes for the Australian market.

Also by Frank Manolson in Pan Books

C is for Cat
D is for Dog

Frank Manolson and **Alistair Fraser**
with Australian notes by Tina Wommelsdorf

Fraser's Horse Book

The Complete Book of Horse Care

Pan Books London and Sydney

First published 1979 by Pitman Publishing Ltd
This edition published 1980 by Pan Books Ltd,
Cavaye Place, London SW10 9PG

ISBN 0 330 26154 1
Set, printed and bound in Great Britain by
Cox & Wyman Ltd, Reading

Contents

Acknowledgements

Top of our list must go Val Watson of Aldbourne who with endless patience and humour typed at least half a dozen versions of this tome.

We hope that our wives won't mind sharing second place. Olive Fraser must have read each version several times and she provided enthusiastic encouragement. Margaret Manolson brewed a lot of tea for our endless consultations while saying, 'Excuse me if I pop out. I don't know anything about horses.'

In the publishing world we would like to thank Simon Master of Pan Books and Navin Sullivan of Pitman Publishing Ltd, both of whom demonstrated confidence in the project before seeing a word. And to Kyle Cathie of Pan, pragmatic editor, who nicely guided our flights of fancy down to solid earth.

In the horse world we have had help from people too numerous to mention. We hope that Caroline Silver of Crooked Soley won't mind if we drop her name. Our gratitude too to Peter Free of Marlborough, now in the rarified atmosphere of Downing College, Cambridge, for his researches.

In the veterinary world our thanks to Gordon Hard, formerly of Melbourne University, Australia, now at Temple University, Pennsylvania, particularly for his help with toxicology; to Professor Angus Dunn of Glasgow for his devastating comments on parisitology; to Peter Rossdale of Newmarket whose particular help is mentioned in the text of the book; to Bob Williams of Ontario, Canada; to Alan Hitchins of London, England and to Duncan McPhedran of the famous Lambourn practice who introduced us to each other.

A special vote of gratitude to Sam Hignett CBE for his forbearance and constructive suggestions.

We hope that Colin Smith FWCF won't feel that the chapter he checked so thoroughly will denigrate his standing as one time Champion Farrier of England and we believe that readers will agree that the illustrations prove that Peter Oliver merits a special medal for services beyond the call of duty to even the family of Fraser.

The section on Restraint was first published in the *Veterinary Record* and is reproduced with permission of that journal's editor.

A. F. and F. M. Aldbourne, Wiltshire, 1979

Author's note

Veterinary surgeons believe that they could keep many more horses actively useful if owners knew more about their animals' health ; so we have written this book about positive health for horses, not to encourage anybody to play at being his own vet, but to help owners to understand their horses' habits and problems and their likes and dislikes, so that both the owner and the horse can get the fullest enjoyment from working together. With this understanding many horse ailments will be avoided altogether while those that do occur will be recognised early enough for veterinary attention to achieve the best results.

Alistair Fraser

Preface

Anyone who has ever owned, ridden or trained a horse knows, or rapidly discovers, the importance of good stable management. Stable management covers many aspects of horse care with the aim of producing the horse in as healthy a condition as possible to perform whatever function is required. It goes without saying that a horse that is suffering in any way or that has not been properly prepared when it leaves the stable will not be able to give of its best.

In simple readable language Fraser's Horse Book describes both the elementary and the more refined details of the day to day care of the horse. In fact anything that anyone could possibly want to know about how to keep and look after a horse, whatever it is being used for, can be found in this book.

As well as describing the commoner diseases and ailments to which horses succumb, some of the rarer ones are also detailed in a readily understandable way making this an excellent reference book – even for the 'knowledgeable'!

Fraser's Horse Book is one of the best horse 'dictionaries' I have ever seen and I'm sure horses the world over will be grateful for its publication! I hope it will enable others to get as much enjoyment from horses as I have.

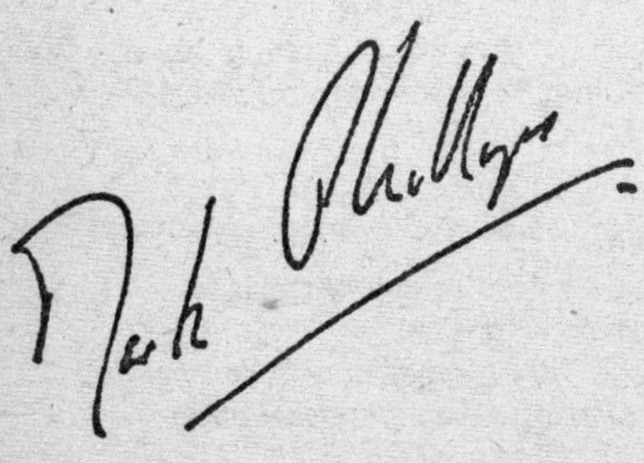

1 The healthy horse

Health

Health in horses is to be distinguished from conformation, which is the animal's inherited structure; from condition, which is related to its fat, flesh and fitness; from presentation, which covers the smartness of its turn-out; and from temperament, its reaction to other horses, people, work and to the usual and unusual events of the day.

Health, in rather a negative sense, consists of freedom from disease and injuries, but there is a more demanding state of positive health that can only be achieved and maintained by intelligent observation and constant care. This responsible attitude towards health requires a knowledge of the appearance and behaviour of horses as well as of the signs of their ailments and diseases – so that early action can be taken to avoid illness or mishaps.

Daily routine A healthy horse shows an interest in anything that is going on: looking, listening and moving responsively. The ears are the most obviously active of the sense organs and they may be seen to be recording events which do not require any other response. Horses spend a great deal of time eating. Left to themselves they graze for about 12 hours out of the 24 in several distinct periods, filling in the remainder of the time resting, though they never remain in one position for long. They rest by dozing, slumbering or sleeping. They doze on their feet with rather a hang-dog air. They slumber on the ground with their legs slightly to one side under the body, with the head raised or with the chin resting on the ground. In really favourable conditions they sleep, flat out on their sides, with the legs stretched out. In this state they really do sleep and may take some rousing, the ears turning being the first indication that they are not as dead as they appear to be. Adult horses get their exercise looking for food. Healthy foals depend on suckling from their mothers for the first few months of their lives but they graze as well from a few days old. They are actively up and about, which includes galloping in circles round the mares for exercise, or they are down on the ground slumbering or sleeping. They never doze on their feet, though in bad weather they may join their elders in adopting a hunched-up, head-down attitude with their backs to the wind and rain and their tails clamped between their hind legs. Stabled horses would follow a similar pattern of feeding and resting but this usually becomes so disorganized by the periods of exercise or work imposed on them by their owners that they give the impression that they are always ready for food. They usually have several resting periods lying down during the night.

Eating Grazing horses select the grasses they propose to eat very precisely with their lips, bite them off with their incisor teeth and grind them up with the molars which move across from right to left and then the other way for a while. They are equally selective when feeding from the manger and leave even quite minute items of which they disapprove at the bottom of the bowl. Eating should be uneventful. Any awkwardness probably means mouth injuries or tooth trouble. The processes of digestion are also uneventful. Horses do not bring up wind or regurgitate their food for a second chew as cattle do. If one listens for the purpose, digestive noises can be heard in a horse's belly consisting of gentle rumbling and intermittent tinkling and splashing sounds that usually pass unnoticed.

Droppings Horses pass wind from time to time depending on their diet. Passing wind frequently or in large quantities suggests indigestion. They pass droppings 10 to 15 times a day, usually a fair quantity at a time. The process is deliberate, the head being lowered, the ears laid back and the tail raised, although, if at work and not permitted to stop, they can pass their droppings while walking or trotting. The frequency, quantity, form, consistency, smell and colour of the droppings vary widely and are most useful indications of the animal's health and management. If the stable is to be put tidy before the veterinary surgeon's visit, it is sensible to collect up recent droppings in a skip for his information. On most stable diets the droppings consist of boluses the size of a lemon that break but retain their form on hitting the ground. The colour varies from yellow-brown to light brown and soon darkens. Horses at grass are likely to pass moister motions with green added to the colour. The smell is slightly sour and acrid. Some undigested droppings smell really foul and the cause should be sought. Whole oats or other unchanged food in the droppings may indicate indigestion or tooth trouble. If sparrows pick over the droppings and they favour one particular horse this is another useful indication that its digestive processes are faulty. Horses that are upset or in a state of fright may pass small quantities of droppings frequently.

Water Horses at pasture drink 2 or 3 times a day, the amount taken at each visit varying extremely according to the weather and the type of grazing. The daily intake may be from 8 to 36 litres (2 to 8 gallons). Stabled horses usually have water available at any time in buckets or water bowls. Buckets have the advantage that they are easily cleaned of foodstuffs that are liable to be dropped in the drinking water. If a constant supply is not given horses should be offered water before each feed.

Hot and exhausted horses that may have become dehydrated drink more freely if they are rested and cooled off for 20 to 30 minutes first, during which time they may be hosed with cold water, scraped over with a sweat scraper and turned loose to dry off or, if the weather is cold, rugged over a layer of straw or some chaff in a sack and walked in hand.

Horses are particular about their drinking water and often refuse to drink water that tastes or smells unfamiliar. It is a great advantage to horses in an exhausted (dehydrated) state to drink 8 or 12 litres (2 or 3 gallons) of water in which a cupful of molasses and a heaped tablespoonful of salt has been dissolved. They soon acquire a taste for this mixture and if they are accustomed to it it helps them to maintain their ability in competitions and overcome the effects of long journeys. Another advantage is that the additives disguise the taste of the local water which horses might otherwise refuse as unfamiliar.

Urine Horses pass their water, also called 'staling', several times a day, raising the tail, lowering the croup and stretching the hind legs apart. They prefer not to stale on hard ground causing splashing and they may retain their urine until they reach soft ground or stable bedding. Mares usually open and close the lips of the vulva after passing the last drop of urine. This should not be confused with the similar but exaggerated action of a mare ready for mating. The quantity of urine passed depends on weather conditions and the loss of moisture by sweating. The colour and consistency vary widely from a pale primrose apparently no thicker than tap water through all the spectrum of bottled beers (except Guinness) and sometimes with an amazing amount of sediment; all these from perfectly healthy horses. If a horse is ill, a laboratory examination of the urine may give useful help, but if the animal is well, peculiarly thick and vari-coloured urine need not be a cause of alarm. Urine approaching the almost black colour of Guinness does indicate disease and must be taken seriously but it will be accompanied by other signs of illness.

Temperature The horse's temperature, taken with an ordinary clinical thermometer, dipped in water or lubricated in vaseline and passed to almost its full length into the anus, is remarkably constant when compared with other animals. If the tail is held turned up with one hand while the thermometer is inserted with the other, one has warning of impending trouble from the horse because it cannot kick without clapping down its tail. Note that this does not apply to mules. The temperature varies around 38°C (100.2°F) seldom rising or falling more than half a degree above or below that figure. It is usually slightly higher in the evening than in the morning. Ordinary exercise, work, and weather conditions have no noticeable effect on a horse's temperature. A deviation beyond the figure given merits an investigation as to the cause, although some horses have a constantly lower temperature and remain perfectly well. It is worthwhile to take your healthy horse's temperature 3 times a day for a couple of days to have its normal temperature established for reference in case of illness.

The heart The heart can be felt beating if the hand is placed flatly on the wall of the chest on the left side close up to the elbow or even between the point of the elbow and the chest wall. The beat can be heard by applying an ear as closely as possible to the same area. The beats can also be heard on the right side but not so clearly, because they are muffled by a lobe of the right lung. They are much more clearly heard by using a stethoscope. Usually each beat consists of two sounds, closely linked, a low note followed by a slightly higher and shorter one, described as lub-dup. In a horse at rest this is repeated 35 to 45 times a minute according to the type of animal; ponies around 45 beats, light horses about 40 and heavy horses down to about 35 beats per minute. Foals soon after birth have a heart rate about twice as fast as older animals and this reduces gradually during the first year of life. The heart beat causes a surge of blood through the arteries which can be felt as the pulse. In horses this is most easily taken on the line of the lower jaw just in front of the cheek where the submaxillary artery turns round the bony edge. The pulse rate is the same as the heart beat by which it is controlled. Veterinary surgeons find the quality of the pulse – tense, hard, full, soft, thready, long or pushing – useful in assessing a horse's reactions to disease or treatment. It is of interest to try to establish normal figures for your own horses.

Heart sounds The two usual heart sounds, lub-dup, may vary by a little in some horses, slurring to lubub-dup or lub-dupup, without indicating disease. Sometimes the heart sounds are confused by murmurs which may be harmless or can indicate disease. Horses' hearts usually have great reserves of power and if a horse is carrying out its work satisfactorily it is reasonable to assume that the heart is capable of responding to the demands being made upon it and of continuing to do so.

Heart rhythm The timing of the heart beat is usually as regular as the tick of a clock. Faltering or irregularities may indicate heart trouble but a great many horses' hearts miss a beat now and again when the animal is resting, a condition in no way detrimental to the heart's health and ability. In humans such a state of affairs might indicate heart disease and this sometimes leads to differences of opinion between doctors who own horses and their veterinary surgeons.

Breathing When a healthy horse is resting it is very difficult to see that he is breathing at all though you may feel the breath if you place your hand lightly over one nostril. The expansion and contractions of the chest are so slight that they are blended with the animal shifting his weight on his legs or twitching a fly off his coat with the small skin muscles provided for the purpose. On a cold day the puffs of steamy breath from the nostrils are readily observed. Resting horses breathe as slowly as 10 to 12 times a minute, once every 5 or 6 seconds. If it is important to see that the animal is breathing normally, the speed and depth of the movements involved in the process can readily be increased by trotting the horse for a couple of minutes. Any disease of the lungs makes a horse breathe faster so, if the breathing is difficult to detect the horse is not likely to have any lung trouble. After severe exertion a horse may breathe at a rate of 100 times a minute, very properly known as 'blowing'. A fit horse will gradually reduce its rate of blowing to a reasonable 20 or so breaths after ten minutes: less fit animals will take longer. Those that continue to blow excessively have been overworked in relation to their condition, or they may have some lung trouble or other disease.

The skin and coat Horses have a coat of fine, short hair in summer. In the autumn they grow a longer and thicker coat which is shed in the spring. The appearance of the summer coat is pleasing, being short, smooth and often shining, and this can be enhanced by correct feeding, suitable exercise and vigorous grooming. The winter coat, left to itself, becomes long, greasy, tangled and dirty, and if the horse is to winter out and not be worked, the coat is best left alone as an excellent protection against winter weather. Under the hair, at any time of the year, the skin should be soft and able to be picked up freely over the neck or ribs between finger and thumb, and be easily movable with the flat of the hand. A 'hidebound' skin that cannot be lifted or moved but is tightly adherent to the tissues below is not healthy and indicates disease or unsatisfactory management.

Horses that are worked in the winter are usually clipped as soon as the winter coat is established and this may have to be repeated two or three times before the new summer coat breaks through. Clipping is not only for smartness. A horse with a heavy coat works less efficiently and sweats into the long coat which is difficult to dry and proper grooming becomes almost impossible. Wet coats, from sweat and rain, expose the animal to chilling from cold winds. Clipped horses are usually stabled; but those that are to be used only occasionally may be turned out in rugs and are often left with the long coat on the belly as some protection. The rugs that are worn by horses that are out at grass are designed to remain in place even if the horse rolls in them. They are waterproof and must be free of external straps and buckles that could catch on fences. The rugs may be blanket-lined or double-lined with a layer of non-conducting acrylic material and another layer of wool next to the skin. They are generally known as New Zealand rugs though there are a number of named varieties incorporating various safety factors. In spite of this they all constitute an accident risk and horses turned out in them should be regularly overseen.

Condition

Condition refers to the amount of flesh a horse is carrying. A thin horse is in poor condition; a well-covered one in good condition; one that is muscled up and ready to compete is in fit condition; while horses in show condition are also muscled up but they carry rather more fat and rounder contours. When the expert asks what you think of his horses it is naive to say they are beautiful but he will take you to his heart if you say they are in beautiful condition.

Horses alter very rapidly in condition. It is mostly a matter of balancing food and work or exercise. Ponies running free on the hills and moors take plenty of exercise searching for their food. They get plump in a good summer and thin in winter even when supplied with extra hay. If they are brought on to better quality pasture they thrive in the winter and get so fat in the summer that they must have their grazing time curtailed to avoid laminitis. Horses, being less hardy, do well enough on good grass in the summer but need extra corn and hay in winter to keep their condition. When work is involved they all need sufficient feeding to meet the energy demand and it is every horse keeper's responsibility to vary the feeding of his animals so that they remain in good condition.

The chief causes of loss of condition are poor quality or inadequate feeding, sharp or diseased teeth which interfere with the amount of food a horse can eat, and worms which steal the nourishment from the horse's stomach and intestines.

Work is an important factor in affecting condition. A well fed but idle horse may have a glossy coat and rounded contours, but the padding is largely fat. Fat horses have big bellies and the muscles of the neck and back are soft when prodded with the fingers. Such a horse put to hard or fast work would soon puff and blow and become tired because of the unaccustomed exercise, undeveloped muscles and a weight of useless fat to carry around. So much fat also interferes with the work of the heart and an actively circulating flow of blood. It is dangerous to put a fat horse straight into unaccustomed hard or fast work. The consequences could be azoturia, acute laminitis, a strained heart or lameness. If fat horses are worked too hard too soon, the fat soon disappears leaving them poorly covered and lacking in muscle.

To prepare a fat horse for work, it should be given increasing exercise very steadily so that the fat gradually reduces and the muscles gradually develop. All the organs are stimulated to lose some at least of their fat and to work harder so that the horse keeps its rounded contours, which gradually change from being based on soft fat to consisting of hard muscle that cannot be prodded, being as hard as a board while the horse is tensed up, though it softens to some degree when the animal relaxes. The bulging belly has reduced and its underline is not nearly so far from the backbone. If this process of making the horse fit is carried even further, the muscles of the quarters bulge individually, with clear grooves between them. Horses in that condition are really fit and require any amount of food and exercise to maintain that fitness and to contain the ebulience that is likely to accompany it. Most people are happy to keep their horses at a lower plane of condition, more suitable for the sort of work that does not involve fierce competition.

Horses at the other extreme of condition, emaciation, also need time and steadily progressive work to restore them to usefulness. The chief sign of emaciation is that the skin appears to be stretched over the bony skeleton with no indication of fat and very little of muscle; skin and bone in fact. This state may be reached by overwork, starvation or disease and provided the disease, worms or infection or poison can be dealt with, it is surprising how much noticeable improvement such horses will show as each week goes by. As soon as it is established that they can eat they should be given gentle exercise, both the food and the exercise being increased as the animal's condition improves until the required state of fitness is reached. Unless the period of emaciation has left permanent effects on the heart or other vital organs, there is no reason why such animals should not proceed to full work once they have been brought back into good condition.

It is interesting to hear horsemen discussing whether they would rather have fat horses to get fit or thin ones. The conclusion generally seems to be that, assuming basic good health, building thin horses up to working strength is easier than transforming fat into muscle.

Conformation

Conformation is the inherited make and shape of a horse which is unalterable except for changes associated with growth. Conformation should not be confused with condition, which refers to the bodily state of the animal – fat or thin or hard and fit – a state which is variable and controllable. In ages past the horse evolved as an animal suited to open country, a long-legged creature of staying power, able to survive against wolves. By selective breeding from different types of wild horse and pony, man has developed massive animals for heavy draught purposes; middle weight ones for lighter draught and for riding; finer horses of some height for speed; and smaller animals, better able to withstand the rigours of hill country and uncertain grazing.

The horse was not designed for burden or draught, and its capacities are limited by heart, lung and muscle power, but especially by the elimination during evolution of all but the middle toe of each limb. The elongated single digit arrangement gives leverage for more power and speed but increases the risk of strains. It also deprives the horse of the cushioning advantages of a spread of toes, leaving it subject to concussion which causes many injuries. Horses that are required to perform heavy or fast work on a hard, uneven surface are liable to be incapacitated by the consequences of jarring and twisting, which may include torn muscles, strained ligaments or tendons, cracked bones and, over the long term, the development of arthritis. It is vital that horses should not add to these risks

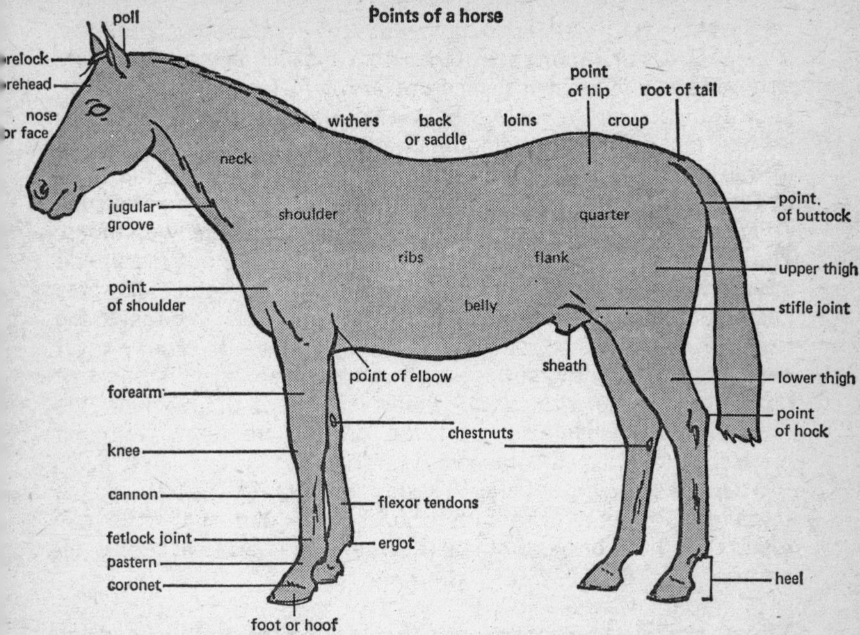

by faults of conformation. Good conformation may depend on the animal's occupation and is sometimes a matter of opinion ; but there is general agreement on faults of conformation which are a disadvantage to the horse whatever work it may perform. Some of these faults are described below.

The whole animal The general view of a horse, whether it is a Shire, a thoroughbred, or a Shetland pony, should give an impression of compactness, the animal's component parts appearing to be closely and neatly packed together. A narrow, gangling, leggy, long-necked animal – a horse aspiring to be a camel or a giraffe – is the opposite of what is required for equine efficiency for any purpose.

The head The shape of the head varies widely from large and square in the heavy horses to fine and tapering in the Arab. Its size should never appear to be out of proportion to the body. A heavy head unbalances the animal by advancing the centre of gravity and throwing extra weight on to the fore legs. The ears vary from small and pricked to large and floppy. They are usually prominent and pointed. Their shape is unimportant but their activity is invaluable as a guide to mood and temperament. The front line of the face may be straight, slightly dished, or Roman-nosed without detriment. Breadth of face is important for the accommodation of the air passages and to give a wide setting to large, kindly eyes. Small, piggy eyes are thought to be undesirable, probably on aesthetic grounds, as they are unusual. They may indicate an ungenerous nature as is generally assumed. The muzzle may be either broad or tapering, but the nostrils should always be wide, since pinched nostrils restrict air intake. In some Eastern countries, horses' nostrils are slit to give more freedom to the passage of air. The upper and lower incisor teeth usually meet exactly on their biting surfaces. Minor deviations are unimportant but if they do not meet at all, being undershot or overshot, the defect is serious because, apart from grazing problems, the molar teeth are likely to be displaced as well, causing the growth of awkward tooth spikes. The lower jaw should widen gently towards the throat giving plenty of room for the larynx. A narrow throttle may restrict the flow of air, particularly when the head is flexed by bit control.

The neck The shape of the neck affects the setting of the head and consequently the whole balance of the horse. The neck should be strong, short and thick in the heavier types, and long and lean without weakness in the lighter horses. It may become crested in entire males and in animals that are over-fat. A ewe neck, concave above and convex below, is seriously deplored as it interferes with the proper flexion of the head at the poll, which is necessary for satisfactory balance and control.

The back and chest The back, from the withers to the quarters, should be wide, strong and either level or slightly dipped. The dip increases with age and may be exaggerated in aged brood mares. An arched or roach back, approved for pack mules, contributes to a stilted action in horses. A short back reduces the capacity for speed, while too long a back, especially if dipped, lacks solidity and resistance to weight bearing.

The chest should be deep through the girth in relation to the distance from its lower line to the ground. A shallow chest above a lot of leg length indicates lack of accommodation for the heart and lungs. In well-developed heavy horses and ponies, bred for work in high altitudes, the chest may be deeper than the length of leg below the brisket. In riding horses the two measures are usually about equal. In thoroughbreds the leg length may exceed the depth of the chest. Foals' legs are disproportionately long, nearly twice the depth of the chest at birth. This enables them to keep up with their mothers for a short distance at least, when escaping from danger. The proportions are adjusted during the first year's growth.

The ribs should be well sprung out from the spine giving a rounded body. The spring of the ribs varies from cobs and some ponies whose bodies are too round for developing speed and too wide for children's riding comfort, to flat-sided animals whose abilities are limited by lack of lung capacity. The ribs in a reasonably short-backed horse will reach well back to the loins giving strength to the junction with the quarters. Long-backed animals may be weakly coupled and appear to be short of a rib.

Between the fore legs there should be room for well-developed pectoral muscles indicating a satisfactory breadth of chest. In very narrow animals the fore legs are described as coming out of one hole. At the other extreme the horse is said to have a leg at each corner, a powerful arrangement suited to animals used for slow and heavy draught work. The withers are not usually noticeable in ponies and heavy horses unless they are in poor condition. In most light horses they are better defined, being associated with the longer striding shoulder movement. Care is needed to avoid bruising them with a low saddle pommel or galling them with stable rugs. Very high withers are objectionable since they are usually associated with a tall and narrow conformation and because they are even more easily injured.

The quarters The quarters should continue the level line of the back without any pinching at the loins, with strong muscles spreading to clearly defined hip bones and rounding off gently to the tail. The quarters and croup are the main source of driving power and they should be long and broad. A short narrow croup dropping sharply to a low-set tail seriously reduces the volume of muscle available for work. A tail set high, as in the Arab, may make the croup appear shorter than it really is.

The fore legs The length and strength of the limbs should be considered in relation to the bulk of the body. Thin legs cannot support a heavy body for long without stress. Short stout limbs are likely to plug on indefinitely at a steadier pace. A horse's abilities are largely controlled by these proportions.

The fore legs viewed from the front should be so straight that a plumbline from the point of the shoulder bisects the limb and foot exactly. The knee and fetlock joints should stand out large, bony and clean, free of puffiness and swellings, points rather difficult to observe in those breeds whose limbs carry a mass of hair or 'feather'. Knock knees, bandy legs and any turning in or out of the fetlocks or feet are objectionable because such deviations interfere with the exact balance of the animal's progression. Their effect can be seen when the horse is trotted and the feet, instead of moving through a single plane, are thrown around in peculiar arcs producing uneven wear of the joints and increasing the liability to injury and strain. Slightly inturned feet are not a serious defect but those markedly pigeon-toed are likely to cause jarring or strain within and above the hooves which are inclined to be blocky. Turned out feet cause strains on the inner side of the limb and are liable to cut or bruise the opposite leg with the edge of the shoe.

On viewing the fore legs from the side, the shoulder blade should slope at about 30 degrees from the vertical. A more erect shoulder shortens the stride and is often associated with upright pasterns and increased concussion. The leg should be strongly muscled to the knee. When the horse is standing with the foot directly below the point of the shoulder the line from the elbow to the fetlock should be vertical. A slight forward projection of the knee is not serious but sagging forward or knuckling over at the knees or fetlocks inhibits any freedom of stride and probably indicates that the horse, whatever its age, is already worn out. A limb bent back at the knee, even slightly, throws serious strains on the lower parts of the limb.

The flexor tendons should run boldly behind the knee and the cannon. Any constriction or 'tying in' below the knee suggests lack of strength and is often associated with long cannon bones. The diameter just below the knee is measured as an assessment of the horse's skeletal development and is known as 'bone'. In the thoroughbred, bone varies from 20 cm (5 in) in fillies to 32 cm (8 in) or more in entire horses. The higher the measurement the stronger the animal is considered to be but quantity does not always mean quality. It is the density of the bone that determines its quality. The cannon bone should appear to be short as compared to the fore arm. Short cannon bones are stronger but a reasonable length is required for speed.

The front line sloping from the fetlock over the pastern should continue down the front of the foot, all at an angle of about 50 degrees from the horizontal. A more upright pastern fails to absorb concussion, while a long, sloping one increases leverage and delays progression. In a well formed foot the walls should be straight and the heels appear to be about one third of the height of the hoof at the toe. The ground surface should be almost circular and slightly concave. Blocky, upright feet exaggerate concussion and compress the sensitive parts within the hoof. Shallow feet are usually flat-soled and shelly, break and bruise easily and are more difficult to shoe and to maintain.

The hind legs The back view of the hind legs should be so straight that an imaginary plumbline from the point of the buttock should divide the leg and foot precisely in two. The legs should be set so that there is ample room for good muscular development inside the thighs. The wide, leg-at-each-corner setting is only suitable for heavy draught animals. The hock and fetlock joints should be bold and clean. Limbs that present the point of the hock or any parts below that joint turning in or out are objectionable as they throw the horse's action out of balance, cause uneven wear of the joints and increase the liability to strain and injury.

From the side the leg should appear well muscled down to the hock. The back line of the hock should be straight. A convex bend reduces its efficiency. When the horse is standing with the point of the hock exactly below the point of the buttock the cannon should be vertical. If it slopes forward the hock is too bent, diminishing drive. If the cannon slopes back the hock is too straight, reducing elasticity of movement. The pasterns and feet should resemble those of the fore limb except that the slope of the front line is more upright at about 55°F, the hoof is slightly narrower giving an oval imprint, and the sole is more highly arched.

Stabled horses

Horses are healthiest if kept out and properly supervised in paddocks. If they are only required for easy and occasional use they can manage very well if they are never stabled. In a field the horse finds its own food, breathes fresh air, beds down comfortably and takes reasonable exercise, galloping about occasionally to dispose of surplus energy. It grows a thick, greasy coat to protect it against the vagaries of winter weather and replaces it with a glossy, short one for summer use.

Horses that are required to work, whether it be hacking, hunting, polo, show jumping, racing or harness work, must be fed concentrated food to produce the necessary energy. Horses must also be able to sweat freely as part of the work production process and this requires that the winter coat should be clipped. Feeding for fitness makes stabling essential; and the loss of the warm coat makes it doubly necessary for horses working in winter weather.

Some owners manage to work their horses from the field, feeding generous rations and replacing the winter coat with New Zealand rugs; but this is an expensive arrangement for horses needed for serious and regular work: most of the extra food is used up in combating cold weather; the rug system is only partially helpful and it is quite impossible to produce really fit horses under these conditions. In consequence, the working horses must be stabled. This involves a lot of extra labour and attention. Food, water and bedding must be supplied; the stable must be roomy, strong, well ventilated and well drained and the horse must be clipped, clothed and (when not working) exercised regularly. In warmer climates horses may be brought up to complete fitness without ever being stabled and they have the great advantage of living continuously in the open air.

The feeding requirements are that the horse should receive enough bulky food to keep its digestive organs active and enough concentrated food to build up its muscular strength and supply the energy needed for whatever work it may reasonably be required to do. In the simplest terms, hay supplies the bulk and oats the energy. A careful balance must be achieved. Horses will not over-eat hay but they will eat more oats than is good for them and the oats must be carefully rationed. The result of over-eating oats is indigestion – and in horses indigestion is likely to lead to serious disease, sometimes with fatal results.

A horse's skin is an important organ in relation to work production. A hard-working horse must be able to sweat freely and this can best be achieved if the hair is kept short and the skin soft and clean. If a horse is worked in its heavy winter coat, the sweat cannot evaporate: the coat becomes soaked through, and exposure to cold (especially to cold winds) leads to chilling, which reduces the animal's efficiency and lowers its resistance to infectious diseases.

Working horses need their coats clipped three or four times during the winter. This and regular grooming keep the skin active and healthy. As long as the horse is at work there is little danger from exposure to cold but a rug should be thrown over it if it is to be kept standing for any length of time; and the rug should be regularly worn in the stable through the winter. In very cold weather horses are often exercised with a blanket over their backs under the saddle.

Canvas rugs are usually blanket-lined to avoid damaging the horse's skin, and extra blankets may be worn under the rug if necessary. Rugs and blankets are liable to gall the withers. They should not be strapped up tight. If the horse has prominent withers, the rug is best fastened with a surcingle that is padded on either side of the spine to allow the rug to be raised slightly over the bones at the withers.

Most horses are clipped all over, leaving the forelock, mane and tail long. Clipping removes the long hair that protects the skin, so some horses have a saddle patch left to prevent saddle galls. As it is covered by the saddle during work this area cannot evaporate sweat anyway. Hunters often have their hair left long on the legs as protection against thorns and rough brushwood. Other horses are sometimes clipped 'trace high' – leaving the hair long on the neck and back but short on the belly and legs, these being the parts most affected by sweating and most difficult to clean and groom in muddy winter weather.

Stabled horses must be exercised regularly. Most horses are stabled because they are in work and they are consequently being given plenty of exercise. Nevertheless, a five-day working week has its dangers. Standing in a stable for three nights and two days without exercise is likely to disturb a horse's digestion, circulation and temperament. The horse should be turned out in a field for a few hours or ridden or lunged for half an hour on Saturday and Sunday. If this is not possible the oats ration should be reduced by two-thirds on Friday evening and through Saturday and Sunday and a laxative mash given each evening. This may reduce the animal's fitness slightly but that is preferable to digestive troubles such as lymphangitis, azoturia or colic appearing on Monday – or having the horse develop filled legs, which increase its liability to injury, especially when, having idled the weekend away, it plunges around on Monday morning expending its pent-up energy.

The fitter the horse the more trouble is likely to build up, unless very great care is taken to counter the effects of even short breaks in the programme of work. This problem is not so likely to arise in those parts of the world where a mild climate allows horses to be out in the paddocks when not actually at work. The constant movement and gentle exercise gives these animals a great advantage over those that must be stabled.

Stable organization

A stabled horse requires a great deal of attention, and stable management consists of ensuring that each horse receives all its requirements. If there are only one or two horses in a stable the owner is likely to see to all the work personally, but in a larger stable with a number of attendants someone is required to accept responsibility for supplies and services and to make sure that each horse is cared for throughout the day.

Each groom or attendant usually looks after several horses. This means that he, or she, waters, feeds and grooms these horses, deals with the bedding, cleans the stable, gets the horses ready for work or exercise, cleans and dries the saddlery, rugs, bandages and grooming kit and shares in keeping the yard clean and tidy. Whether or not the attendant takes part in training, exercising or working the horse depends on the circumstances of the stable.

Each attendant should notice any unusual circumstances and report it to the supervisor. This includes any food left in the manger indicating loss of appetite, any shoe defects, loose shoes or sharp nails, any signs of illness, injury or disease, torn clothing, defective saddlery or stable damage.

The head groom or supervisor is responsible for the day's ventilation of the stable; for clothing requirements according to the weather; and for maintaining supplies of bedding, oats, hay and other foodstuffs. He is also responsible for issuing the manger food to each horse. In some stables he takes the early morning feed to each horse himself. This gives him an opportunity of checking round the whole stable and all his charges at a time when he is likely to be free of distractions and enables him to assess each horse's condition and make adjustments to its daily food scale. He is likely to issue the other two feeds to the attendants from the food store. A suggested work and feeding timetable is:

7 a.m.	Manger feed: 1/6th of daily ration Hay: usually some left from evening feed
8–9 a.m.	**Morning stables** Stack bedding, clean stable, groom, saddle-up
9–12 noon	**First work period**
12 noon	Manger feed: 2/6ths of daily ration Hay: 1/4 of daily ration. Clean tack and yard

12.30–2 p.m.	**Lunch break**
2–4.30 p.m.	**Second work period**
4.30–5.30 p.m.	**Evening stables** Groom, put down bedding Manger feed: 3/6ths of daily ration Hay: 3/4 of daily ration Clean tack and yard

The supervisor is also responsible for arranging clipping and mane and tail trimming by the attendants, for regular and emergency shoeing by the farrier, for vaccinations, worming routine, tooth rasping and emergency attention by the veterinary surgeon, and for maintaining the first-aid and veterinary aid boxes. He should also keep a register recording each horse's manger ration, work done, shoeing, vaccinations and veterinary items. He will also have the important task of allocating work to the attendants in relation to time off, holidays and illness.

Grooming

The necessity for grooming Really good grooming makes a horse attractive to the eye, but all that hard work is not just for appearance. Grooming is also necessary for a horse to be able to perform its work efficiently. The skin and hair are responsible for conserving heat in cold conditions and, more urgently, for losing heat when the animal becomes hot from work; and it is grooming that keeps the skin in a fit state to perform these functions.

Heat conservation Long-term heat conservation is arranged for by the growth of a thick coat on the approach of winter. If the horse is to winter out and is not to be put to any strenuous work, the coat should be left ungroomed. Grease from the skin-glands and dirt from lying and rolling on the ground accumulate in the matted hair and form a nearly waterproof wind-cheater, a most satisfactory protection against foul weather. Any interference with this heavy coat by grooming would spoil its usefulness. Horses with a full winter coat cannot cope with strenuous work. Working horses need to sweat. With a thick coat they cannot sweat properly and they rapidly become exhausted. If horses are to be used in the winter their coats are clipped short, and protection against bad weather is supplied by stabling and rugs. In the spring the winter coat is shed, pushed off by the new short coat growing in for summer use. This may occur gradually, the change being hardly noticed, or piecemeal so that the animal has a rags-and-tatters appearance for a week or two. Brushing out the old coat and better feeding will hasten the process. Healthy, well-fed horses shed their winter coats earlier and more quickly than animals that are in poor condition for any reason.

The hairs of the summer coat lie flat against the skin, all in the same direction over wide areas. This presents a smooth and often shining surface to the skin, but these hairs are capable of standing on end almost vertically and the horse's nervous system can effect the change in a moment. A horse's coat, smooth and shining in the stable, can suddenly go dull if the animal is brought out into a cold wind. The erected hairs trap air in the coat and reduce the chilling effect of the wind, achieving a degree of short-term heat conservation. This is the same principle as that used by birds which fluff out their feathers on a cold day to appear twice their usual size. In warmer, sheltered conditions the hair (and the feathers) rapidly flatten to a smoother surface. The coat of an unhealthy horse will not lie down. Worm infestation, faults in feeding and indigestion are soon reflected in the state of the skin and the hairs stand up, giving a 'staring coat'. Insect bites have the same effect locally, causing what appear to be raised spots but, on investigation, these are usually found to be small groups of hairs standing up around each bite.

Heat loss The value of grooming is directly related to the need for horses at work to lose heat by sweating. A dramatic illustration of this need is presented by horses which are unable to sweat.

In tropical conditions, when both the air temperature and the humidity are high, some horses slowly develop a condition known as a dry coat and completely lose the capacity to sweat. Such animals are useless for work, rapidly becoming short of breath and running a high temperature. If they are pressed to exert themselves they collapse. It seems certain that the non-sweating is entirely responsible for this state of affairs because if the same horses are moved to a more temperate climate, they recover their ability to sweat after some time and are able to work normally. They also sometimes learn to sweat again in tropical conditions, helped by frequent cold water hosing and carefully graded exercise.

A horse doing fast work generates a great deal of heat from its muscular activities and this heat must be dispersed by the production of sweat, and its disposal by running off or by evaporation. This process can be observed at the side of any polo ground on a hot day when the ponies, at the end of a chukka, are sweating so freely that a sweat-scraper draws it off – literally in streams.

The mechanism of this cooling process is that the sweat glands which lie in enormous numbers in the thickness of the skin take up fluid from the network of small blood-vessels that surround them and pour it out as sweat on to the hair to evaporate. A clean, healthy skin with a good circulation of blood is necessary for this arrangement to work satisfactorily and demands regular and careful grooming.

The health of the skin Grooming alone will not ensure a healthy, active skin. Feeding and exercise are also important. Proper feeding ensures that the skin is well nourished, with enough moisture and fat in its composition to keep it supple, while exercise ensures the ability of the horse's heart to keep a full circulation of blood through the vessels of the skin. Warmth increases the blood supply to the skin. Cold decreases it, so a horse that is chronically cold cannot nourish the skin and hair adequately. The skin can be warmed by higher atmospheric temperature, by clothing or by exercise.

A healthy skin feels soft and smooth and it can be moved over the underlying tissues or picked up in a fold between the thumb and finger, quite easily on the neck and rather less easily over the body and ribs. This free movement of the skin is reduced a little as a horse becomes really fit because the underlying muscles enlarge and harden and there is rather less fat in the tissues; but with a horse in that condition there is no doubt about the healthy appearance and texture of the skin. The hair lies smooth and clean and the skin is supple and free of scurf.

By contrast, a neglected horse is likely to be hidebound; that is, the skin, lacking in moisture and fat, feels dry and clings tightly to the connective tissues below. It cannot be moved over them or be picked up in a fold. The hairs stand up, bristly, dry and dull in colour, deprived of nourishment by a poor blood supply; and if they are rubbed against the grain a grey streak of scurf and dirt appears. The skin's activities are reduced by the lack of circulating blood and many of the grease glands and sweat glands cannot function because their openings are blocked by scurf and dirt.

The process of grooming Active horses require grooming thoroughly once a day. This usually takes place before the horse goes out to work in the morning but the time may vary with the stable programme. Another cleaning process, less thorough than grooming and known as quartering, may be required if grooming cannot be arranged immediately before going out to work. The proper grooming routine can be arranged at a more convenient time.

Grooming tools and grooming routine The equipment needed for grooming consists of:

water brush	stable rubber
dandy brush	face and dock cloths
body brush and curry comb	hoof pick
hay wisps	hoof dressing and brush
comb	grooming tool bag

Grooming takes place in the following way:

The water brush is used to wash off obvious dirt and stains.
The horse's body and legs are brushed over with the dandy brush.
The body brush is then used over the head, body and legs to clean scurf from the roots of the hair.
The horse is then dressed over with hay wisps for the massaging effect.
The mane and tail are combed out.
A stable rubber gives a final polish to the coat.
The eyes, nostrils and dock are wiped with the cloths.
The soles of the feet are picked out and washed and the hoof walls are oiled.

The whole process takes from 30 to 45 minutes according to the thoroughness with which it is undertaken.

The water brush This is a small brush set with stiff yellow bristles which is used for wetting and brushing out stains or patches of droppings or other dirt that may be clinging to the coat. Such patches should be dried off with the stable rubber before grooming with the dandy and body brushes begins.

The water brush is also used for wetting the mane or tail to help to straighten out tangles of hair and for washing and cleaning the soles of the feet after they have been picked out.

The dandy brush Dandy brushes are made up of stiff yellow bristles about 8 cm (3 in) long, set rather widely in a wooden handle. This brush is used to clean off mud, dirt and loose hair from the horse's coat as a preliminary to the more vigorous massaging application of the body brush. The dandy brush should be used with some care, as the bristles are hard and sharp. As the bristles are set apart, the brush is to a certain extent self-cleaning and it is to be used in short strokes ending in a flick to rid it of the debris it has picked up. It should be washed after use. The dandy brush is not usually used on the face or inside the thighs. It may not be advisable to use this brush at all on thin-skinned, sensitive animals.

The body brush and curry comb The body brush is a broader brush than the dandy and is set with fine bristles about 2 cm ($\frac{3}{4}$ in) long and very close together. It has a strap across the back to help the hand to retain its grasp. This brush is used with pressure with a long sweeping movement to clean out contained matter, dust, scurf and loose hairs from the coat. After each stroke the body brush should be drawn across the curry comb to clear the brush of the debris it has picked up. The body brush is used over the whole horse – head, neck, body and limbs – but it is not suitable for the mane and tail.

The curry comb is a metal square fitted with a handle, carrying on its face five or six vertical metal strips with fine-toothed edges. Its purpose is to clean the body brush and it is not for use on the horse. The curry comb should be knocked on the floor from time to time to rid it of the debris it has collected. If the same spot on the floor is used to clear the curry comb a small mound of scurf accumulates. This evidence of thorough grooming is often carefully protected until it has been duly noted by the stable owner or manager on the usual round of inspection. In some well disciplined stables a definite number of scurf heaps have to be produced from each side of a horse before it is passed as properly groomed.

There are now rubber curry combs which are more versatile and may even be used directly on the horse to remove dried mud and winter coat.

Hay wisps Hay wisps are made by twisting hay into a rope. Just over a metre (4 ft) of the rope is doubled, knotted near the loop and independently knotted again close to the first knot. The knots are folded on to each other and the loose ends are tucked into the loop. This makes a firm bundle that can be gripped by the hand. The wisp is used over the neck, body and upper parts of the legs as a massager to stimulate circulation in the skin. The wisp is banged on to the horse and swept with firm pressure for a short stroke in the direction of the lie of the hair. Wisping is hard work but there is nothing to equal it for improving the condition and appearance of the coat.

Wisps are also useful for drying a wet or sweating horse though a good handful of folded straw may be just as useful for drying a horse off.

The comb The usual comb is a metal one with wide set teeth 2.5 cm (1 in) long. After brushing them thoroughly the comb is used through the mane and tail to lay the hairs straight, to clear tangles and to remove loose hair. It should then be possible to plunge the comb to its full depth through the mane from above or below or into the tail and draw it through the hair with no obstructions. Wetting and brushing tangled knots of hair with the water brush may help to clear them. The wet parts should be dried with the stable rubber.

The stable rubber The stable rubber is a strong cotton or linen towel used as a fine polisher after wisping over the horse. It is also used for drying off any parts that have had to be washed. A clean rubber is often used, laid over the horse's back to act as a saddle cloth when horses are being exercised, to keep the saddle clean from scurf and sweat.

The face and dock cloths Any pieces of flannel or towelling are suitable. The face cloth is used slightly damp to wipe any dust or discharges from the corners of the eyes and from the nostrils. The other is similarly used under the dock and around the anus and vulva. The cloths should be washed and boiled daily.

The hoof pick This is a metal rod with a blunt pointed hook at one end and a ring at the other. The hook is for cleaning out the feet after grooming and every time the horse leaves the stable to make sure that there are no accumulations of droppings or other matter in the arched sole which might pick up stones that could bruise the sole. The feet should always be picked out when returning to the stable; otherwise a stone picked up while at work may bruise the foot while the horse is stabled or loose in the paddock. The hoof pick should be used from the heels towards the toe, cleaning out the frog clefts and the edge of the shoe. Used in the other direction the hoof pick might catch up in the frog or pull off large flakes of sole. The ring on the hoof pick is for tying it by a length of string to the grooming tool bag, as no other piece of stable equipment is so frequently borrowed and so easily lost.

The hoof dressing The purpose of a hoof dressing which is an oily or greasy mixture is to keep the horn from becoming brittle. It also gives the feet a pleasing shine. The walls of the feet carry a natural varnish or periople secreted from the coronet rim as the horn grows down. This prevents the horn from drying out and becoming brittle, but the periople layer is thin and suffers from wear and tear and some inevitable interference by shoeing. The oily hoof dressing replaces the periople to some extent. Hoof dressings are mostly based on animal oils, neatsfoot oil or lanolin. Some are clear, others have oil of tar added to give the feet a boot-black shine. A prescription for hoof dressing, for anybody who cares to make it up, is given below. For most people it is easier to buy it at the saddler's.

Hoof dressing:

Tallow wax 1.5 kg (3 lb)	Boil together until thoroughly mixed
Neatsfoot oil 570 ml (1 pint)	Add turpentine 285 ml ($\frac{1}{2}$ pint)
Oil of Tar (optional) 100 g (4 oz)	Boil together for another ten minutes
Powdered Resin 225 g ($\frac{1}{2}$ lb)	Stir until cold

Do not use black fast drying varnish, sometimes sold as a hoof dressing. It dries out the horn and interferes with the normal expansion of the hoof which requires moisture.

Grooming kitbag labelled for each horse All the requirements for grooming may conveniently be carried in a canvas bag. There should be a full set of kit allocated to each horse and used on no other. This is a simple, hygienic arrangement that will reduce the spread of infectious diseases from horse to horse.

Washing the legs There are differences of opinion about dealing with horses that come back from a day's work with muddy legs. Horses' heels at the back of the pasterns are covered with very thin skin that can chap readily and develop cracked heels or mud fever, even more readily if the heels are white haired, and these conditions are likely to develop if the legs are washed in cold water and not properly dried. The theorists, knowing that this can happen, play safe and say that the heels should never be washed. They advise that muddy-legged horses should be covered with stable bandages overnight and the dried mud brushed off next morning. In practice, different methods are used according to the type of horse, the work the animal is doing and the local variety of the soil. Some soils produce mud fever very easily and some don't; some horses' heels are not sensitive. No conscientious groom feels inclined to put his horse away dirty overnight. The sensible course is to wash the mud off with warm water and bandage the clean wet legs and heels. This avoids the risk of mud fever and chapping and presents clean dry legs in the morning with a reasonably clean set of bandages. It is often wise to leave the longer hairs at the back of the fetlock, instead of clipping them for the sake of appearance. They channel the water to drip off without touching the pastern.

Drying off sweating horses Horses that are sweating from severe exertion may continue to sweat for a long time during which they are at risk of becoming chilled from draughts or cold winds. If left alone they may continue to sweat or they may dry off and then break out and sweat again from time to time.

The horse should be taken into a stable or other shelter and as much sweat as possible should be stroked off with a sweat scraper. The animal is then wiped over gently with hay wisps to soak up the moisture or rubbed over with towels. A layer of straw or a bag one quarter full of chaff can then be laid over the horse's back and covered with a sheet or a light rug and the horse should be walked around. In hot weather the walking should be in the shade if possible. In half an hour the rug and straw can be removed and the horse wisped or towelled again. If sweating continues the animal should be walked around again for half an hour. When sweating has stopped the horse may be left rugged up over a layer of straw and there should be an inspection from time to time in case sweating has broken out again. In warm weather a few buckets of cold water poured over the horse's back or better still, water from a pressure spray are found helpful in speeding the cooling process.

Sweat scrapers A sweat scraper is a thin strip of steel or brass, 5 cm (2 in) wide by 38 cm (15 in) long, bent on edge to a semi-circle and held in that shape by spokes to a handle. The curved metal strip is drawn over the horse's skin and scrapes off the sweat that has accumulated on the surface.

Quartering If grooming cannot be fitted in before a horse goes out to work, a minor dressing over – quartering, which might well be called a lick and a promise – is substituted, leaving the full grooming process for some other time in the day.

For quartering, the horse is dressed over with the dandy brush or, for thin-skinned horses, the body brush. The eyes, nostrils and dock are wiped over and the feet are picked out and oiled.

Manes and tails The crimped hair of the foal's mane and tail is replaced by straight hair while it is a yearling. The resulting straight mane and tail hair is not shed with the summer or winter coat but continues to grow through the horse's life.

The mane is usually encouraged to lie to the off-side of the neck. The length of the hair of the mane is a matter of choice. It is usually trimmed to hang as a fringe 12 cm (5 in) long. This is effected by pulling out any hairs that grow longer than the required line, a few at a time, or by trimming with a razor comb which is less distressing to animals with sensitive skins and looks almost as neat if it is well done. The hairs are most easily pulled if they are selected by combing down until all except a few have escaped the comb. The remaining few are twisted over the back of the comb to obtain a grip and then pulled sharply. This does not worry the horse if only a few hairs are pulled at a time. It is better to keep the mane tidy by frequent attention rather than having a major trimming that can build up to a painful process.

Tails lose their purpose, which is to repel the attacks of insects, unless they reach to the hocks. Some show animals are turned out with the end of the tail cut straight across so that the full tail ends suddenly and horizontally at the lower level of the hock joint. Most horse owners prefer the tail to be narrow at the top, full past the thighs and narrowing to a blunt end at the hock joint. This is the natural tendency of the tail but the effect is enhanced if some of the short hairs at the side of the top of the tail are pulled to give a narrow upper tail and some of the longer hairs taken from the sides of the bottom of the tail, leaving the tail's middle section full. The upper part of the tail is often bandaged in the stable so that the narrow effect of that part of the tail is not spoiled by projecting hairs. Horses living out should not have their tails trimmed. The broad tail protects against insects and acts as a blanket against cold wind and rain.

Tails reaching well below the hock are quite attractive but are a nuisance in work, collecting up the mud from splashing hooves. Polo ponies usually have the dock bandaged with the long tail hair folded up into the bandage. This avoids the tail hair interfering with the sticks during play. Driving horses sometimes have their tails similarly bandaged out of the way to prevent entanglement with the reins.

For beautification at shows and other occasions horses may have their manes woven into neat plaits tied up at intervals of a few inches and the hair of the tail woven into a continuous plait from the top of the tail to the end of the dock, leaving the remainder of the tail free. For exotic display the plaits are embellished with the addition of coloured ribbons. The correct colour of the mane tapes for dressage horses is white.

Clipping Clipping off a horse's winter coat is carried out because the animal would rapidly become exhausted if worked hard in a heavy coat of hair that prevented heat loss by sweating.

The first clip is done when the winter coat is established in October and clipping may need to be repeated if the winter coat continues to grow.

Usually, one more clipping is needed after Christmas but some horses continue to replenish the heavy coat and may need clipping at six-week intervals.

Electric clippers with a 7.5 cm (3 in) or 10 cm (4 in) head are used and the whole area of the horse's skin may be clipped except for the nostrils, lips, the eyelids, inside the ears, the mane, forelock and tail, the back of the pasterns and the almost hairless parts between the hind legs and under the tail. The clippers are always run against the natural lie of the hair. Running with the hair they would slide over the surface. In general this means clipping up the limbs, up the sides of the body and neck, up the back towards the ears and up the face also towards the ears.

Horses in regular fast work through the winter need to be clipped out as described but the full clipping is not always used. Hunters often have the hair left long under the saddle for comfort and on the legs to halfway up the forearm and lower thigh, as a protection against brushwood and thorns. Horses used for heavy draught work are often trace clipped, the long hair being taken off between horizontal lines from the point of the shoulder to the back of the thigh and from halfway down the forearm to the lower thigh.

Hunters frequently have the mane and forelock clipped. This is known as hogging and it must be realized that the mane will not grow again, other than as a bristly stubble, for many months. The new growth is just long enough to be plaited after a year.

Clothing Horses that work in the winter and are clipped need rugs to keep them warm when they are not at work. The rugs replace the warmth of the winter coat, keeping the body warm even though the horse is breathing cold air and, as the circulation of blood is better in a warm skin, they keep the coat healthy, enabling the horse to work more satisfactorily.

Stable rugs The usual stable rug is made of coarse unbleached hemp or hessian lined with grey woollen blanketing, cut to cover the body from in front of the withers to the tail and to extend forwards from the shoulders, to buckle across the breast. A strap below the buttocks stops the rug slipping forward and it is kept in place by a canvas strap around the girth or by a surcingle. The only problem the rug is likely to cause is rubbing over the withers which may develop into a gall. This can be guarded against by padding under the canvas strap on either side of the withers or by using a surcingle that has an inbuilt metal loop that lies over the withers and avoids pressure there.

Blankets At night as the weather gets colder one or more woollen blankets may be put over the horse's back under the stable rug. These usually have a breast strap to stop them slipping back and sometimes a strap under the girth, but otherwise they depend on the stable rug to hold them in place.

Day rugs Day rugs are usually of blanket cloth which is not so serviceable as hessian but looks smarter, especially if bound with coloured webbing and bearing the owner's initials on the flanks. Day rugs are put on for stable visits or are taken to events where it is necessary to have some clothing to keep the horse warm between events in which it may be appearing, especially if the horse is being put to strenuous exercise.

Sheets Sheets are light covers of the general design of a stable rug and are made of cotton material or nylon netting. They are used in hot weather to cover a horse that is cooling off after severe exertion, giving protection against draughts without interfering with the loss of sweat.

Hoods Hoods, enclosing the head and neck with openings for the muzzle, eyes and ears, are useful for horses travelling in cold weather or to complete a warm covering for a sick horse. They have another use in making a good covering for dressings that may need to be applied to injuries around the head, especially those affecting the eyes.

Tail bandages When travelling any distance by horse box, rugs not only keep the horses warm, they also act as considerable protection against damage if the horses are thrown against the vehicle. The tail is usually bandaged because horses often lean back against the tail-board and rub hair off the top of the tail. Tail bandages slip very easily but can be prevented from doing so if a small tuft of hair is turned up on each lap of the bandage as it is spiralled down the tail. The tie fastening the bandage must not be so tight that it affects the circulation of blood in the dock. This should be checked and the tail re-bandaged after a few hours, as serious injury and even the loss of the tail may result from this tourniquet effect. It should be remembered that ties tighten if they get wet. Leather tail guards lined with lamb skin are safer than bandages for travelling. The guard has crupper straps to fasten to the roller or surcingle.

Leg bandages Leg bandages are a great help in keeping horses warm. Woollen bandages about 2 m (7 ft) long are used from the pasterns up to the knees and the hocks. They are usefully applied in exceptionally cold weather, to dry the legs overnight after washing off, to act as leg guards while travelling by horse box or as comforting warmth for a horse that is sick.

The bandage should be rolled up from the taped end with the taped surface inside. The free end is placed above the fetlock and the bandage is unrolled round the leg to cover the free end and then spirally down the leg covering two-thirds of the higher portion of bandage at each turn and keeping the top edge of the bandage tight. When the fetlock has been well covered the bandage should be spiralled upwards keeping the lower edge tight. This should expose the tapes when the bandage reaches just below the knee or the hock. The tapes should be passed in opposite directions around the leg and tied with a reef knot on the inside of the leg over a thick layer of bandage to avoid the knot causing pressure on the limb. The knot should never be in front to press on the cannon bone or behind, pressing on the tendons. The ends of the tape should be tucked carefully away.

Identification

Horses of the same breed, conformation and colour with no clear distinguishing marks can easily be confused. This may lead to problems of ownership; accidental or deliberate falsification of pedigrees; or to criminal substitution of one horse for another in competitive events. Some means of differentiating these animals is obviously necessary and a number of methods of identifying horses have been used. The simplest methods apply indelible marks to the animal by branding or tattooing. All other methods require documentation in the form of description, photography or laboratory records.

Branding Hot-branding and freeze-branding clearly identify the animals by permanently altering the hair growth on the branded lines or by scarring the skin. These methods are not universally acceptable because they blemish the animal and are to some degree painful.

Numbers hot-branded on to the hooves are also used but they require repetition every six months. Renewal may be forgotten, so that the brands grow out and are lost.

Tattooing Tattooing inside the upper lip is used in some countries. This is a very satisfactory method although the tattoo marks may fade or be maliciously superimposed.

Blood-typing The most certain identification of a horse is by blood-typing. The blood-typing now available is so detailed that each horse's record is unique, being comparable in accuracy to finger-print identification in man. Once the laboratory has blood-typed a horse, that animal can always be identified by a blood sample. The method is infallible but has the disadvantage of requiring laboratory expertise. The blood-typing method can also establish parentage if blood samples from the various horses concerned have been or can be examined. Several breed societies are now including blood-typing in their records to confirm and maintain their accuracy.

Photography Some breed societies issue identity cards with photographs of the horse in various aspects. This is satisfactory in the case of Appaloosa, Pinto, Knabstrup and other multi-coloured breeds whose patterning of colours is difficult to describe and unlikely to be closely repeated. Other societies depend on photographs of the chestnuts inside the fore and hind limbs which, it is stated, are never the same in two horses. The disadvantage of photography is in establishing standard techniques which require trained personnel to impose.

Descriptions and diagrams (including hair-whorls) The method which appears to receive most international approval is the issue of an identity book which contains a written description of the horse confirmed by an outline drawing on which distinctive marks are recorded. While some animals may be identified by clear markings, there are many breeds of horses, ponies, donkeys and mules which are naturally whole-coloured, without any white or other markings. However, in all cases there are hair-whorls, which are whirlpools of hair growth, present on the forehead, on the crest on either side of the mane and in various places on the neck, body and limbs. These are permanent and are located so erratically that describing the position of at least five of them, combined with indicating them by small St Andrew's crosses on the outline drawing, enables animals of identical colour and similar conformation to be distinguished from each other with complete accuracy.

The description of a horse The description of a horse is usually set out as follows: Name, age, colour, breed or type, sex, height, parentage, natural markings, hair-whorls and any acquired marks.

Name Registered horses are always listed in their society's records by name. Such horses may also have a stable or pet name. For ease of identification both names may sometimes be used on certificates. The registered name is the only official one.

Age A horse's age is most easily assessed by observing variations in the teeth as described in the section on telling the age by the teeth.

Colour A statement of coat colour is not always dependable, as changes occasionally occur according to the season of the year or with advancing age, especially in grey horses which become whiter at each change of coat. The colour of foals may be misleading. A check should be made at 9 months, at which age the foal coat has been shed and the permanent colour established. An *International Guide to the Identification of Thoroughbred Horses* (published by the French Racing Authority) lists the following colours with the limited description suitable for each colour:

Black Black pigment is general throughout the coat, the limbs, the mane and the tail. There is no pattern factor other than white markings. Description: black. Abbreviation: bl.

Brown There is a mixture of black and brown pigment in the coat with black limbs, mane and tail. Description: brown. Abbreviation: br.

Bay-brown The predominating colour is brown with a bay muzzle and black limbs, mane and tail. Description: bay-brown or dark bay. Abbreviation: b. (as for all bays).

Bay This varies considerably in shade from a dull red approaching brown to a yellowish colour approaching chestnut but it is distinguished from chestnut by the fact that the bay has a black mane and tail and almost invariably has black on the limbs and tips of the ears. Description: bay or light-bay. Abbreviation: b.

Chestnut Yellow coloured hair in different degrees of intensity. The darker types have a chestnut mane and tail which may be lighter or darker than the body colour. The lighter coloured chestnuts may have a flaxen mane and tail. Description: dark chestnut, liver chestnut, chestnut, light chestnut. Abbreviation: ch.

Grey The body coat is a varying range of black and white hairs with black skin. There may be a dappled pattern. As the horse increases in age the coat grows lighter in colour. There are variations according to age and season, all of which are described as grey. Description: grey. Abbreviation: gr.

Roans There are three sorts of roan distinguished by the body colour which is permanent. The blue roan has a body colour of black or black-brown with a mixture of white hair which gives a blue tinge to the coat. Generally on the limbs from the knees and hocks downwards black hairs predominate. There may be white markings. Bay roans or red roans have a body colour of bay or bay-brown. There is a mixture of white hairs which give a reddish tinge to the coat. From the knees and hocks down black hairs usually predominate. There may also be white markings. Strawberry or chestnut roan : the body colour is chestnut but there is a mixture of white hairs. Description : roan, blue roan, bay roan, red roan, chestnut roan, strawberry roan. Abbreviation : r.

Colours not included in the International Guide are : Albino : white hair on a pink skin ; Cream : a pale coat on a pink skin ; Palomino : a golden coat with a flaxen mane and tail ; Dun : mouse coloured ; Piebald : black with large areas of white ; Skewbald : any colour, not black, with large areas of white.

Breed or type If a horse is recognized as being of a certain breed, its breed should be stated. This classification is not essential to identification but is useful as a general guide. Most of the known breeds of horse and pony are described in the section on breeds.

If the horse is cross-bred it can be so described or it may be classed according to its occupation : as a hunter, polo pony, a riding horse, a child's pony and so on.

Sex Male horses are described as colt foals, yearling colts, two-year-old colts and so on until they are castrated, when they become geldings. Colts which are not castrated but are used for breeding become stallions when they start their stud duties. Those that are not used at stud remain colts indefinitely, though in some breeds from four years old they are called entires or simply horses.

Females are filly foals, yearling fillies, two-year-old fillies and three-year-old fillies, but they become mares when they are in foal or when they reach four years of age.

Height The height of a horse is the distance of the highest point of its withers above the ground. Measurements are made in hands and inches, a hand being 10 cm (4 in). The hand as a unit of measurement derives from the width of a man's hands which, placed one above the other, flat against the horse's shoulder and withers with the fingers horizontal, present a convenient way of comparing one horse's height with another. Such rough measurements do not start from the ground but from a known height such as the top of a walking stick or the measurer's top waistcoat button. More precise measurements are made with a measuring stick marked in hands, inches and eighths of an inch. This is placed vertically at the side of the horse and then a sliding bar which projects horizontally is gently lowered to reach the withers. The measuring stick must be fitted with a metal base and the cross bar with a spirit level. Any county council's Weights and Measures department will check and certify a measuring stick's degree of accuracy for a small fee.

To obtain an accurate measurement the ground on which the horse or pony is to be measured should be level and the animal should be standing with all its four limbs perpendicular. The thickness of the shoes should be deducted from the height.

Measuring for show purposes by registered officials is done with all four shoes removed.

Natural markings Most marks are clearly defined. Those that are not may be described as edged irregularly. Those that have a definite border of mixed hairs are described as bordered.

White marks on horses are usually described as follows:

Star A white patch of hairs on the forehead. Its size, shape and position should be described. A star may be qualified as faint, small, large, elongated, irregular bordered, of mixed hairs, crescent opening to the left or right or conjoined with a stripe.

A few white hairs on the forehead These should be described as a few white hairs on the forehead and NOT as a star.

Stripe A white mark down the face not wider than the nasal bone. If it is joined to a star they should be described as a star and stripe conjoined. If not joined it is an interrupted stripe. If there is no star the point of origin of the stripe should be defined. Stripes may be qualified as narrow, broad, interrupted, irregular, bordered, of mixed hairs, faint or broadening.

Blaze A white area over the forehead and extending beyond the width of the nasal bones.

White face A white area covering the forehead and the front of the face.

Snip An isolated patch of white hairs between the nostrils.

White muzzle A white area embracing both lips and extending to the nostrils.

White on the lips The area should be carefully described.

White on the coronet is described as a white coronet or as a white mark on the coronet, describing its position. Black or chestnut marks on a white coronet should be mentioned.

White on the heels describe one or both heels as white.

White on the pastern describe as a white pastern.

White extending on to the fetlock is described as a white fetlock.

White extending towards the knee is described as white to one-third of the cannon, white to half the cannon or white to two-thirds of the cannon.

White extending to, or over, the knee or hock is described as white to (or over) the knee (hock). The terms sock or stocking should not be used as they do not clearly indicate the extent of a white mark.

Flesh marks Flesh marks are patches of skin in which there is no pigmentation.

Hair-whorls The hair-whorls which are usually sufficient to establish identity beyond doubt are those on the forehead – of which there may be one to four – and those on the crest of the neck one on each side of the mane. The distance of these crest whorls from the poll, which may be quite different on one side from the other, should be recorded. Hair-whorls other than simple ones may be described as crested or tufted. When there is a line of hair laid against the normal growth of the coat leading from the hair-whorl this is described as a hair-whorl, feathered up or down for so many inches.

Other markings

The Prophet's Thumb Marks Small depressions in the skin due to fibrous insertions in the underlying muscle sometimes seen on the neck or shoulder area are known as the Prophet's Thumb Marks. Their location should be described.

Eye colour Wall eyes. Horses in which the iris is lacking in pigment are wall-eyed. Those whose eyes lack pigment around the cornea are said to show the white of their eyes.

Acquired markings Patches of white hairs resulting from galling scars and tattoo marks should be recorded. Docking and stitched vulvas should also be noted as aids to identification.

An example description

(name) **Golden Arrow,** (age) 1970, (colour) bay, (breed or type) hunter, (sex) gelding, (height) 15.75 hands, (parents) by **Robin Hood** out of **Nancy Gold.**

(natural marks) Head Star, a three inch triangle irregularly bordered with the upper edge broken by two finger-like projections of bay hair.

Body Round patch of black hair 10 cm (4 in) across on left quarter.

Limbs Left fore pastern white; right hind white to half cannon on the inner side sloping to centre of the fetlock on the outer side.

(hair-whorls) Two forehead hair-whorls, one of them just to the left of the centre of the star, the other slightly lower, halfway between the edge of the star and the left eye. Left-side crest-whorl 10 cm (4 in) from the poll; right-side crest-whorl 40.5 cm (16 in) from the poll and feathered 17.5 cm (7 in) towards the poll. One whorl in the right jugular groove.

(acquired marks) A saddle mark each side of the withers. Scar across the back of the right fore pastern sloping down from the outside to the inside of the leg. V-shaped notch 2.5 cm (1 in) deep out of the inner edge of the left ear.

Telling the age by the teeth

The number of teeth A horse may have as many as 42 teeth: 12 incisors, four tushes, 24 molars and two rudimentary molars or wolf teeth. In some horses the wolf teeth do not appear at all and as mares seldom grow any tushes, it is quite usual for mares to have only 36 teeth.

Arrangement of teeth in lower jaw

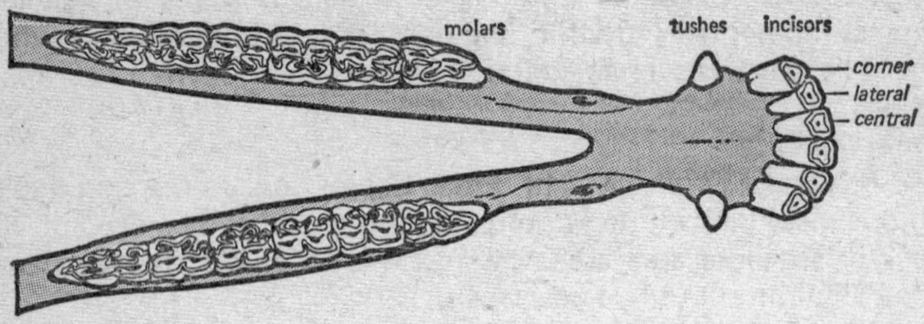

There are six incisors forming a semi-circle across the front of each jaw. These are used for grazing and they can also inflict a playful nip or a savage bite. There is then a gap of about 10 cm (4 in) to the first of the molar teeth. The tushes grow in this space, one on each side of the upper and lower jaw a short distance back from the corner incisor tooth. In past ages the tushes were fighting teeth not unlike a boar's tusks but now they seldom reach more than 2.5 cm (1 in) above the gum line in colts and geldings. Some mares grow very small tushes.

The molars are large teeth with corrugated biting surfaces or tables 2.5 cm (1 in) square. They lie closely applied to each other, a row of six on each side of the upper and lower jaws. Their purpose is to masticate the food and they are well named as grinders. The rudimentary molars, also known as wolf teeth, if they are present, grow one on each side of the upper jaw in front of the first molar, sometimes up against that tooth and sometimes a short distance from it. They vary in diameter up to 1.25 cm ($\frac{1}{2}$ in) and seldom show more than 1.25 cm ($\frac{1}{2}$ in) above the gum. Like the tushes, they are relics of the past and serve no purpose now.

The eruption of the teeth In a young horse all 12 incisors and the first three molar teeth in each jaw are temporary or milk teeth which are replaced at varying intervals by permanent teeth. The rest of the teeth, the three molars at the back of each jaw, the tushes and the wolf teeth are permanent teeth from the time they appear.

The six incisor teeth in each jaw are identified as a central pair, flanked by lateral teeth which in turn are flanked by the corner teeth. The temporary central incisors are present at birth, the laterals appear at one month and the corner teeth at nine months. The three temporary molar teeth in each row are present at birth or come through a few days later.

The permanent incisors replace the temporary ones as follows: the centrals at 2½ years, the laterals at 3½ years and the corners at 4½ years. The permanent molars appear in a peculiar sequence. The fourth molar erupts at one year, the fifth at 2 years and the first and second replace temporary teeth between 2½ and 3 years. The third molar replaces its temporary tooth at four years and the sixth comes through at about the same time.

The wolf teeth come into view at the age of one year and the tushes appear in male horses when they are between three and four years old.

The age of a horse Horses, like humans, must have a date when they add a year to their age. As the actual dates of birth are not often available for reference, it is customary to take 1st May as the date of birth in the Northern hemisphere. Thoroughbred horses which are bred as early in the year as possible date their births in the North from 1st January. In the Southern hemisphere the horse's birth date is 1st August.

Telling the age by the teeth Variations in the incisor teeth can be used as a guide to a horse's age with considerable accuracy up to eight years and less precisely up to 30, after which the demands for this information are likely to be few and far between.

The points to be observed are the erupting of the temporary incisors from birth to two years old, the erupting of the permanent incisor teeth from 2½ to 5 years and changes in the marks on the biting surfaces or tables of the lower row of incisors from six to eight years. Various changes in the incisor teeth are used to make an assessment of age from nine to 30 years. These are Galvayne's groove, the length, breadth and alignment of the upper row of incisors and the angle of projection of the lower incisors.

the teeth at birth

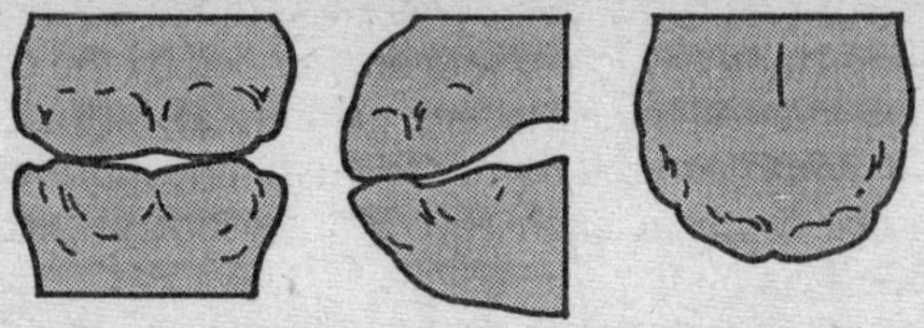

Tooth changes from birth to 2 years At birth the foal has the two central incisors present in both the upper and lower jaws. They may be covered by a thin membrane but this is worn through almost immediately.

the teeth at 1 month

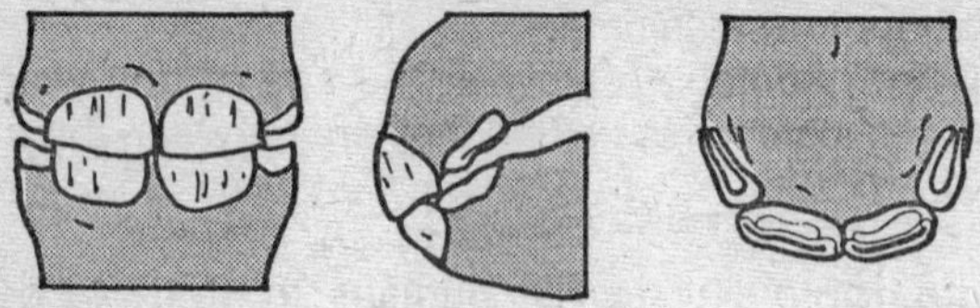

the teeth at 5 months

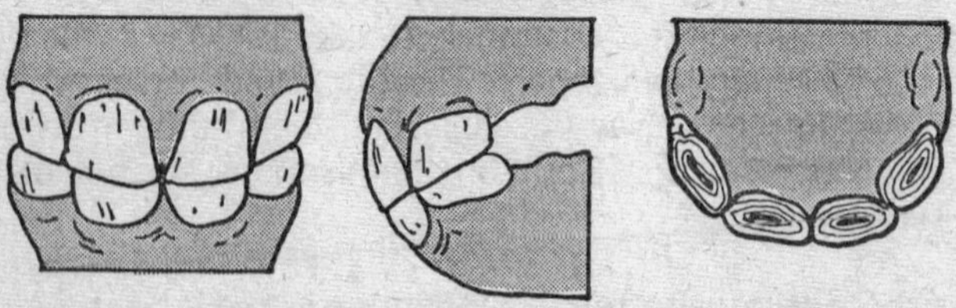

At one month the adjoining lateral incisors appear through the gum but they do not meet the opposite teeth until five months, by which time the corner incisors can be felt under the gums.

the teeth at 1 year

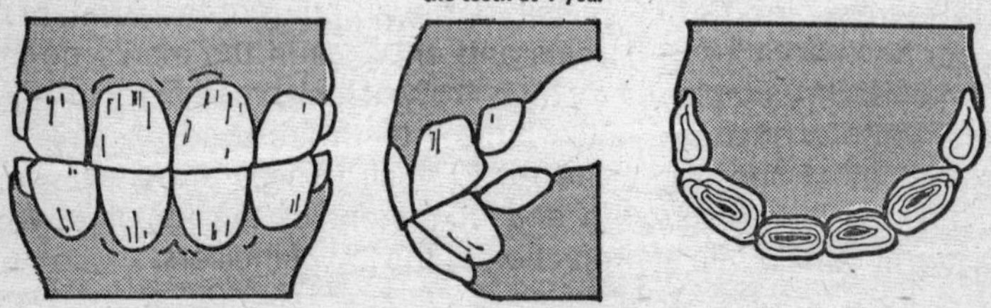

At one year the corner incisors are well through the gums but it takes until 18 months before they meet their opposing teeth and even then their extreme corners are not quite in contact.

the teeth at 2 years

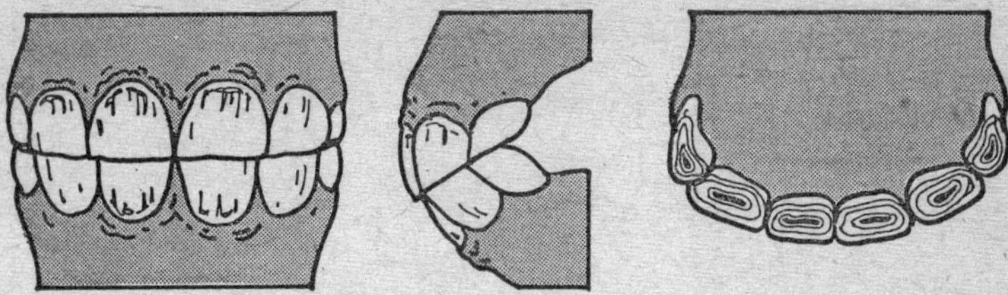

At two years the six upper incisors meet the six teeth in the lower jaw in a level line from corner to corner. The central pairs, shortly to be replaced by permanent teeth, have had their roots absorbed and are beginning to separate at the gum line.

the teeth at 2½ years

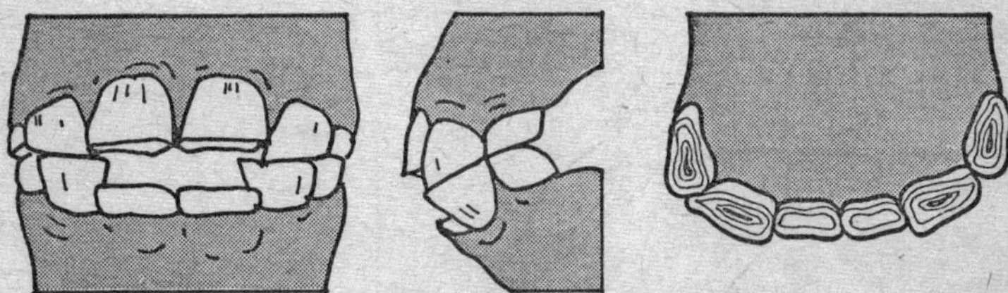

Tooth changes from $2\frac{1}{2}$ to 5 years At $2\frac{1}{2}$ years the temporary central incisors are pushed out by the erupting permanent teeth. These latter can be seen partly filling the gap between the remaining milk teeth.

the teeth at 3 years

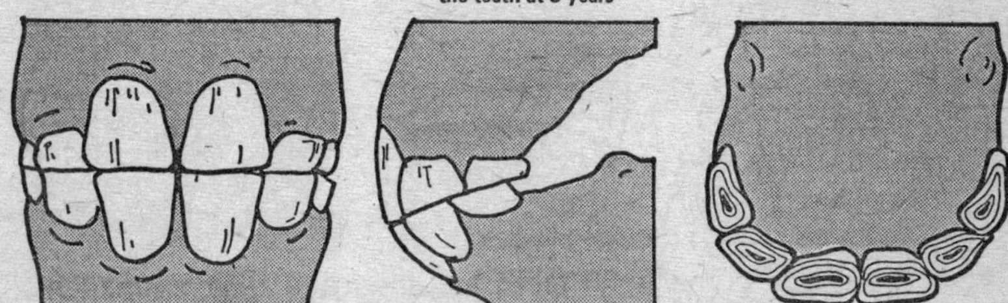

At three years the upper and lower permanent central incisors meet when the mouth is closed. Each jaw has two large and rather yellow central teeth flanked by the remaining white milk teeth. The lateral incisors are beginning to separate at the gum line.

the teeth at 3½ years

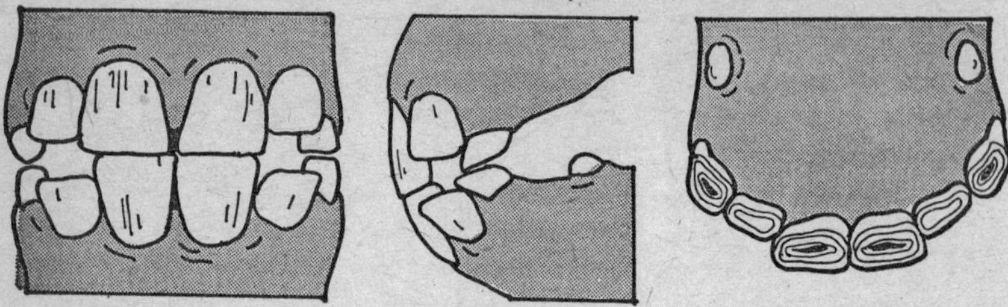

At $3\frac{1}{2}$ years the temporary laterals are shed and their permanent replacements are visible. In male horses the tushes may appear about this time.

the teeth at 4 years

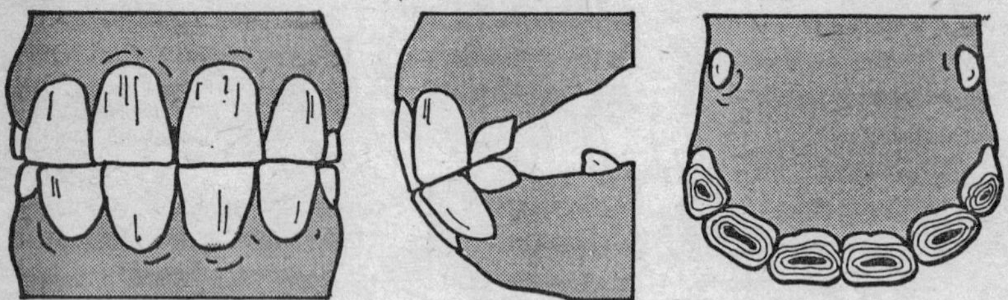

At four years the permanent lateral incisors meet.

the teeth at 4½ years

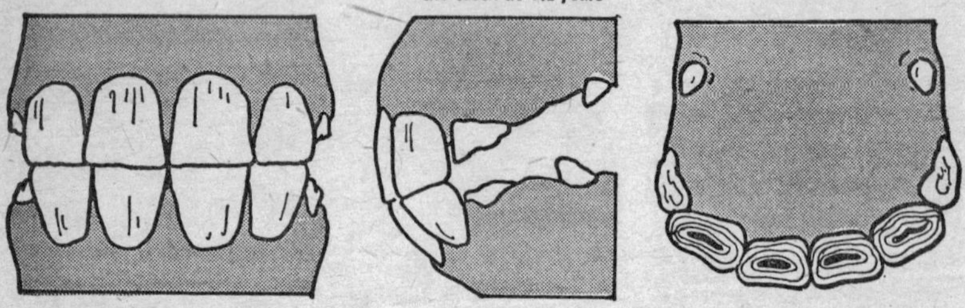

At $4\frac{1}{2}$ years the corner milk teeth are shed and their permanent replacements come into view.

the teeth at 5 years

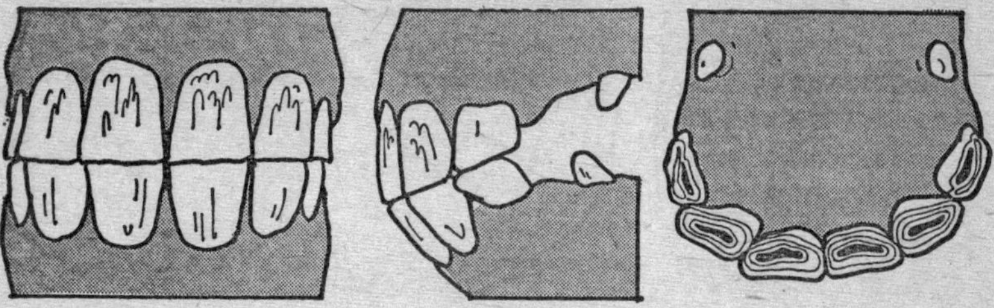

At five years all 12 permanent incisors are well developed, although the corner teeth are only just in contact when the mouth is closed. There can be confusion between a horse which has 12 temporary incisors neatly aligned at two years of age and one which has 12 permanent incisors meeting in a similar way at five years. Temporary incisors, the milk teeth, are white or only slightly tinged with yellow and they have a narrow base or neck, spreading to a wider crown. The permanent incisors are larger, broader and, as they have no neck, they look more solid. They are darker in colour and show vertical grooves on their outer surface.

At the age of five, the central hollows on the tables of the incisor teeth are all dark and clearly defined. These are known as 'the marks'.

the teeth at 6 years

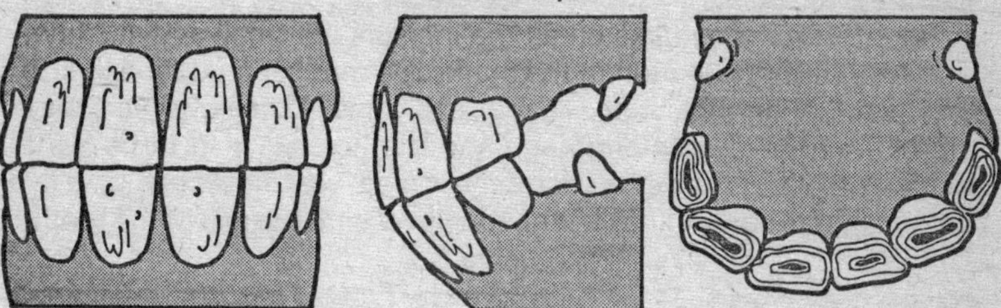

Tooth changes from six to eight years At six years the table or biting surface of each of the incisor teeth has a ring of smooth worn tooth, partly or completely surrounding the mark. The marks on the central pairs of incisors are smaller and shallower than those in the adjoining teeth.

the teeth at 7 years

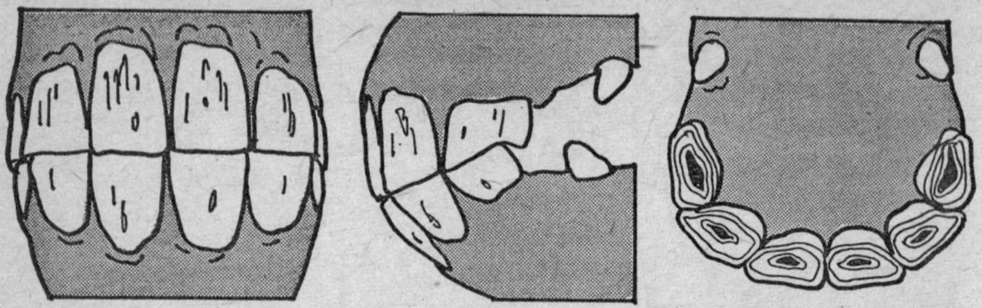

At seven years the marks on the central and lateral incisors are noticeably smaller and more shallow than those on the corner teeth. Each of the upper corner incisors overlaps the back of the opposite tooth in the lower jaw and develops a small downward projection, the seven-year hook.

the teeth at 8 years

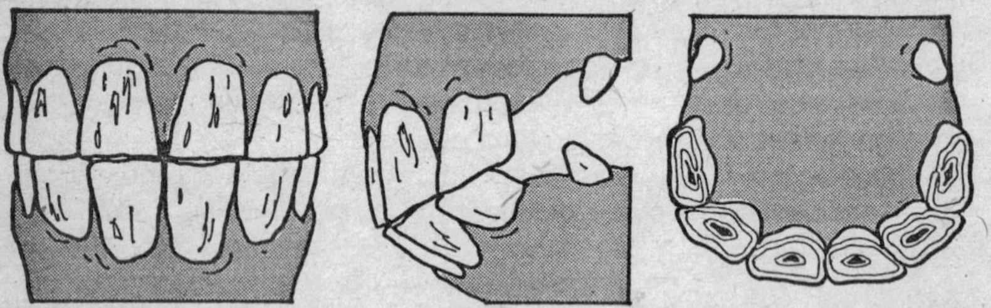

At eight years the marks on all the incisors are small and shallow. The only further variation in the marks is a gradual reduction in size and eventual disappearance at about 15 years. After eight years they are of no help in estimating age and the horse is said to be 'past mark of mouth'. At eight years, the seven-year hook has usually become quite small or has been worn level with the rest of the tooth.

the teeth at 10 years

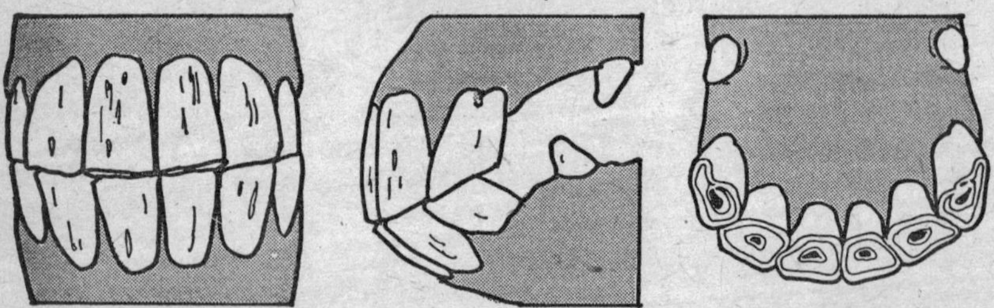

Tooth changes from nine to 30 years The estimate of age from nine to 30 years is based on Galvayne's groove, on changes in the lower

incisors affecting the tooth tables, the length and breadth of the teeth and their angle of projection from the jaw and on the alignment of the rows of incisor teeth.

Galvayne's groove is named after Sydney Galvayne, an Australian horse-breaker, who first called attention to it in the middle of the nineteenth century. The groove, slightly darker than the rest of the tooth, appears at nine years of age as a small mark, which is the beginning of the groove, just below the gum line of each of the upper corner incisor teeth and it grows down with the tooth.

the teeth at 15 years

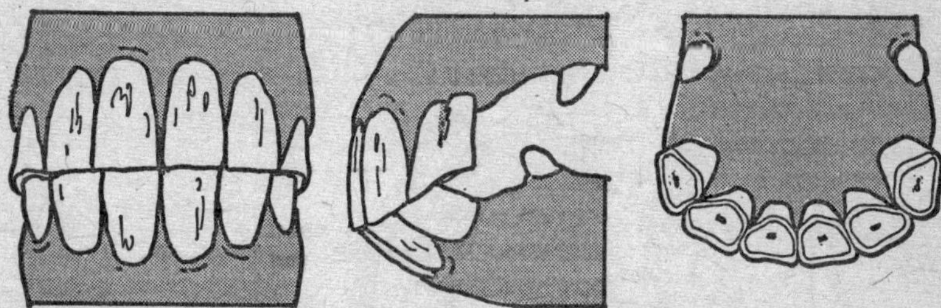

At 15 years the groove is halfway down the tooth and at 20

the teeth at 20 years

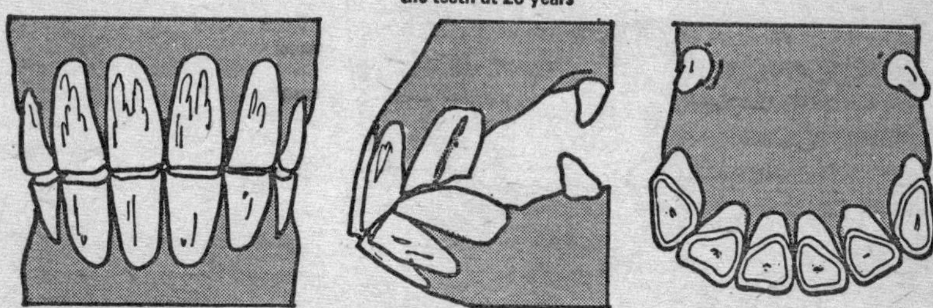

it reaches the biting edge. This is the full length of Galvayne's groove but the tooth continues to grow.

the teeth at 25 years

At 25 years the groove is only present in the lower half of the tooth ...

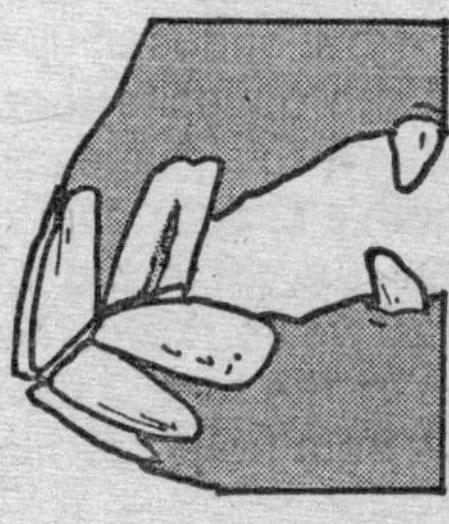

the teeth at 30 years

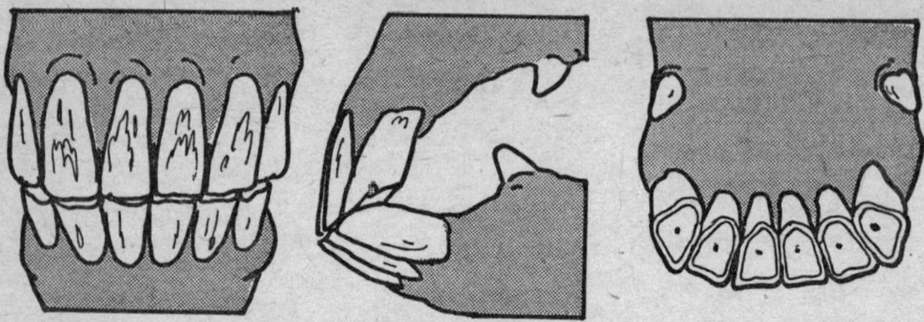

and by 30 years it has grown out completely.

An incisor tooth, sectioned

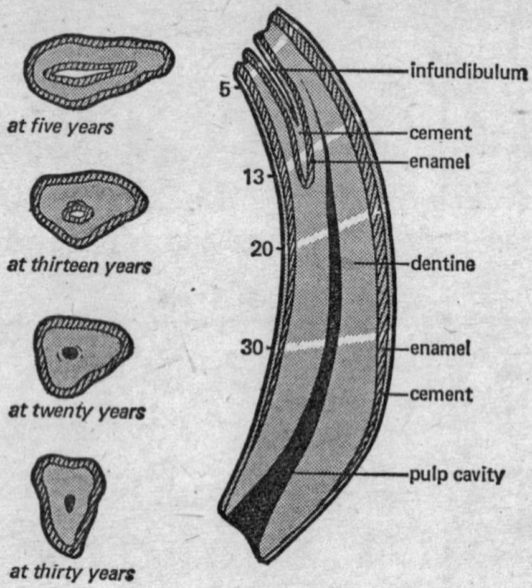

The shape of the tooth tables Each young incisor tooth presents an oval biting surface or table, broad from side to side and narrow from front to back. The tooth tapers away to a small root that is narrow from side to side and deep from front to back. During the horse's life each tooth continues to grow and is almost equally rapidly worn away by friction against the opposite tooth. As the tooth wears away, its table alters gradually to a shape resembling the root.

Up to 10 years, the tooth's table is oval with the long axis from side to side. By 15 years the table has become triangular with rounded edges and by 20 years the corners have become more sharply angular. At 30 years the tooth table is shaped as a narrow wedge with the long axis from front to back. Inevitably this leaves gaps between the teeth though they are not as wide as might be expected because the lateral and corner incisors partially close the gaps by sloping towards the central teeth more and more after the age of twenty.

At about 15 years the mask, with its border of enamel, grows out and disappears. Shortly before this happens another dark spot appears a little nearer the front of the tooth. This is the star which is the pulp cavity of the tooth and it persists for the rest of the horse's life. (See section diagram opposite.)

The length and breadth of the lower incisors The teeth grow throughout the horse's life and are worn down by friction. Usually growth and friction break even. Occasionally, friction exceeds growth and the old horse's teeth become stumps. Sometimes growth wins and the teeth lengthen. They certainly appear to lengthen in most horses because the gums recede, leaving more of the tooth exposed. This gives rise to the expression 'long in the tooth', indicating advancing years. Another factor making the teeth appear longer is that they are actually narrower. The broad flat face of the young tooth is replaced by a round and narrow shaft. The teeth at 30 are likely to be half as long again as they were at the age of 10 and the shafts will have lost at least one-third of their width.

The angle of projection of the lower incisors The upper incisors manage to keep a profile that is close to a vertical line throughout their whole life. The lower incisors up to ten years of age project from the jaw at about 45 degrees above the horizontal but from then on they gradually lower this angle so that at 30 years they project at only 25 degrees. This difference of 20 degrees may not seem striking but it alters the shape of the tooth closure very noticeably and may be dramatized by noting that it is about the same deviation as driving a car up a 1 in 2 slope or on level ground. (See illustrations opposite.)

The alignment of the incisors Up to the age of 10 years the incisor teeth form a semi-circle in each jaw. At 30 they are nearly in a straight line. The alteration is gradual in the earlier years, most of the re-alignment taking place after the age of 20. (See illustrations opposite.)

The physical alterations described vary quite widely from horse to horse; and, while none of them can be depended upon for defining the exact age, if they are each carefully observed and assessed a very fair estimate may be deduced.

Buying a horse

Horse dealing is reputed to be fraught with dishonesty and this perfectly reasonable assessment needs to be put into perspective before the problems of buying a horse fall into a pattern that can be understood.

Each horse is a complex individual with its own status of health, training and temperament. It is quite impossible for a seller to describe a horse fully and accurately to a purchaser, so he presents the horse for sale, points out its creditable features and forgets its failings. Nobody but the buyer knows what he wants from a horse, and it is accepted that it is he who should assess the horse's suitability and discover its undesirable characteristics. Consequently, horse selling is usually conducted over a period during which the buyer has time to inspect and try the animal and he would be unwise to accept as true anything that is said by the owner or his friends about a horse that is for sale. Among people who sell horses, whether they are ruthless dealers or your dearest horse-riding friends, there is no guilt associated with telling blatant untruths and no embarrassment in being exposed as a liar. The horse-deal is a privileged transaction and casts no shadow on the character of an upright and moral person whose word, in any other context, may be taken as his bond.

Surtees, writing in 1854, allowed John Jorrocks to say: 'Honesty is of no use to 'oss dealers. Every man supposes them to be rogues and treats them accordingly.' To this day any mention to a lawyer of the sale of a horse produces the phrase *caveat emptor*, or 'buyer beware'. There are honest people who sell horses honestly – but how is one to find them? Price appears to be the controlling factor. One is unlikely to be deceived at the top-rank bloodstock auctions where horses are confidently sold 'as described' at prices that average over £5,000 and may top £100,000. Reputations and business interests are at stake, and if a purchaser justifiably claims to have been misled the deal is erased and the horse quietly put up for sale again later in the day. At the other end of the scale the compulsive trickster brightens his routine of selling patched-up £100 hacks to a gullible public with the considerable achievement of selling a really bad one to an equally dishonest colleague.

As well as having time to examine and try out a horse, the potential buyer has other defences against a horse dealer's salesmanship: a safe hold on his purse; the assurance of warranties; two Acts of

Parliament; and professional help from his veterinary surgeon.

The prime safeguard is not to pay until all the preliminaries are over and the buyer is ready to commit himself irrevocably to owning the horse. All assurances of money back if not satisfied must be ignored. Once the horse is paid for, no matter how unsuitable it may be, the buyer is unlikely to see his money again. He will be offered another splendid horse instead, that costs rather more and is unlikely to be any better than the first one.

Warranties Warranties are statements of fact about a horse by the seller. They may be by word of mouth or in writing. If they turn out to be untrue the buyer can claim compensation. It might be thought that warranties would handicap the seller's confidence in his horse's perfection until one considers the consequences of making a claim. First, the buyer must establish that a warranty has been given. Written warranties are easily produced as evidence, but to prove spoken warranties the buyer must find witnesses to convince the court that a particular statement was made by the seller. Second, the buyer must employ a veterinary surgeon to examine the horse and confirm that it is not as warranted and third, a solicitor and probably a barrister as well will be needed to prepare and conduct the case. In the event of a verdict that the horse does not meet the warranty, the seller will be ordered to pay the buyer a sum of money representing the difference between the value of the horse as received and its value had it been as warranted. The horse remains the buyer's property. The court may order each party to pay its own costs or the loser in the case to pay all of them. Warranties are important when buying very expensive horses but in the range of a few hundred pounds they are not much protection.

If a buyer can persuade the seller to put in writing that the horse is sound and may be returned if it proves not to be so on a veterinary examination, that warranty is valuable – though no payment should be made until the vet's report has been received.

Some of the established horse auctions use warranties very helpfully. Vendors are invited to warrant their horses in terms that are clearly defined in the auction catalogue. If a buyer observes within a reasonable time, also clearly stated, that the horse he has bought does not answer to the warranty he can, on payment of a fee, have an immediate veterinary examination; if his complaint is upheld, the sale is nullified and the auctioneer returns the purchase price which has been paid.

The Misrepresentation Act of 1967 and the Trade Description Act of 1968 are both designed to protect a buyer who can prove that he has been misled and suffered loss in consequence of a vendor's statement. However, recovering the loss over a horse once again requires a veterinary examination and a legal process which take up so much time, trouble and cash that any advantage is likely to be nullified. Tangling with the law can usually be avoided altogether if a veterinary surgeon is asked to express his opinion on a horse before it is bought.

Veterinary examinations The time to arrange for a veterinary examination is when the buyer has found a horse that appears to be what he requires. The seller should be asked if he will agree that the horse should be examined. If he refuses then the deal is likely to be off. If he accepts and permits the examination to take place at his stable it is the buyer who should arrange the examination. The veterinary profession's advisers do not attach value to certificates arranged and paid for by a vendor. The buyer should explain to his vet what he requires of the horse.

The veterinary examination is an established process that occupies an hour or more, depending largely on the distance from a place suitable to exercise the horse strenuously. The report will identify the horse, note its age, and list any signs of disease or injury observed, with comments on their significance and a conclusion that the horse is, or is not, suitable to be purchased. The vet can only advise on the animal's health, that is its freedom or otherwise from disease or injury. He is not professionally concerned with the horse's condition, training, temperament or vices. These are to be discussed with the seller and assessed by the buyer.

The veterinary routine of examining a horse for a purchaser is considered to be adequate to reveal if the animal is healthy or not, but if a buyer requires for any reason that the horse he is interested in should be the subject of specialized examinations these can always be arranged. The vendor's permission would have to be obtained. Equipment and expertise are available at equine hospitals for radiography, electrocardiography and a wide range of laboratory techniques which are used for the investigation of diseases and injuries.

Freedom from documentation Before discussing where you find your horse, it may be of interest to mention that horse ownership is free of bureaucratic control. Since the British army became mechanized and farmers took to tractors, horses are no longer vital to defence and the economy. Nobody knows how many horses there are. Fortunately, there are not enough to make a census, registration and taxation worthwhile. No tests, licences or permits are demanded (for the one exception – permits for colts over two years – see page 133). Horses involved in international sporting events need passports, and breed societies must naturally keep registers of their members' horses, but in general you can buy a horse, ride it away and keep it at home without signing anything more than the cheque in payment.

Where to buy a horse Horses or ponies may be bought from bloodstock agencies, dealers, trainers, breeders, riding schools or friends; at sales, markets and fairs or through advertisements in the horse publications or the local papers.

The approach to a bloodstock agency is rather like buying a house. You declare what outlay of money is intended and state that you require a string of racehorses or a stud farm, a horse qualified to run in the Derby or something less ambitious. On their side the agency will arrange visits to premises or animals that are on offer or they will undertake to buy suitable horses at future sales. They have pedigrees, performance and potential at their finger tips and can arrange for health reports, accommodation, transport and insurance. If you wish, they will put your purchase in the charge of a trainer or send it to a stud farm. You pay commission and expenses.

A possibly less costly approach to racing is to contact a public trainer direct. It is not difficult to get an introduction but it is wise to find out a little about the trainer before you consider becoming one of his owners. Trainers are public figures in racing circles and their abilities are commented upon daily in the racing news. A trainer prefers that a potential owner should discuss his intentions before buying a horse. Some trainers buy horses at bloodstock sales and include them in their training programme with the intention of acquiring owners for them. This arrangement has the advantage that the horse has been selected by an experienced man as one likely to be a credit to his stable. The price he has paid for it is known and he will charge a reasonable profit. There will also be a monthly bill for training and for such extras as transport, veterinary and farriery expenses and entry money for races – totalling £2,000 or so a year at the time of writing. It is not advisable to anticipate covering any of this outlay by winning races. Prize money is a bonus soon dispersed in statutory percentages to the jockey, your trainer and his stable staff and the cost of sundry celebrations. It is possible to own a horse jointly with a group of friends, which can be a slightly less expensive way of becoming part of the racing scene.

Auction Sales Auctions usually confine themselves to a narrow range of horse types. The big bloodstock sales at Newmarket, Doncaster and Dublin sell thoroughbreds in various categories: brood mares and foals, yearlings and horses in training. Ascot sells mostly thoroughbreds, Leicester mostly hunters. The horse publications are replete with advertisements for sales of all sorts of horses and ponies all over the country. Send for a catalogue and read up the sale.

The catalogues are important. They give the terms on which horses are sold and these may appear to be complicated but a little study will reveal the logic on which they are based. They also give details of the horses for sale: age, colour, sex and height with a varying amount of information about each animal's career and successes, and similar information about near relatives. This last is to convey that the horse is well connected, to stress the point that good horses come from good horses. Do not be over impressed. Bad horses are not likely to breed good ones, but the best can produce some very odd progeny.

Buying horses at public auction demands experience. Most of the buyers are in the horse business already and have their trained powers of observation to help them. They know the habits and characters of many of the horses and of their vendors and they have a sixth sense and a bush telegraph system to warn them about certain entries. It is as well to have the help of somebody in the know before waving your catalogue at the auctioneer.

Private sales Buying a horse or pony from an acquaintance is a good deal easier than coping with the rules, regulations and risks of a public auction. The most likely vendors are owners of riding schools. Probably you know which animal you want. You are once again advised to have the horse examined by a veterinary surgeon. However well you know the animal it is useful and sometimes surprising to learn its age and current state of health. The vet may give his full approval, but he may find something that causes him to advise you against purchase or he might even recommend that you buy the animal in spite of signs of disease because he doesn't consider them significant. Have a word with him. He will have sound reasons for his advice and you will find them interesting.

Advertisements Buying from an advertisement raises problems of time and distance but you will meet interesting people and must expect some surprises because the horse in the stable may be difficult to match with the advertised description. Carefully studying advertisements and reading between the lines may save journeys. 'Suitable as a child's second pony' may mean it is unsafe as a first pony because it has a mouth of iron and a habit of bolting. 'Keen pony' may be acceptable if your daughter is an Amazon. 'Not a novice's ride' is fair warning and you should let the vendor have a good ride round first before you climb into the saddle. 'A pony of courage for a strong rider' could also be crossed off your visiting list unless you seek unpopularity mixed with danger. You might telephone to enquire why some horses are advertised as unbroken or untried. Are they lame, vicious or just pampered? There may be a very good explanation but they would sell much better if there was some indication of ability and temperament.

Have a good look at the horse, see it ridden first and ride it yourself later. This way safety lies and it gives you a chance to assess the animal's movements, temperament and the state of his training. Accept with equanimity the welcoming sherry and the later grumblings about time wasting that are often meted out if you decide not to buy. It saves embarrassment if you position your car for a reasonable getaway when you arrive. If you do approve of the horse, ask if you may decide after receiving your vet's report. Don't say you will buy if the report is satisfactory. That raises high hopes and may later lead to quibbles as to what is meant by satisfactory. Do not worry about the two other people who are likely to buy the animal that afternoon or other efforts at salesmanship. If it is sold to somebody else there are plenty of other suitable horses about.

Prices The activities of dubious dealers are restricted by the considerable prices now paid for horses or ponies which are lame, vicious or otherwise unsuitable for riding, by licensed exporters who slaughter such animals and send the meat to Europe for human consumption. This trade removes these creatures from the indignities of being sold and re-sold around the markets and it also has the effect of maintaining a price level for any horse or pony which is healthy and amenable.

The price of a riding horse is related to its age and size. It is best to buy one at 5 to 8 years of age, old enough to have learnt its job and young enough to have a number of years of useful work ahead of it.

Younger or older animals should be cheaper. At the time of writing the price of an 11-hand pony is about £200, 12-hands £250, 13-hands £300, 14-hands £400. For horses the cost is likely to be £500 at 15-hands and £700 at 16-hands. These prices assume a reasonable state of training and ability. Horses and ponies with British Show Jumping Association grading are naturally at a premium and are likely to share in the hunter and point-to-point range of £750 to £1,500 and away up from there into five figures for outstanding animals. Prices for thoroughbreds depend on breeding, conformation and racing form. Foals can be bought for as little as £200 and up to £5,000, yearlings from £500 to £10,000. Horses in training average around £7,000 with the 1978 top price in Britain £118,000. Recent bloodstock sales in the USA averaged £14,000 each for more than 1,000 horses, with one in-foal mare changing hands at £300,000.

Thoroughbreds reach their highest value in their early years. Horses that race on the flat have mostly retired by the time they are 5, while hurdlers and steeplechase horses seldom run beyond 12 years of age. Riding horses and ponies may well live till they are 30 but they begin to age at 14 or 15 and their value drops steadily from the time they are 8 or 9. They are most valuable at 6 years old, mature and well trained.

The figures given above are current averages. Widely varied prices are paid according to the type of horse, its age, health, condition, temperament and, possibly the most expensive item, its training. If the price asked veers significantly away from the average the reason should be sought. Cheap animals advertised to go to good homes are likely to have something seriously wrong with them. The owners of wildly expensive ones can usually justify the price with rosettes and certificates galore.

Horse owning and horse riding are expensive hobbies, but they exercise the mind as much as the body and create escapist interests that never pall. Twist your bank manager's arm and join the people who know about horses. When they are not trying to sell you one they are the best company in the world.

Insurance

Horses are costly to replace if they become incapacitated or are stolen, or if they die; they can run up expensive veterinary accounts if they are lame or ill; and if they cause an accident or injure anybody their owner may be liable for huge compensation.

All these risks can be covered by insurance. An insurance broker will know the companies specializing in horses and will probably have proposal forms giving exact details of their terms. The premiums charged are a percentage of the animal's value and the rate varies with the purpose for which the horse is used. For riding horses and ponies the premium to cover death, or loss by theft or straying (with 100% compensation) would be about 3%, while 6% would cover death or loss as above, as well as permanent incapacity (100%), veterinary fees up to £100 for each incident, and third party liability up to £500,000. A veterinary certificate of health may be required for horses valued at over £500 or over 12 years old. Owners are expected to look after their horses properly and this includes regular treatment for worms at least four times a year.

The premiums are higher for horses used for hunting, eventing and hurdle-racing (death 6%, including incapacity clauses 9%) and higher still for steeple-chasing (9% to 13%) but it is interesting that horses for flat-racing can be insured at very low rates ($2\frac{3}{4}$% to 4%) since they are constantly under expert care and are never required to jump obstacles.

Early veterinary attention and notification to the insurance company are important in the event of any illness or a mishap to the horse. Early notification gives the company an opportunity to advise owners who may be in doubt about the proper course to adopt in the particular case and to ensure that proper remedial measures are being taken.

Early veterinary attention is obviously advisable for the sake of the horse and because the company is guided by the veterinary surgeon's report that accompanies any claim that may follow. The company may not accept liability if the horse has been ill or injured for a considerable time before they are notified. It is the owner's responsibility, not the veterinary surgeon's, to inform the company of any incident that might lead to a claim.

Restraint

Trained horses are always handled or worked under the minor restraints of a halter, head-collar or a bit and bridle or by being tied to the manger or to a ring in the wall. They vary in temperament. Most of them will stand to be clipped but some will fidget so that clipping is almost impossible. Shoeing is usually managed without extra restraint but blacksmiths sometimes need more control with awkward horses. Vets carry out many of their examinations and treatments without trouble if their patients are firmly held; but when they have to deal with horses in pain or distress more definite control is required to enable them to do their work without too much risk. The horse is likely to be more nervous because the blacksmith and the vet are strangers and are doing unaccustomed things.

The necessity for grooming has established ways of approaching the various parts of a horse. The trained animal will not usually resent a stranger's approach if he is accompanied by its owner or usual attendant and if he goes through a part of the established grooming routine in a gentle and orderly manner. The prudent stranger, too, will know the value of keeping the horse informed of his whereabouts and intentions by quiet conversation.

The stranger should pay due regard to the horse's attendant, whether he (or very likely she) be the horse's owner, a trained groom, or a garden help otherwise unfamiliar with horses. It is the attendant who knows the animal's habits and temperament and he is likely to be the only person available to exercise such restraint as may be necessary to assist the stranger. It is, therefore, essential to establish a satisfactory relationship with the attendant; otherwise the visitor may be left to discover for himself that the horse has peculiar abilities such as an unerring aim with the hind foot in a forward direction.

The habits and temperament of the horse are of great importance in the context of restraint. On this subject Leahy and Barrow, in their book *Restraint in Animals*, state that 'horses, due to their size, strength and speed, are potentially dangerous animals. They are able to inflict fatal injuries easily and they cannot be controlled by force alone. They are not necessarily hard to handle, however, if the pecularities of their nature are understood and the many differences between individuals noted and respected.' Basically, horses are nervous animals, suspicious of anything unusual, and their inclination is to escape by flight, preferably in company. When cornered they protect themselves by kicking, striking and biting. They can be attracted because they strongly desire food at all times (unless they are sick) and they rapidly become accustomed to almost any regular treatment; that is to say, they accept, if they do not enjoy, routine. They retain their fear of the sudden and the unfamiliar. Any horse is liable to inflict injuries, particularly to the unwary, by what may be considered as normal actions, such as stepping on a man's foot or squeezing him against a wall when turning in a confined space; or injuries may be caused by the horse's normal reaction to stimuli, such as kicking out when being groomed or biting when the girth is being pulled up. Such injuries can usually be avoided by a knowledge of the usual approach to horses. Awareness is particularly necessary when approaching animals in peak condition such as thoroughbreds in training, or hunters and polo ponies ready for work. These horses are often difficult simply because they are bursting with energy. They rush about in the box, but will usually subside as soon as they feel a rope over their necks, or they may require a smack on the quarters with the head-collar. A twitch handle in the right hand may be used to keep quarters at bay while the head is approached. When such horses are caught the safest place to be is at the left shoulder, and grasping a hank of the mane with the left hand may be a help in remaining in that correct relationship with the horse even though he is plunging about. Sometimes a horse that is in a headshy mood will allow a front foot to be picked up. He then gives in as this is part of the grooming routine.

There are many horses which are in some degree vicious and not all of them lay their ears back to give notice of their intentions. Some are just more frightened, or more sensitive, or more defensive than is usual and they may strike at a twitch or plunge away when a foot is picked up or kick forward with a hind foot. Some submit humbly to the applied controls and then, when all is confidence and progress, they burst into violent resentment in a maelstrom of twitch, ropes, legs, instruments and people. Perhaps this is particularly true of thoroughbreds. The only way to avoid this mishap is to anticipate that it is likely to happen. The horse may appear to doze but the attendants must not. Horses should not be tied to fixed objects or even more damage will be done when they 'blow up'. Such occurrences are even more dangerous when the horse is under the influence of a tranquillizer, because too much confidence may be placed in the drug's efficiency.

Some horses are actively agressive, kicking without warning or attempting to corner somebody where he can be kicked, struck at, bitten and trodden on. Such dangerous animals require the most intelligent approach and they can often be dealt with if handled quietly. If met with shouts, sticks and beatings they become impossible to approach and more confirmed in their vicious behaviour. While the vet may think such animals would be better destroyed, the owner may be most anxious to keep them, as they are often of high courage and consequently exceptional performers.

Young or unbroken horses are usually frightened of being handled but are seldom vicious. Closely packed in a mob they are not inclined to kick, and if a halter (which is simpler) or a head-collar (stronger) can be slipped on while the animals are packed together, the single animal can be pulled to a corner and held for treatment. He will be less distressed if not separated too definitely from his companions.

Horses usually grow up in some proximity to people and the establishment of their relationship with man is a gradual process. The army allows several years for the training of a cavalry horse and a similar period is usually devoted to horses that are being trained for riding. There is a military system for use when transport animals might be needed in large numbers, whereby horses, mules or ponies may be trained for work in six weeks. A quick resumé of this method as applied to animals rounded up on the open lands of South America and Australia may throw some light on the working of the equine mind.

A herd of these animals is driven into a corral and then into a crush where the leading horse is fitted with a strong head-collar. From this moment he becomes an individual. He is then led or pulled to a standing where he is tied by his head-collar rope and supplied with water. Movement of animals is effected by men in sufficient numbers to overcome any attempt at refusal by simple traction. No animal is ever struck or beaten. Attendants constantly visit and supply fodder to the tethered animals so that they rapidly learn to appreciate, instead of fear, man's approach. These men carry $1\frac{1}{2}$-metre (5 ft) poles, with a loop for fodder so that they can feed the animals with more safety and accustom them to being touched (which the horses seem to dread more than anything else) at first by the poles and, after a few days, by hand. As soon as possible the feeding of tit-bits is accompanied by a pat on the neck so that eventually, by conditioned reflex, the pat on the neck conveys a sense of satisfaction to the animal and is used as a reward. Grooming follows and hobbles are put on the pasterns so that the horses can be tethered by shackles and their feet trimmed and shod. The horses are led about, by force if necessary, and are saddled. At this stage some of them fling themselves down and refuse to rise. Closing their nostrils by hand has them on their feet in 30 or 40 seconds and they seldom repeat the manoeuvre.

The horses are then introduced by stages to a variety of conditions covering the whole range of experiences likely to confront a transport animal on active service, on the assumption that what is familiar is no longer frightening. The horses are conducted through rivers and trenches, over rattling bridges and rocky gorges, are familiarized with railways and aircraft and are fired upon, bombed and met by galloping horses and motor cyclists with open exhausts. Most of the animals supported by their human leaders and the company of their kind, face and overcome these chaotic conditions in calm anticipation of the usual meal after parade. An animal refusing to face up to any obstacle is promptly hooked on to a gang of men who march him through, over or past it. He is then faced with it again, and, after one or two attempts, finding that it is harmless, he fears it no more. In six weeks about 95 per cent of the animals are ready for issue to troops. The remaining 5 per cent go through another course and if still not successful they are rejected. Nearly every one of the rejected animals is found to have indications of some previous major physical injury.

It appears that horses, mules and ponies can be taught rapidly to accept almost any conditions by the judicious application of force, combined with intelligent feeding and handling and without resort to any form of punishment.

Restraint by contrivances It is inevitable that some veterinary interference with horses will be painful so that restraint is needed to control the animals. If inadequately controlled the horse is liable to fidget, snort, plunge and work himself up into a state of fright that would never have developed had he been firmly held from the first. On the other hand it is undesirable to apply any method of restraint that is more severe than is necessary in the particular case. The natural inclination of horses to run from trouble, makes them difficult to deal with in the open, even if attempts are made to hold them in a corner of a field or yard. They are usually much quieter in a shed or stable. Too little space for manoeuvre is dangerous. The best conditions are in a roomy loose-box with enough bedding on the floor to prevent the horse slipping.

A good attendant holding the horse firmly with a head-collar and conveying confidence by talking to the animal, is excellent restraint – but other means may be required : a twitch or a rope gag to distract the horse's attention, hobbles when dealing with the feet, a tail rope or service hobbles when approaching the hinder parts of awkward horses, or stocks, particularly when dealing with untrained animals. Horses may be controlled completely by being cast and tied with ropes, but this is rarely necessary since the same result can be achieved more readily by methods of general anæsthesia which require the services of a vet.

Head harness Horses cannot be dealt with unless some harness is put on the head. There are stables where the staff are on such familiar terms with the horses that they present them without halter or head-collar. Such people usually leave the stable door open and the horse is caught down the road and brought back with somebody's belt round its neck. A leather head-collar is stronger than a halter, does not pull tight, and gives hand holds for the attendant. It should always have a rope shank attached so that, if the horse throws his head up violently, no control is lost as the attendant has a length of rope to pay out. Horses are often fastened to the wall or manger by a chain from the head-collar. This should be replaced by a piece of rope when the horse is being held. The chains are too short for proper control and they can cause severe injuries running through the attendant's fingers or flung across his face. Horses should not be examined while tied to a fixed object. A rope with a knot at the end is usually sufficient and it allows the attendant to give and take with the horse. If more purchase is required the rope may be run through a ring on the wall. *Ropes should never be wrapped around the hand or the fingers* as the horse may apply such force from his end that it is impossible to let go when urgently necessary to do so. A bit and bridle may be used for restraint if the mouth is not being examined.

To examine the mouth and for attention to the teeth a head-collar is better than a halter or a bridle as the mouth can be opened more readily. Most horses do not resent their teeth being examined or rasped once they realize what is going on. They object even less if the hands and rasps are dipped in salt water. The tongue held outside the mouth at the side of the face crosses over the molars and prevents the horse closing his mouth while the teeth at the opposite side are being dealt with. Divergent views are held on the subject of mouth gags. Some vets always use a gag when rasping teeth. Others maintain that a gag should only be used with a general anaesthetic. The gag adds considerably to the horse's capacity for causing injury.

The twitch A loop of 30 cm (12 in) of cord threaded through a hole 2.5 cm (1 in) from the end of a metre-long (4 ft) piece of broom handle and applied to the horse's upper lip as a tourniquet is a long-established method of applying restraint. It has the merits of being simple, effective, easy to apply and comparatively safe for the horse and the operator. Attempts to produce a more elegant or more durable article by substituting chain for the cord or by adding metal bands to strengthen the handle are not be to encouraged. The chain can cut into the horse's lip and the metal bands can cause injury if the twitch strikes somebody on the head as it may do if the horse breaks free or strikes the twitch with a fore foot. The twitch is very useful when stomach-tubing young or unbroken animals as it reduces their inclination to throw themselves over backwards. Twitching the ear should be avoided as it may paralyse the ear or make the animal bridle shy. In very difficult horses the ear twitch can be applied as a brief means of control while another twitch is put on the upper lip.

The rope gag A nylon calving rope passed over the poll and under the upper lip and then threaded through its loop at the side of the face acts similarly to a twitch when pulled tight as a running noose. A piece of rubber tubing slipped over that portion of the rope that presses on the under part of the lip reduces any risk of injury and does not seem to interfere with the effectiveness of the gag.

The tail rope There are times when it is useful to have a purchase on a horse's tail. A rope from the tail passed over a beam or a partition and held by two men enables a third to examine the scrotal or mammary region of an animal that is inclined to kick. Horses are said to be unable to kick if the tail is held up in the air. This is certainly not true of mules. If the horse's tail is pulled up by the rope so

The tail rope

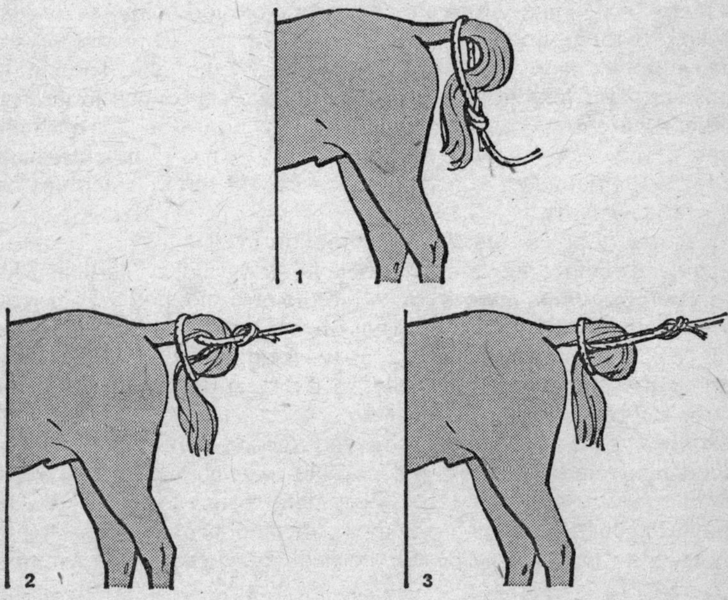

that his hind feet are only just on the ground his activity is severely curtailed. Damage to the horse's tail or spine is most unlikely. If the horse raises his feet from the ground throwing all the weight of his hindquarters on his tail, the rope should be slackened to keep his feet on the floor. The tail rope should never be tied to a fixed object. The tail rope can be used also to raise and steady a hind foot. A rope from the tail is run through a hobble on the hind pastern and passed over the horse's back to an assistant who can pull and hold the foot off the ground. A tail rope can be applied by making a loop with the end metre (3 ft) of a piece of rope. Fold the tail under at the last coccygeal vertebra and place the loop over the folded tail. Pass one hand through the bend of the tail and draw the loose rope end through. Arrange the loop 12 or 15 cm (5 or 6 in) from the fold of the tail and pull tight. The tail can be released by pulling it straight and slipping off the rope.

Service hobbles Service hobbles are designed to limit a mare's ability to kick the stallion during mating. The various patterns of service hobbles all act by limiting the mobility of the hind legs by attaching them by ropes to a band around the horse's neck and most of them are fitted with some form of quick-release device. A simple method is to take a 10-metre (30 ft) rope and make a loop of 1 metre (4 ft) in its centre. Place the loop around the horse's neck. Take one rope-end between the forelegs to the left hock where a half hitch is made above and another below the joint. The end is then brought forward and threaded through the neck loop. The other rope-end is dealt with similarly on the right side. The ends are held at the neck or may be tied to the neck loop with quick-release knots. Alternatively the ropes can be passed through hobbles on the hind pasterns.

Service hobbles offer some protection to vets making rectal or vaginal examinations, though a bale of straw is often sufficient for this purpose or the mare is backed to the box door and the surgeon works around the door post. These examinations should never be made over a half-door. The mare may kick right over the door damaging herself or suddenly collapse inside the door breaking the operator's arm.

Stocks Stocks used to be standard equipment in any establishment working a number of heavy horses. They were chiefly for the benefit of the farriers, but vets found considerable use for them. Stocks have declined in numbers with the disappearance of the heavy horse but they are still of value, particularly when dealing with untrained animals. Most ranches have a crush used for singling horses. This has all the advantages of stocks.

The simplest form of stocks are two rows of three rounded poles 10 to 13 cm (4 to 5 in) in diameter, the rows and the poles being half a metre (2 ft) apart. The poles are sunk or driven into the ground to a depth of 1 metre (1¼ yd) leaving 2 metres (2½ yd) above ground, with no cross bars, side rails or other complications. These stocks present minimum offence to a nervous hourse and a minimum of obstruction to approach any part of the animal.

The horse is led between the rows of poles and is held with his head between one end pair. The middle pair of poles controls lateral movement. This amount of control is sufficient for simple dressings. The height of the poles and the smooth round finish make it unlikely that even an unruly or frightened horse can hurt himself. If it is necessary to control the head, leading ropes from the head-collar can be wrapped around the two front poles. The neck area is exposed without obstruction. If required, one or more of the feet may be hobbled and roped to the corner poles so that any part of the animal may be approached safely. A fore or a hind foot may be held firmly to a middle pole by a hobble and rope, or a hind foot may be held to one of the corner poles at a convenient height.

Stocks can be fitted with side bars, overhead cross bars for pulling up the head, attachments for slings, or with rings for threading and tying ropes. All these may be useful for special requirements but all add risk when dealing with young awkward horses.

Casting horses The simplest method of casting a horse with ropes is to take a 9-metre (30 ft) rope and make a 1-metre (4 ft) loop in its centre. The loop is placed over the horse's head as a necklace and the rope ends are passed between the forelegs, one round each hind pastern and then back through the necklace. Pulled sideways the ropes draw the hind feet under the horse and he goes down in the dog-sitting position from which he can be pushed over on to his side. This was often sufficient control for the lethargic farm horse and was an easier approach to the feet than could be obtained by holding up the heavy limb of an animal that might be unable or unwilling to stand steadily on three legs. Very much more control is needed if a light and lively animal is to be cast with ropes. Hobbles should be used around the pasterns to prevent scoring of the heels. The top of the necklace should be tied to a surcingle to avoid the risk of the neck rope slipping over the horse's head. A 20-metre (60 ft) rope is required, and after the horse has been cast each hind leg should be flexed at the fetlock and hock joints, tied in this position with two figure-eight loops and then tied to the necklace. Each fore limb is to be flexed also and tied and bound to the necklace. This involves a lot of knots and a number of men and is excellent with a trained team. Simpler methods are based on a strong leather surcingle with metal rings and a breast strap that together replace the necklace, but they too require some good rope work. The English hobbles and chain which draw the feet together, so that the horse can be pulled over, involve no knowledge of knots – but they are fraught with some danger as the horse may injure himself as he pitches over on to his shoulder. When he is down, the hind limbs should be flexed by a rope or strap from one cannon to the other around his back, but before this can be applied, the horse has some freedom to struggle and may injure himself. This risk is lessened if the horse is prevented from arching his spine by keeping his head up and his tail raised.

Fortunately, nearly all the risks involved in casting horses are eliminated, if the services of a vet are available, by the present use of premedication and intravenous anaesthetics; hobbles now are simply used to keep the feet tidily out of the way of the operator and to prevent the horse from attempting to rise from recumbency too soon.

Roping horses There are many ways of controlling horses by ropes. Galvayne's method of putting horses down by strapping up a foreleg and pulling the head round to the girth on the opposite side is simple and effective and is a most satisfactory way of establishing mastery over a horse in that even a vicious animal, thrown several times by this method, will concede that man is the master and will behave better in consequence. Another and possibly more effective way of subduing an awkward horse is by the 'Flying W'. A surcingle is required with a ring at its lowest point. Two ropes run separately from this ring through hobbles on the fore pasterns, then back through the ring and together to the attendant's hands. Any misbehaviour on the part of the horse, while he is either stationary or moving, is met by a pull on the ropes which brings him down on his knees.

Comment is sometimes made on the remarkable facility with which the gauchos of South America can rope up their horses in ingenious ways for various purposes. As well as admiring and envying the men's ability, it should be remembered that their horses are familiar with ropes, lassoos and hobbles and consequently are not as frightened by controls applied in that way as many of our horses would be if confronted with them without adequate introduction.

Restraint by medication

Physic Horses accustomed to strong work and eating the large quantities of food that are required to keep them in fit and vigorous condition are usually more difficult to manage and control than when they are not in full training. The management of these vigorous animals becomes even more difficult if they are not able to be exercised because of labour troubles, bad weather or injuries. If the confinement is of short duration the excess energy can be released when exercise is resumed, as is seen in many stables where the horses are more than usually fresh on Monday mornings. If the horse is likely to be denied his exercise for more than a day or two his rations should be reduced and he will benefit from a dose of physic.

It is usual, to prevent griping, to prepare horses for physic by feeding them on mashes for two days before dosing them. Your vet will dispense the physic. As well as purging the animal, one effect of the physic is the rapid reduction of the horse's excitability; and, if he is confined to the stable because of injury, the early administration of physic is not only of benefit to the horse in preventing digestive disturbances, but the calming effect is most valuable.

2 Breeds

Cold-blooded horses 101

Ponies 107

Donkeys 124

Mules 126

The horse's family tree 129

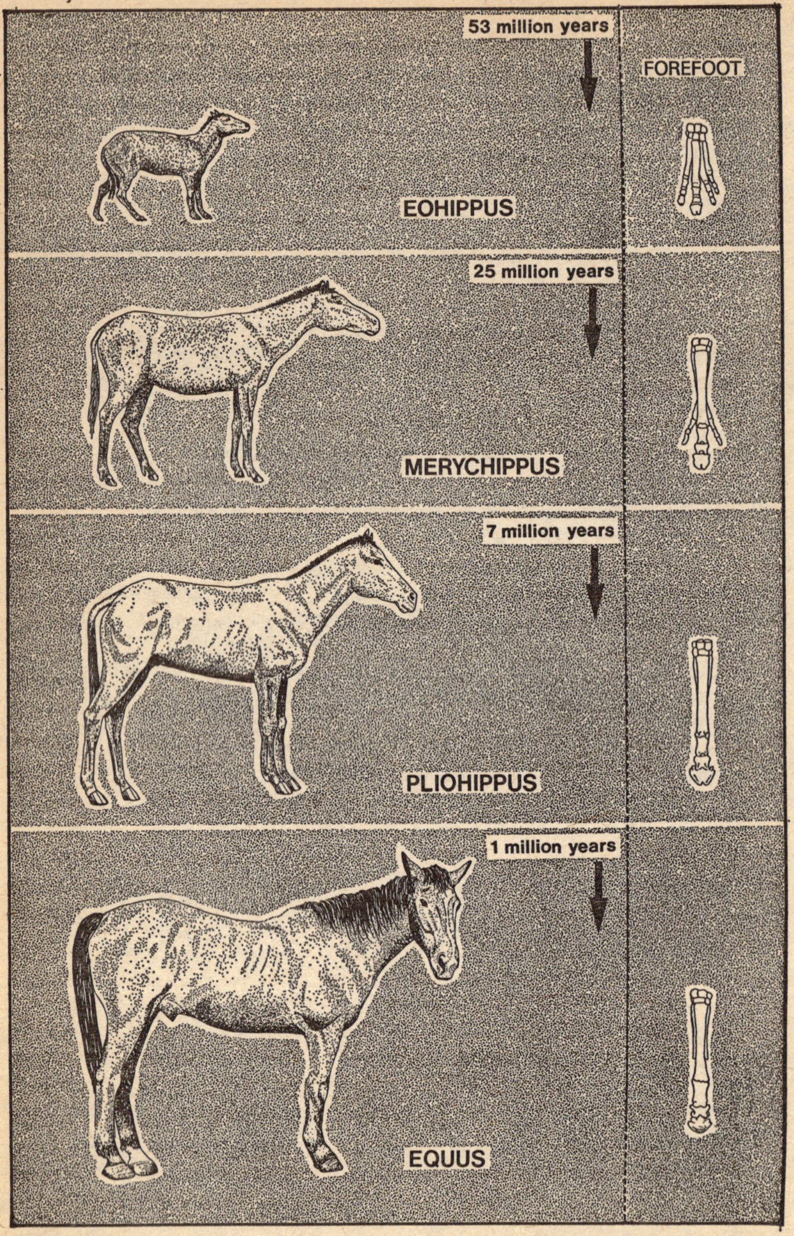
53 million years
FOREFOOT
EOHIPPUS
25 million years
MERYCHIPPUS
7 million years
PLIOHIPPUS
1 million years
EQUUS

Ancestry of the horse

The ancestor of the modern horse was a small short-limbed animal with four toes and probably padded feet. It is called *Hyracotherium* and lived in the Eocene period. It had short jaws, low-crowned teeth and lived on tit-bits found in shrubbery. During the many millenia of the Eocene, Miocene and Pliocene periods, the third bone of the foot became longer and stronger and evolved as the hoof. The first bone was completely lost. The second and fourth became the vestigial splint bones. Later, during the Oligocene period, horses evolved longer limbs and changed from browsers in the bush and forests to the fast-footed prairie animals we know today. The jaws became longer. The teeth became longer. It evolved into an efficient herbivore who not only survived, but thrived on the toughest of grasses.

Although the horse was originally a native of North America, by the late Pleistocene period it was extinct on that continent. But in early Eocene times it had migrated to the Old World and became established in Asia, Europe and Africa. All the domestic horses that we know today (*Equus caballus*) are thought to have originated from the wild stocks of those horses who established themselves in the Old World.

Later development In more recent times it is thought that three basic types evolved – the Steppe, the Forest and the Plateau. The Steppe, a zebra-like equine with a large head and slender limbs surmounted with an upright mane is thought to resemble Przewalskis's Horse which those of us who don't travel widely in Mongolia can only see in zoos.

The Forest was a thicker and, some unkind people suggest, a stupider progenitor of our heavy, cold-blooded draught horses.

The Plateau was a finer, faster type (some say the Tarpans of today are direct descendants) thought to be the ancestor of our pony and a faster, lighter horse.

There is no problem breeding between various types of horse, so one must assume that in fact all our modern breeds contain some of each. Certainly, no one has been able to prove otherwise. However, postulating percentages of Steppe, Forest and Plateau in our modern breeds is a harmless and diverting occupation.

Today there are almost 200 recognized breeds – of which more than sixty are ponies, more than eighty are classified as warm blooded and almost thirty are distinct heavy-draught, cold-blooded types.

Possibly the most universally recognized prototype of each are the Shetland pony, the thoroughbred and the shire. One can fairly comment that Britain has had more influence on the development of the modern horse than any other nation.

But what is a breed? Some, like the Arab, the thoroughbred, the Morgan and the Clydesdale, are so readily recognized or so well documented that few would argue. At the other end of the scale are 'breeds' like the Java pony and the Sumatra pony whose only apparent differences are the islands on which they are found. Certainly authentic pedigrees are not available. In between there is a vast range in which variations of colour or origin seem to be the only criteria for differentiating.

In many places the definition of a breed appears to be: 'a breed becomes a breed when three people form a society and agree to call it a breed.' That may be cynical. But it is a fact that some breeds are established. They have three well-defined criteria: they breed true; their ancestry is recorded; they are recognized by experts. There are other breeds which, to put it kindly, are in a transitional state. They are still evolving or being developed, and with sufficient enthusiasts will become established. And there are others which few recognize for the very real reason that their only claim to fame is their name.

To avoid argument, all 'breeds' are classified in this section as either ponies or horses. The horses are called warm-blooded or cold-blooded. We're perfectly aware that many a pony has a thoroughbred grandfather. We're also aware that no creature registered as a thoroughbred today could possibly have a pony grandmother. One is not detracting from either, just – hopefully – stating the facts.

Insofar as possible we have also tried to group breeds geographically. Possibly we have placed too much emphasis on the British breeds. It's quite obvious that there are more horses in Spain or in Russia than there are in Britain. But who outside of those countries breeds Orlov trotters or Andalusians in appreciable numbers?

Possibly American breeds are not sufficiently detailed. No disparagement is intended. After all, if one has a combination of large numbers of enthusiastic devotees in the wealthiest country on earth, combined with scientific skills of the highest order, it is likely that their evolving breeds will in the generations to come have a greater universal influence than the older established European breeds.

But, essentially, this is a book of facts. Enthusiastic devotees of the newer breeds might find this boring. But they may accept that knowledge of the development of other, older breeds could aid their aspirations towards perfection.

May the obvious be repeated? Horses, like cats, are much of a muchness. All are easily recognized. Despite man's interference, neither the cat nor the horse has been appreciably altered. The dog, by contrast, has been changed into so many shapes and sizes that a stranger from outer space could scarcely be expected to believe that a Pekinese, a Great Dane and a Pug were branches of the same family tree. Let us hope that the horse can overcome man's genius for meddling and remain simply a horse.

For simplicity we have divided this rather general breed outline into three basic sorts – warm-blooded horses, cold-blooded horses and ponies – followed by a note on donkeys and mules. The body temperature of a cold-blooded horse is the same as that of a warm-blooded horse. They tend, however, to be more equable – even docile; but the differences will become more apparent as you look up different breeds. Ponies are horses under 14.2 hands. In some cases all three types almost overlap. In other cases the differences are dramatically clear. Because this is a reference book, the breeds are listed alphabetically, except where it seems more sensible to group some under their places of origin.

Finally, may we state that this is simply an outline. There are many books – and good ones – on individual breeds. It is to those and to the breed societies and enthusiasts one must go for the involving – and evolving – facts of each breed.

Warm-blooded horses

The English Thoroughbred Thoroughbred horses are clean-limbed, fine-boned, light horses – the usual colours being brown, bay, chestnut and grey, often with white markings on the face and on the lower extremities of the limbs. The height varies from 14.5 hands to 17 hands. The breed was created between 1650 and 1750 from crosses between English racing horses of which there are no descriptions or records and a number of stallions originating in the Middle East. These were variously described as Arabs, Barbs or Turks but seem all to have been Arabs, a breed established for many hundreds of years. This outcross of the Arab to English running horses was fortunate in producing a larger, stronger and faster type of animal than the Arab. Under Royal and aristocratic patronage this soon became established as the English Thoroughbred.

Many breeds of horses have originated from the prepotency of one particular sire which consistently bred good quality offspring. In the case of the thoroughbred the honours appear to be divided between three imported sires to which every thoroughbred pedigree can be traced: the Byerley Turk, a horse captured from the Turks at Buda to become Colonel Byerley's charger in further affrays before taking up stud duties in 1690; the Darley Arabian, bought in Asia Minor by Mr Darley's brother to race in England but, not being very successful, retired to stud in 1710; and the Godolphin Arabian, said to have been pulling a cart in Paris before being bought by Mr Coke in 1729.

Thoroughbred horses are claimed to be the fastest in the world. This may be disputed by the American Quarter Horse in short sprints and the Arab over exceptionally long distances. However, the thoroughbred is certainly the most popular horse for flat racing in Europe, the Americas, South Africa, Australasia and Japan.

The thoroughbred horse has been bred to a consistent pattern throughout its 300 years of existence with no throwbacks which might reveal other origins than from the Arab line. The laboratory techniques of blood-grouping are now so precise that an individual horse's pedigree can be determined precisely. It may eventually be possible by these methods to relate some of the characteristics of thoroughbred blood to those of breeds other than the Arab, and so solve the mystery of the blend that produced the thoroughbred horse.

English Thoroughbreds readily transmit their fine conformation and lively temperament and have been used to improve the quality of many other breeds. Crossed again with Arabs a new breed, the Anglo-Arab, evolved in France in the 19th century and is now extremely popular, especially in that country and in Poland.

The Arab Archaeologists have revealed that a light-framed horse was one of the articles of diet of European man 25,000 years ago, but it was not until 5,000 BC that the Tartars of Asia tamed them for riding. Although horses were used in many countries for their milk, for food, clothing and transport it was only in the Middle East that the horse became so highly esteemed that individual ones reached values comparable to a king's ransom. The horse now known as the Arab was evolved for speed and staying power with its distinctive features: fine-boned limbs, dished profile, large eyes and wide open nostrils; the neck being arched, the back short and the tail carriage high. This type has bred true for centuries with carefully treasured pedigrees reaching back to two outstanding horses, Hoshaba the sire and the mare Baz, which were contemporary with Noah's grandchildren about 2,200 BC.

The tough physique and the mental alertness of the Arab blend readily with breeds of a coarser nature and improve their quality. The most outstanding cross was developed by blending Arab blood with English running horses that had long been used for racing and of whose origins nothing is known. The result was the English Thoroughbred, now the world's paramount racehorse. Indications of Arab blood are found in the horses of many countries where Arab sires have been used to improve the quality of native stock. This is particularly noticeable in the pony breeds, many of which owe something of their temperament and conformation to Arab influence.

Akhal-Teke An ancient Russian breed from southern Turkmeina, developed from the Turkoman or Turkmene breed, they are a hardy breed which can survive in desert conditions with little food and water.

Today they are bred for racing and jumping, and excel in dressage. Many are kept wearing the traditional seven blankets and eating light high-protein food, such as eggs and butter with barley and bread dough fried in butter. They have a lean, narrow body. Some say they look emaciated. Others proclaim they have the grace of a greyhound. All agree they can be very temperamental. Their height is between 14.2 and 15.2 hands. The most desired colour is a pale honey-gold with black points, but grey and bay are also common.

Albino These horses have been bred since about 1910 in the United States. Most are descended from an albino sire named Old King, foaled in 1906. He had a pink skin and snow-white hair and mane, with no dark spots, and these are now the main characteristics of albinos; they also have either pale blue or dark brown eyes. They are handsome horses, often used in circuses and on ceremonial occasions. The fact that neither nature nor most breeders of other species of domesticated animals find albinos a type worthy of promulgation might be seriously discussed by enthusiastic supporters of the breed.

Alter-Real Founded in 1747 when 300 Andalusian mares were taken by the House of Braganza to form a stud at Vila de Portel in the Alentejo Province of Portugal. They were used by royalty in the

18th century but in Napoleon's time were outcrossed to foreign breeds, reducing the quality. Since 1930 the breed has been improved by selective breeding under the direction of the Ministry of Economy.

The Alter-Reals are similar in appearance to the Andalusian breed. Their height is 15 to 16 hands. The usual colours are bay and brown and occasionally grey. Enthusiasts declare them to be among the most intelligent, willing and obedient of saddle horses.

American Quarter Horse The oldest of the American breeds. It was developed in Virginia, to race on rough 'race-paths' which are about 400 m ($\frac{1}{4}$ mile) long. They originate from Arabs, Barbs and Turks, bred with English horses, imported in the 17th century.

Quarter horses are very versatile, able to race, work with cattle and take part in rodeos. They are now very popular – there are over 800,000 horses registered in more than 40 countries – the largest equine register in the world.

They are muscular creatures with massive hindquarters and back. Height between 15.2 and 16.1 hands. The main colour is chestnut, but other solid colours are acceptable.

American Saddlebred (Kentucky Saddler) Developed by the American settlers, who needed adaptable horses which could be used under saddle and in harness, they have five characteristic gaits: the walk, trot, canter, slow gait and rack. The rack is an even, four-beat gait in which each foot pauses in mid-air before coming down. All five gaits are precise and graceful, well suited for the show ring in which the horses compete in two classes: three-gaited and five-gaited.

Height of 15 to 16 hands. The colours may be black, brown, bay, grey or chestnut, usually with white markings.

American Standardbred A thoroughbred which has been modified by an admixture of Hackney, Barb, Morgan and Norfolk Trotter blood, not to mention a dash of Canadian. Selection for over a century has been exclusively for performance and endurance. Hence today one may see ungainly representatives of the breed (most are heavier in the limbs and more muscular than their cleaner looking thoroughbred cousins) but it is unlikely that one would find a track failure perpetuating its kind. In America, trotting and pacing races (the latter is the lateral movement as opposed to the diagonal) are almost as popular as racing under saddle. Trotters must do a mile in 2 minutes 30 seconds; pacers in 2 minutes 25 seconds. The fact that they better these times heat after heat is sufficient testimony to their endurance. The sport and the breed thrive.

Andalusian Like its country of origin, this breed is big, proud and occasionally gracefully brutal. It has a rather longer history than many breeds. Until recent years it was bred on a scale that Hollywood might envy but could never simulate. It is claimed that there were horses on the Iberian peninsula before the encroaching seas created the Straits of Gibraltar. The first records of imports is that of 2,000 mares brought by Hasdrubal of Carthage. Until the Roman invasion of 200 BC these ran wild and interbred with the native horses. During their occupation the Romans tamed and selectively bred from these herds. For some 600 years after the Roman retreat the horses were left to nature's own selective processes. Then northern European Barbarians brought in some taller horses to help 'vandalize' the area. The Moslems came in 711 AD and stayed for 700 years. Those uninvited guests brought 300,000 Barb horses and in their spare time started the stud at Cordoba. In the 15th century, Carthusian monks in Jerez started the line known as Andalusian-Carthusian or Carthusian.

They are nearly always grey but they may be black. To the northern European and American eye they may seem slightly coarse-headed. One may argue in favour of their appearance, but not their character.

Average height 16 hands.

Anglo-Arab Developed in several countries by breeding English Thoroughbreds with Arabs. The horses have characteristics of both breeds. They are elegant lightweight animals, suited to dressage, eventing, jumping, hunting and as hacks.

Studs in south-west France and at Janon in Poland are particularly well-known.

Height about 16 hands. Common colours are bay and chestnut, but any solid colour may be acceptable.

Appaloosa The colour or breed depends on where you live. In America this is a breed developed by the Nez Perle Indians from Spanish stock imported in the 16th century. They ranged in the fertile area fed by the Palouse River in the North-west States.

In other parts of the world it remains but a colour. Their origins remain obscure. Paintings over 3,000 years old of similar horses have been found in China and Persia, and they are depicted in cave paintings at Pêche Merle.

There are six basic patterns: frost, leopard, snowflake, marble, spotted blanket and white blanket. The main ground colour is roan, with any colour spots, provided that they conform to the recognized patterns.

Height between 14.2 and 15.2 hands.

Barb Native to Morocco and Algeria this is one of the foundation breeds formerly widely used to improve other stock. Barbs were originally crossed with Spanish horses in AD 800, at the time of the Moorish invasion, giving rise to the Andalusian. They first came to England in 1662 when Charles II took over Tangier as part of his dowry, and were extensively used to improve English racehorses.

Barbs are exceedingly tough horses, able to survive on very poor food.

Height of 14 to 15 hands. The colours found are dark bay, brown, chestnut, black and grey.

Bavarian Warm-Blood A new name for an old breed; developed from the Rottaler (which originated in the Rott Valley in Lower Bavaria) by the introduction of thoroughbreds, Cleveland Bays, Normans and more recently Oldenburgs. The process has taken a couple of centuries. They have a characteristic chestnut colour and the docile, willing temperament of their war horse ancestors.

Beberbeck The Beberbeck stud near Kessel in West Germany was started in 1720 and sold to Poland in 1930. Initially, Arab stallions were used on local mares, then thoroughbreds were introduced. The principle was that mares produced by a thoroughbred were bred to local stallions. The result is a horse with many thoroughbred characteristics but with the strength, endurance and versatility of its native progenitors. Equally at home under saddle as a cavalry horse and in harness as a farm worker.

Most are bays or chestnuts. Most exceed 16 hands.

Brumby This is called the wild horse of Australia. In fact it is feral (domestic gone wild). The origin of its name is not known, but may come from one of the following sources: a horse breeder named James Brumby; *baroomby*, the aboriginal word for wild; or 'Baramba', a creek in Queensland.

The breed is derived from horses which were turned loose during the gold rush of the 1850s. These horses bred in the wild, but only the most intelligent (or vicious if you like) survived. Brumbies today are difficult to catch and most are impossible to train.

Soon after the First World War more horses were turned loose, due to mechanization and the Brumby became a pest. They have been reduced in number by subtle techniques developed by the Australians. These include shooting, trapping and hunting them with jeeps and light aircraft.

Budyonny This breed was founded by Marshal Budyonny, during the Russian Revolution. Thoroughbreds were crossed with Dons at the army stud at Rostov. This produced a good cavalry horse which was selectively bred. The breed was recognized in 1948.

Today the Budyonnys excel in steeple-chasing and show-jumping.

Average height 16 hands. Their main colours are chestnut and bay, often with the beautiful golden shading shown by many Russian horses.

Calabrese This is a medium-weight saddle horse, bred in the wildest part of Italy. It has a strong but compact body, with a small head. It may be any solid colour.

The height is about 16 hands.

Campolino Similar to the Mangalarga but slightly heavier. It is used for riding and light draught work.

Named after Sr Cassiano Campolino, who founded the breed about 100 years ago.

Charollais, Nivernais, Bourbonnais (halfbreeds) These are three very similar French halfbreeds, known collectively as the Demi-Sang Charollais. They were bred from the horses of Lorraine, Doubs and Saône, crossed with thoroughbreds and Anglo-Normans. Formerly used as cavalry and artillery horses, today they are prized as hunters.

Height 15 to 16.2 hands. Any solid colour.

Cleveland Bay Claimed to be among the oldest of established English breeds. It was known as the Chapman Horse in the 17th and 18th centuries, and used by travelling merchants in the north of England. The nearly extinct Yorkshire Coach Horse was an 18th-century development of the breed. Today they are in great demand as ceremonial coach horses.

The colour is usually bay or bay-brown. White hairs on the heels are acceptable but other white markings are not desirable. The height is between 15.2 and 16.1 hands.

Criollo Derived from Spanish, Arabs and Barbs ridden by the Conquistadores in the 16th century. Some 300 years of selection by man and nature has produced this small South American horse which by any standard is a symbol of toughness and endurance.

In the Argentine, much of the breeding stock is selected by a test in addition to inspection by the owner. The test is standard: the horse covers 750 km (470 miles) carrying 110 kg (17 stone) in 15 days, with no accompanying vehicles carrying food or water. They survive on the countryside. One assumes that those who don't pass the test are either culled as breeders or sold to those who believe that words, descriptions, pedigrees and appearance are more important than performance.

There are several types of Criollo: the Criollo in Argentina and Uruguay, the Crioñlo of Brazil, the Costeño and Morochuco of Peru, the Caballo Chileno of Chile and the Llanero of Venezuela. They are all descended from the same Spanish stock.

Height 13.3 to 15 hands. Colours include a characteristic dun with a dorsal stripe and zebra-striped legs, chestnut, greys, blacks, palominos, and mixed colours like blue and white.

Danubian This 20th-century breed was developed from Nonius stallions and Anglo-Arab mares. They are bred on a state stud near Pleven which supplies foundation stock for the horse population of northern Bulgaria. They are mainly used as draught animals but are more than adequate under saddle. They are strong and active horses with massive shoulders and powerful hindquarters.

The height is about 15.2 hands. The usual colours are black and dark chestnut.

Døle – Gudbrandsdal This Norwegian breed is similar in appearances to the Dales pony and the Friesian; all three derive from the same stock. It is widespread in Norway and varies from heavy draught to thoroughbred types. They are used for many purposes, including farming, lumbering and saddle but since the Second World War demand has decreased. Today, government studs produce lighter horses for riding.

The height is between 14.2 and 15.2 hands. The most usual colours are black, brown and bay.

Døle – Trotter Developed from lighter Dole horses in the 18th century because of a demand for horse-drawn vehicles. Odin, imported in 1834, was the most influential stallion.

Although similar in appearance to the Fell pony, the Trotter is noted for its free and active movement and readily adapts to harness.

Average height above fifteen hands.

Don Formerly used by the Cossacks in the central Asian steppes. It was important as a cavalry breed in the 19th century and was used against Napoleon's army in 1812. Improved later in the 19th century by the introduction of Turkoman, Karabakh and Karabair blood. Today it is a quality saddle horse with great hardiness and endurance.

Height between 15.1 and 15.3 hands. Colour usually chestnut, bay, grey or golden.

East Bulgarian Developed at two state studs: the Vassil Kolarov farm near Shumen and the Stefan Karadja stud at Dodrudja. Four foundation breeds were used: thoroughbreds, half-breds, Arabs and Anglo-Arabs. By 1950 the type was fixed, and since then the only outside introductions have been thoroughbreds. It is used in sports such as dressage and eventing, and also competes successfully in endurance courses such as the Grand Pardubice in Czechoslovakia. It is expected to work on the farm as well.

The height averages 15.3 hands. Its colour is usually chestnut or black. The appearance is definitely Anglo-Arab.

East Friesian This was the same as the Oldenburg until the division of Germany at the end of the Second World War. Since then the East Friesians have developed separately, with the introduction of Arabian and Hungarian-Arab blood. They have produced a more refined breed equally at home under saddle or in harness.

It may be any solid colour. The height varies between 16 and 16.2 hands.

Einsiedler Named after the Benedictine abbey of Einsiedeln in Switzerland, where there has been a stud since 1064. Closely related to the Anglo-Norman. It is used in many sports, including jumping, dressage and trotting; it is also used in light farm work and in the Swiss Cavalry.

The height is about 16 hands. The most common colours are bay and chestnut.

Frederiksborg Originated at the stud of that name founded by King Frederick II in 1562. Foundation stock was mainly Andalusian and Neapolitan. Judicious breeding produced offspring that were in great demand as carriage and saddle horses, but injudicious selling depleted the stud to such an extent that in 1839 it had to close. Later, outside blood was introduced. Today the breed is popular throughout Denmark as a light draught and harness horse as well as under saddle.

Height between 15.2 and 16.1 hands. Colour usually chestnut.

Freiberger Saddle Horse Developed recently at Avenches in Switzerland. It is based on the old Freiberger cold-blood which in former years was widely used in agriculture. However, as much as 90% Arab blood has been used to produce the modern, elegant riding horse which appears to have lost none of the strength and hardiness of its cold-blooded ancestors.

Height 15.2 to 16.1 hands. Any solid colour but greys and blue-roans are the most common.

French Saddle Horse (Selle Française), **Anglo-Norman, Norman** These three breeds are not exactly the same, but have all developed from similar stock. There is no definite dividing line between them.

In France about a thousand years ago, there was a heavy draught-type known as the Norman. The modern horses are descended from these, crossed with German and Scandinavian stallions in the 17th century and English blood in the 18th and 19th centuries. These formed the French saddle horse and the Anglo-Norman which, today, are selectively bred for the saddle.

The Anglo-Normans are popular for cavalry work and in show-jumping. They are being given a new name: the French Saddle Horse.

Usual colours are chestnut or bay, but they may be any colour. The height is between 15.2 and 16.3 hands.

French Trotter (Demi-Sang Trotter) A development of the Anglo-Norman. The first trotting races were held in Cherbourg in 1836 and were widespread by the mid-19th century. A stud book was opened in 1922 for any horses which could trot 1 km ($\frac{5}{8}$ mile) in less than 1 minute 42 seconds. The most important stallions in the breed then were Young Rattler, Normand, Lavater and Fuchsia. They have produced a tall, lightweight breed capable of carrying up to 75 kg (160 lb) over quite long distances. This is because some French trotting races are run under saddle rather than in the shafts.

Usual height about 16.2 hands. Colours: black, bay, brown, chestnut, grey and roan.

Friesian Said to be one of the oldest breeds in Europe. It comes from the province of Friesland, where horses have been used for over 3,000 years.

In the 19th century the Friesian was bred towards a lighter, faster type of horse, suitable for racing. In the process it lost much of its ability as a farm horse. This nearly caused the extinction of the breed, and just before the First World War only three Friesian stallions were left. The breed was revived by Dutch farmers, and became important in agriculture in the Second World War. Today it is popular in harness, in circuses and under saddle.

It has a pleasant temperament, is willing and hardworking, and has the ability to survive on poor food. The colour must be black – no other colour is allowed. The height is about 15 hands.

Furioso These horses have been bred in Hungary since the middle of the 19th century. The initial stallions were Furioso, an English Thoroughbred, and North Star, a Norfolk Roadster. They were bred with Nonius-type native mares.

Popular in their native and adjoining countries where they are used for dressage, cross country, jumping, steeplechasing and carriage.

The colours are black, dark bay and bay-brown, often with white markings. The height averages 16 hands.

Gelderland Originates from native Dutch horses crossed with Andalusians, Normans and Norfolk Roadsters. Recently the breed has been improved. Today it is an excellent carriage horse and good showjumper.

It has a stylish action and is docile and good natured. Its height ranges from 15.2 to 16 hands. Chestnut and grey are the most usual colours.

German Trotter These were developed in the second half of the 19th century from Russian Orlov Trotters. They have been improved by the introduction of American Standard and French Trotter blood. Eligible for the standard register if they can cover 1 km in less than 1 minute 30 seconds. A special register is open to horses who cover the distance in less than 1 minute 20 seconds. The record is 1 minute 17.3 seconds, held by Permit.

Groningen Originally a Dutch farm horse developed from heavier Friesians and East Friesians. It is useful as a heavy saddle horse, and also has the showy action desirable for a carriage horse.

The height is between 15.2 and 16 hands, but it may be taller. The usual colour is black but bays and dark browns are acceptable.

Hackney The Hackney horse's immediate ancestor is the Norfolk Roadster. This breed was started in 1729 for farmers who wanted fast and strong riding horses. The Hackney was developed from these.

The action of the Hackneys is extravagent – even spectacular. The shoulder movement is free, giving a springing walk. The fore-legs are thrown well forward, with no side to side movement. The tail is set and carried high.

The height varies between 14.3 and 15.3 hands in Britain, and up to 16 hands in the USA. The main colours are black, bay, brown and chestnut.

Hanoverian One of the older warm-blooded German breeds. Descended from the Hanoverian Creams (or Isabellas, as they were also called). They were justly famed as ceremonial carriage horses. Today they command top prices as dressage horses and show-jumpers.

Height 15.3 to 17 hands. All solid colours.

Hispano (Spanish Anglo-Arab) Bred from Spanish Arab mares with thoroughbred stallions, in the Estremadura and Andalusia areas of Spain.

An agile horse used in the testing of young fighting bulls and in hunting, jumping and dressage.

Height about 16 hands. Colours are bay, chestnut or grey.

Holstein Before Columbus discovered America, the Germans were improving their Marsh Horse. In those days they used it as a war horse. Between wars they used it for carriage and agriculture. Andalusian, Oriental, Neapolitan and later thoroughbred blood was introduced. Today, as carriages and wars are relatively rare, the Holstein proves his worth at show-jumping and three-day events.

Height 15.3 to 16.2 hands. Any solid colour, but blacks, bays and brown are most common.

Iomud Developed by the Iomud tribe, in Northern Turkmeina. Adaptable; able to live in extremes of temperature ranging from fierce summers to severe winters. It has the courage and endurance necessary for long distance and cross-country races.

Height between 14.2 and 15 hands. Most common colours are grey, then chestnut and bay.

Irish Cob Strong, reliable horses which have existed in Ireland for many centuries. In the 18th and 19th centuries they were in great demand for pulling carts to market and for tradesmen's delivery carts. Today the few remaining representatives of the type are considered ideal hacks for the heavy rider.

Height between 15 and 16 hands. May be any colour, but the most common are black, bay, chestnut and grey.

Irish Draught Horse Large, powerful horses with massive shoulders and hind quarters. They may be classified as cold-blooded horses, but they possess so many of the characteristics of top riding horses that one may be better to leave the final decision to their Irish admirers. Certainly, when crossed with Arabs and thoroughbreds many produce top hunters and jumpers.

Height 15 to 17 hands. Colours bay, brown, chestnut and bay.

Irish Hunter A type rather than a breed, but recognized internationally as a classical hunter and show-jumper. Although they are of obvious thoroughbred descent, their verbal 'pedigrees' may contain whimsy, fantasy and a dash of reality. The breed has achieved its fame by results rather than paper.

They stand 16 to 16.3 hands. Any solid colour.

Kabardin This Russian mountain breed comes from the northern Caucasus area. It is extremely sure-footed and courageous, able to tackle narrow, steep mountain paths. The breed results from crossing native Mongol horses with Persian or Arab blood. It has been improved with Turkoman stock.

Height between 14.2 and 15.1 hands. The colour is usually bay, but may be black, dark brown or grey.

Karabair An ancient mountain breed from the Uzbekistan area of Russia. It is used in central Asia for farming and in many equestrian games. The breed is divided into three types: the fast Strong-Saddle, the massive Harness, and the Saddle-Harness.

The colour is usually grey, bay or chestnut. The height is 15 to 15.3 hands.

Karabakh An ancient breed from the Karabakh Mountains. It was known 1,500 years ago and is thought to contain Turkoman, Arab and Persian blood. It became popular in the 18th century but is now relatively rare.

Height between 14 and 14.3 hands. Colours dun, chestnut and grey, usually with a golden sheen.

Kladruber A Czechoslovakian breed of Andalusian origin. They were first bred by Emperor Maximilian II in the 16th century, at a stud in Kladruby in Bohemia. The breeding was done very selectively and new blood was only introduced from Lipizza and Piber studs.

Today the Kladruber is a tall horse, from 16 to 17.2 hands, but otherwise similar to the Lipizzaner. Its usual colour is grey, but may occasionally be black.

Knabstrup This Danish breed dates back to the Napoleonic Wars, when a spotted mare called Flaebehoppen was mated with a Frederiksborg stallion. The colt, named Flaebehingsten, became the foundation stallion of the breed.

Today, unhappily, Knabstrups are selected for breeding according to colour rather than type. The colour is roan, with an Appaloosa pattern. Height is about 15.3 hands.

Kustanair The Kustanair was improved from the hardy horses running wild in Kazakhstan. They were crossed with thoroughbreds and Dons to produce a taller breed divided into three types: the massive Steppe, the light Saddle, and the Basic (which is between the two). They are good horses under saddle and in harness.

The usual colours are bay and chestnut. The height is between 15 and 15.2 hands.

Latvian Harness Horse A typical northern European Forest horse which has been known and used for at least a couple of thousand years. Recently, Arab, thoroughbred, German Saddle and heavy breeds have been introduced. Today they are divided into three types: 85% are considered all-purpose; the others are either taller and heavier harness types or lighter trotters. In the north it is still widely used as a draught horse but is considered all-purpose. In the south it is more commonly saddled.

Height 15.2 to 16 hands. Colours bay, dark brown and chestnut.

Libyan Barb These horses come from Arab and Barb stock. They are not bred selectively but are much used in north Africa as a saddle horse and for any general work. They are handy, have great stamina and can survive on poor food.

The colours and height are similar to the Barb.

Limousin Halfbred An all-purpose quality saddle horse developed from local stock and thoroughbred, Arab and Anglo-Arab stallions. Sometimes used for farm work but the farmers tend to prefer the oxen of the same name. This may be partly due to the fact that they mature relatively late. It is said that they can hardly be used for hunting before the ripe late-adolescence of seven years.

Any solid colour but bays and chestnuts predominate.

Lipizzaner An Austrian breed developed in the 16th century. The original stock was Andalusian, bred at the Lipizza stud, so the breed today is very similar in appearance to the Andalusian. The Lipizzaners today are well known at the famous Spanish Riding School of Vienna, founded in 1758, where they are trained in 'Airs' and other advanced exercises.

They have a height of between 15 and 16 hands. The colour is almost always grey, but may be bay, chestnut or roan.

Lokai A tough Russian horse from the mountain areas of Uzbekistan and Tadzhistan. It was developed by the Lokai tribe of Uzbekistan in the 16th century, for pack and transport work. Since then it has been made taller and more handsome by the introduction of Iomud and Karabair blood.

It is used in the Russian game of *kop-kopi* (goat snatching), in which a mounted man carrying a goat is chased by others who try to take the goat.

The Lokai is usually bay, grey or chestnut. There may be a golden sheen to the coat. The height is between 14 and 14.3 hands.

Lusitano A Portuguese breed of obscure origin probably derived from Andalusian and Arab stock. Certainly it has been recognized for several centuries.

It is much used in the bull-ring now, by the mounted bullfighters known as *rejoneadores*. They are responsive to a high standard of training. They are also noted for their exceptional bravery – which one doesn't commonly associate with intelligence.

The height is between 15 and 16 hands. The colour is usually grey, but may be any solid colour.

Mangalarga A Brazilian breed derived from Andalusian and Portuguese stallions bred with Crioñlo mares about 100 years ago. Similar to the Criollo but generally lighter in build. An elegant riding horse. Many are easily taught a gait known as the 'Marcha', a movement between a trot and canter.

Height about 14.3 hands. Colours: Bay, chestnut, grey and roan.

Maremmana (Maremma) An indigenous Italian breed, strong and hardy, used as a heavy saddle or light draught horse. It is ridden by the Italian mounted police and the *butteri* (cowboys) who herd cattle. It is also used as a light agricultural horse.

Height about 15.2 hands. All solid colours.

Masuren Aside from memories and corpses, the Nazis left some good Trakehner horses in Poland in 1945. These have been judiciously bred with no outside introductions to produce the Masuren which is indistinguishable from its German cousins.

Mecklenburg Originally a heavy horse more suitable for draught, this East German breed has been modified over the last century. The idea was to produce an animal suitable for the cavalry or artillery when duty called and equally suitable for general use in the odd lulls between. The area after which the breed is named has lush pastures – possibly not ideally suited to the English Thoroughbreds who have occasionally been introduced. Many Hanoverians have been reared there and to some eyes the breeds are almost indistinguishable. Today it is a good-boned saddle horse.

15.2 to 16.3 hands high, and all solid colours are recognized.

Metis Trotter American standardbreds were crossed with Orlov Trotters in 1950 to produce this breed which is obviously still evolving.

Like the Orlov its average height is 15.3 hands. Common colours are grey, black, chestnut and bay.

Mexican Native (Native Mexican) This is a small saddle horse containing blood from North and South American horses: Andalusian, Arab, Criollo and Mustang.

It is a tough, hardy breed, adapted to a harsh climate by natural selection. Its height is about 15 hands. It is found in any colour.

Morgan One prepotent sire called Justin Morgan, after his owner, was the founder of this deservedly popular breed. His origin is obscure but we know that he was born in New England towards the end of the 18th century and every Morgan today can trace its origins back to him. Besides founding the breed he did heavy farm work, won weight-pulling contests, harness and saddle races. Although the modern Morgan is taller and more refined than Justin Morgan they have retained the endurance and the skills of their progenitor.

Height 14 to 15.2 hands. Colours bay, black, brown and chestnut.

Murgese This Italian saddle horse comes from the famous horse-breeding district of Murge. The original breed died out about 200 years ago, but it has recently been revived. It is a light draught or saddle horse. It shows an Oriental appearance, but is not yet uniform in type.

The colour is usually chestnut. The height is between 15 and 16 hands.

Mustang (Bronco) A North American 'breed' derived from the Spanish horses brought by the Conquistadors in the 16th century. The name is a derivation of the Spanish *mestengo*, meaning 'stranger'. Mustangs have roamed wild on the plains of Western America for 300 years. During this time natural selection has changed them from the finer aristocratic Arab types to the tough, hardy horses of today.

The Mustang is on the decline today but has been given certain areas where it may roam freely, so it may continue as a North American 'breed'. Quite obviously there are no definitive standards, but heights average about 14 or 15 hands and all colours are acceptable.

May one note in passing that the majority end up being slaughtered for dog food.

New Kirgiz An all-purpose saddle and harness breed developed about fifty years ago by using 50% Don, 25% Kirgiz and 25% thoroughbred. 'Stamina', 'free-moving' and 'sure-footed' are the characteristics of this breed.

The smallest representatives just reach pony height. The largest go to 15.25 hands. Bay, grey or chestnut are the common colours

Nonius Originated on the Mezohegyes stud in Hungary. Descended from Nonius, a French stallion, who was foaled about 1810 in Normandy. Today the Nonius is also bred in Yugoslavia, Rumania and Czechoslovakia. It is an all-purpose horse used for sport, carriage work and farming.

The breed is divided into two according to height: the Large Nonius is over 15.3 hands, the Small Nonius less than 15.3 hands.

Oldenburg This, tallest of all German breeds, has been evolving since the early 17th century. The original draught Friesian type has been modified by the use of at least ten other breeds including Andalusians, thoroughbreds, Barbs and Cleveland Bays. Formerly a carriage horse, today it is an all-purpose saddle horse quite obviously more suited to the taller rider.

Height from 16.2 to 17.2 hands. Blacks, browns and bays predominate but any solid colour is acceptable.

Orlov Trotter On state farms in the USSR there are thirty-odd thousand representatives of this breed. Many can cover a mile in just over two minutes. Count Alexius Grigorievich Orlov (born 1737) developed the breed by crossing his Arab stallion Smetanka with a Dutch mare. The colt Polkan was crossed with another Dutch mare to produce Bars First, who was the foundation sire of the breed. Later, more Dutch, Arab and English blood was introduced.

Their average height is 15.3 hands. The most common colours are grey or black.

Palomino The colour has been recognized and highly regarded for centuries. What better image than an armoured knight riding on a golden horse? But is it a breed? Despite half a century of enthusiasm in America and despite the existence of dozens of Palomino Clubs with thousands of horses, the fact is that the true golden sheen is not easily reproduced in the progeny. Many that could better be described as chestnuts, yellows, or even dirty whites, join the parades.

In Britain the colour is more popular with owners of ponies. In America the enthusiasts aim for a quality riding horse of Arab, Barb, Morgan or Quarter Horse type.

The Association of Palomino Horse Breeders of America set their heights at 14.2 to 15.3 hands.

The colour ideally should be gold. No markings other than white. Mane and tail white with not more than 15% dark or chestnut. Dark eyes are obligatory. Quite wisely they have decided that anything else would be a step to albinos.

One is almost obliged to comment that where colour is the prime object in selective breeding, other standards may be neglected.

Paso Fino Bred mainly in Puerto Rico and equatorial South America from horses brought in by the Spanish explorers in the 16th century.

The breed is famous for its natural four-beat gaits: the paso fino (the slowest), the paso corto (used for covering long distances) and the faster paso largo. Some say the gait is characteristic, others enthuse that it's inherent.

Height about 14.3 hands. They may be found in all colours.

Peruvian Stepping Horse (Peruvian Paso) Basically a criollo type with a unique gait known as the paso. This is a movement adapted to carry a rider for long distances. The forelegs are moved in an extravagant paddle, while the hind legs move in a long straight stride, giving an ambling gait at about 18 kmph (10 mph). Originally bred some three centuries ago from Barb and Andalusian stock it is virtually unknown elsewhere.

Height 14 to 15.2 hands. They may be any colour, but bays and chestnuts predominate.

Pinto A breed based on colour. The horses have black and white patches all over the body. There are two distinct patterns: Overo and Tobiano. The Overo pattern has white patches originating at the belly and extending upwards. The back, mane and tail are usually dark, with dark and white alternating on the legs. The Tobiano pattern does not have a particular place of origin. The white and coloured areas are larger and not so patchy. The legs are usually white. It is reputedly a 'breed' that originated in America. Certainly it is popular there. Standards are not exacting.

The height varies so widely that no limits are laid down.

Pleven Originally bred at the Georgi Dimitrov stud. Now bred throughout Bulgaria. Developed from about 1900 using Anglo-Arab stallions and, later, Hungarian Gidran stallions, with local mares. In recent years English Thoroughbred blood has been introduced. A lightweight all-purpose animal, well suited to jumping.

They are about 15.2 hands high. The colour is bright chestnut.

Salerno A quality saddle horse, from the Maremma and Salerno regions of Italy. Like people of that salubrious area, it is attractive, intelligent and responsive.

The height is about 16 hands. It may be any solid colour.

Sardinian This is a hardy island breed, used by mounted police and as a general saddle horse. It can be used in jumping, and has taken part in international competitions for the Italian army.

Its height is between 15 and 15.2 hands, but it may be smaller. The most usual colours are bay and brown.

Shagya Arab Some of the original mares were not Arabs. The breed was started in the 1830s at the Babolna stud in Hungary, when five Arab mares and nine stallions were brought in. The breed is named after the best of these stallions. Today the stallions are still named Shagya followed by a Roman numeral which shows how many generations separate them from the original Shagya. They are highly rated and used throughout Europe and America; and they are versatile.

The Shagya Arabs are almost always grey. Their height is about 15 hands.

Sokolsky A powerful, thick-set and good-natured beast of burden. Highly valued on small farms throughout Poland and Russia for its frugality and its willingness.

Most are closer to 15 hands than its maximum 16. All solid colours but most are chestnuts.

Swedish Halfbreed (Swedish Warm Blood) Started 300 years ago by crossing Oriental, Andalusian and Friesian stallions with local mares. In those days they were used for the cavalry. Today the cavalry use tanks: the horses compete in the Olympics.

By any standards they are a big breed – averaging 16.2 hands. Chestnuts, bays, brown and greys are common.

Tarpan Today recorded as a Polish breed. Like Przewalski's horse (the Mongolian wild horse) it is also named scientifically after the man who devoted much of his life to the study of the progenitors of our modern horses. Superficially it resembles the Mongolian but many authorities suggest it has been reconstituted from domestic stock. Unless you're very serious it would be inadvisable to study the subject at close quarters. They can be effectively aggressive.

Height around 13 hands. Colours dun to brown with a dorsal stripe. Like the Mongolian, zebra-stripes may occur on the limbs and body.

Tennessee Walking Horse (Plantation Walking Horse) Like the

Morgan, all are descended from one stallion. He was a standard-bred named Black Allan (foaled 1886) of Hambletonian and Morgan ancestry. They have developed a unique four-beat gait, known as the running walk. The forelegs move in a high straight walk, while the hind have a long striding action. They are said to be the most comfortable of all riding horses, and the gait is so characteristic of the breed that foals at foot have been seen doing it quite naturally. Some assume this to be imitative behaviour, others would say it's part of an innate pattern due to generations of in-breeding. It may be a bit of both.

Height 15 to 16 hands. Any solid colours.

Tersky A Russian breed, developed in the 1920s and officially recognized in 1948. It was bred in the Tersk stud in the northern Caucasus, from Russian-Arab (Streletsk) stallions with pure-bred Arab and Kabarda mares. Today the Tersky is a hardy horse, used in flat-racing and cross-country.

Its height averages 15 hands. The colour is grey.

Toric Developed at the end of the 19th century in Estonia. The basis of the breed was the local Klepper horse, crossed with Arab, Ardennais, East Friesian, Hackney, Hanoverian, Orlov Trotter, thoroughbred and Trakehner. It is a handsome, light draught horse popular on the farms of northern Russia.

The main colour is chestnut, but may be bay. The height averages 15.1 hands.

Trakehner (East Prussian) These horses were originally bred at the Trakehnen stud, founded in 1732 by Frederick William I of Prussia. It is now administered by the Polish government. The breed originated with local and Schweiken horses, but latterly Arab and thoroughbred blood was introduced. Today they are bred privately in West Germany where they are known as East Prussians. Enthusiasts claim it is far and away the best German breed. It is certainly versatile, being used for dressage, farm work and as military mounts.

The height is between 16 and 16.2 hands.

Waler More a type than a breed. At its best, a quality riding horse. At its worst, a biggish horse of indifferent quality. As Australia has no indigenous horses it is thought that the originals were Spanish horses brought in about 1795. Salubrious New South Wales is famous for all sorts of athletes. By 1810 there were 1,134 horses. By 1821 the figure was 4,564. Later, Arab and thoroughbred blood was introduced to produce what some experts called the best riding horse in the world.

But three historical events led to the decline of the breed. The gold rush of the 1850s created a demand for indifferent draught horses and this resulted in an inevitable lowering of quality. The First World War literally wasted 120,000 of the best. Although they were highly reckoned in India, the Middle East and Europe, Australian quarantine laws decreed that they be shot. And, of course, the motor car which eclipsed the horse in much of the world made its impact in Australia.

Height about 16 hands. Found in all colours.

Wurttemberg A product of the Marbach stud founded in 1573. They used local mares, Arab stallions and introduced East Prussian, Anglo-Norman, Suffolk Punch and a few other unrecorded breeds. They were either very bad judges of horseflesh or perfectionists, because it wasn't until 1895 that they opened the stud book. Today the breed is still principally bred at the original stud. A willing worker ideal for mountain farms, it is equally at home in harness or under saddle.

The average height is about 16 hands, which is rather remarkable when one considers that most mountain bred equines are ponies. Black, bay, brown and chestnut are the usual colours.

Cold-blooded horses

Ardennais An ancient breed. Some say it was praised by Cæsar. It was used by Marshal Turenne in the 17th century as a cavalry horse and as an artillery horse by Napoleon in 1812. Today it is on the decline as mechanization replaces its agricultural and military roles.

A massive, compact horse, extremely strong, but also calm and gentle. Ten-year-old children can handle the stallions.

Height about 15.3 hands. Usual colours are bay, roan or chestnut.

Auxois An old breed from north-eastern Burgundy. It has existed since the Middle Ages, but since the 19th century has become a heavier draught horse because of crossings with Percheron and Boulonnais stallions. Today the Auxois also contains much Ardennais blood. In appearance it is similar to the Ardennais and Trait du Nord.

A strong, heavy horse up to 16 hands high. Usual colours are red roan or bay.

Boulonnais Similar to the Percheron. It comes from northern France and contains Oriental and Andalusian blood introduced in the Middle Ages. Today it is bred in two types: the medium-sized Abbeville and the large, heavy Dunkirk type. Both are active, hard-working farm horses but they have been used as carriage horses because of their speed and endurance.

They stand between 16 and 17 hands. The usual colour is grey but chestnut and bays are not uncommon.

Brabant (Belgian Heavy Draught) Said to be descended from the large horses of the Quarternary period, and the Ardennais. During the Middle Ages it was used as a war horse and at that time was closely related to the Flander's Horse, which does not exist today. Since the Reformation, the Brabant has been selectively bred and even inbred for outstanding qualities. Now it invariably breeds true. It has had more influence on the development of many other heavy breeds than its present numbers would suggest. Powerful, willing and good tempered.

Height is up to 17 hands. Traditionally the colour is red roan with black points, but it may be chestnut, bay, brown, dun or grey.

Breton There are three sorts of 'native' cold-blooded horses in Brittany. The draught was produced by using Percheron, Ardennais and Boulonnais. The Postier Breton, a medium-height coaching type, shows the influence of Hackney and Norfolk Trotter blood. The lighter, rare type called the Corlay was heavily influenced by Arab and thoroughbred blood.

From 14.3 hands upwards depending on type. Most are red roans or blue roans, but chestnuts and bays are not uncommon.

Clydesdale Developed in the mid-18th century in Lanarkshire. Local mares were crossed with heavy Flemish stallions to produce a horse capable of pulling large loads on the improved road surfaces. During the heyday of the heavy draught it was exported all over the world. A strong, active horse, it is characterized by heavy feathering and long, clean action. Both these factors have advantages for work on hard surfaces, but are obviously not adaptations one would choose for heavy pulling on low-lying farmland.

Height averages 16.2 hands. The most common colours are bay and brown with much white on the face and legs.

Comtois Bred in the Franche-Comté region of France, near the Swiss border. A sure-footed mountain breed, strong and active. Brought to the region about the 6th century. Since the Middle Ages has been considered an ideal military horse. Now largely supplanted by the helicopter.

Height between 14.3 and 15.3 hands. The most common colour is bay, then chestnut.

Dutch Draught Horse This breed is only about fifty years old. It was developed from the old Zeeland horse, crossed with Ardennais blood. It has been carefully bred for quality and purity of line. Horses attaining high standards may be entered in a special stud book. The Dutch draughts are quiet, kind horses with great stamina. They are extremely massive and strong.

They reach a height of 16.3 hands. The usual colours are chestnut, bay or grey.

Finnish The Finnish possesses characteristics of both warm-blooded and cold-blooded horses. It is descended from two breeds: the Finnish Universal and the Finnish Draught. Traditionally, the horses are selected for breeding by their performance, rather than appearance. This has produced a breed known not only for its speed, strength and stamina but also for its kindness and gentleness. It is used for all-purpose agricultural work, timber hauling, takes part in trotting races and is not bad under saddle.

Height is about 15.2 hands. The usual colour is chestnut but may be bay, brown or black.

Italian Heavy Draught Developed from the Breton in north and central Italy. An active, willing worker, its compact body is so like that of the ideal steer that many if not most are bred for the slaughter-house.

Height 15 to 16 hands. Characteristically it is an attractive if not striking dark liver-chestnut with a chestnut-blond mane and tail. Chestnuts and roans are not uncommon.

Jutland This breed has existed in Denmark for about 1,000 years. It was ridden by the Vikings and was the Danish war horse in the Middle Ages. Today it is primarily an agricultural horse and owes some of its development to the Suffolk Punch, imported from England.

It is a kind, gentle horse which is very easy to handle. It is a typical draught horse with massive features but short legs.

Height between 15.2 and 16 hands. The usual colours are chestnut or roan. Bays and blacks occasionally.

Lithuanian Heavy Draught Developed over the last 100 years in the Baltic States. The native Zhmud horse was crossed with imported Swedish Ardennes to produce a compact, hard-working draught horse. The breed was first registered in 1963 in two types: the basic and the lighter.

Height between 15 and 15.3 hands. The usual colour is chestnut, often with flaxen mane and tail. Blacks, bays, greys and roans are acceptable.

Murakoz Originally bred on the banks of the River Mura in southern Hungary. As well as native Hungarian it contains Ardennais, Percheron and Noriker blood. A strong, active breed, well suited to heavy agricultural work. It became very popular in Hungary during and after the First World War, when twenty per cent of the horses in the country were Murakoz. During the Second World War numbers inevitably declined. It is doubtful if there will ever be a resurgence.

Height about 16 hands. The usual colour is chestnut, with flaxen mane and tail but blacks, greys, bays and browns are not unusual.

North Swedish Descended from native domestic horses of north

Sweden. It was only established as a breed about 1900 when Døle-Gudbrandsdal stallions were introduced to upgrade the local stock. By 1944 the breed had 400 breeding stallions and 15,000 mares, producing about 8,000 colts a year.

Farmers reckon it highly. It is frugal, long-lived and willing. They also consider that it is resistant to most diseases of the horse – a claim which scientists view with some scepticism.

Height 15.1 to 15.3 hands. Colours may be black, bay, brown, chestnut or dun.

North Swedish Trotter Basically the same as the North Swedish breed. Some of the North Swedish horses were found to do well at trotting, so were selectively bred for this purpose. The Trotters are lighter in build, more energetic and have a better stride than their North Swedish cousins (or progenitors, if you prefer) but their reputation is parochial. They simply can't run as fast as other European or American trotters.

Percheron This French breed has developed from Oriental and Norman horses, crossed many centuries ago. Today they are popular all over the world, but can only be entered in the Percheron stud book in France if they were bred in one of the Departments: Sarthe, Eure-et-Loir, Loir-et-Cher or L'Orne.

In Britain the Percheron is often crossed with thoroughbreds to produce good heavyweight hunters. They are active, energetic horses but very easy to handle. The body and legs are immensely strong and powerful, so the Percheron is an ideal horse for heavy farm work. Absence of feather on the feet is a characteristic of the breed in Britain and America, but they're not quite so fussy in France.

Height is between 15.2 and 17 hands. Usual colours are grey or black.

Pinzgauer Noriker (South German cold-blood) An ancient breed, first bred by the Romans in the Kingdom of Noricum, part of present-day Austria. Further development of the breed took place during the Renaissance in the Pinzgau district of Austria, when Andalusian and Neapolitan blood was added.

Today it is still in demand in the mountain regions of central and southern Europe, as it is a very sure-footed breed well adapted to hill and mountain country.

Height is between 16 and 16.2 hands. Main colours are bay or chestnut, with flaxen mane and tail. Spotted, dun and skewbald are acceptable.

Poitevin Originally brought to the Poiters area of France from the flat lands of Northern Europe; it was used to help drain the marshes. When that job was done it might have died out, but for the fact that it produces mules of repute. Even admirers of the breed don't boast about its intelligence.

A heavy horse with massive legs and very large feet. Height between 16.2 and 17 hands. The usual colour is dun but it may be bay or brown.

Rhineland Heavy Draught (Rhenish) Developed at the end of the 19th century for use in agriculture and industry. It became the most popular of German breeds but latterly, with the general decline of the heavy breeds everywhere, it is seldom seen.

A good-natured, gentle, powerful giant. Height between 16 and 17 hands. The colour is chestnut or red roan with blond mane and tail, or red roan with black points.

Russian Heavy Draught This native Ukrainian is the closest creature to a pony among the draught breeds. Developed in the last 100 years from local mares crossed with Swedish Ardennes, Percherons and Orlov Trotters. Powerful but lively, it is widely used on farms throughout western Russia.

Height averages only 14.2 hands. The most usual colours are chestnut, roan and bay – invariably solid.

Schleswig Heavy Draught Although some authorities state this is a 19th-century breed, others say it has been known since the Middle Ages. At the end of the 19th century it was specially bred into a heavy draught type suitable for farming and industry. It contains much Jutland and Suffolk blood, and also Breton and Boulonnais. Today it is mainly bred in the western part of the Schleswig province of Germany.

Height between 15.2 and 16 hands. Its colour is almost always chestnut, with flaxen mane and tail.

Shire Draws gasps of admiration wherever it's shown. Possibly the gentlest horse in the world – certainly the tallest. Among the few people who consider it a viable commercial breed are the brewers. Long may they and the breed thrive! Probably developed from the old English Great Horse which originated in northern Europe, it attained its present unique stature in the counties of Cambridge, Lincoln and Huntingdon when our grandfathers were boys. Some postulate that an admixture of thoroughbred blood was the factor that gives it its height, its bearing and its free-flowing movement.

Height up to 18 hands. Bays and browns with white markings are the most common colours. Occasionally blacks and greys.

Suffolk Punch The indigenous Anglian horse. It has existed since at least the 16th century, when it was mentioned in Camden's *Britannia*. Development of the breed took place at the end of the 18th century. Today all trace back to a horse called Blakes Farmer, foaled in 1760.

The Suffolk is a universally popular horse, well suited to agricultural work and economical to feed and keep. Farmers who have no use for a draught horse find them a joy to have around.

Height between 16 and 16.2 hands. Colour is always chestnut, but seven shades exist: red, gold, copper, yellow, liver, light and dark.

Swedish Ardennes Bred in Sweden from Ardennais horses imported from Belgium, crossed with native north Swedish horses. Similar to the Ardennais horse, since it is bred in similar climate and terrain. It is the most popular Swedish heavy draught horse, formerly much in demand for general farm work. About sixty per cent of the country's horses are Swedish Ardennes. Today, like all heavy breeds, it is declining in numbers. It is still used for hauling timber.

Height is between 15.2 and 16 hands. Colours are black, bay, brown or chestnut.

Trait Du Nord A 19th-century development of the Ardennais, containing Belgian and Dutch heavy draught blood. The breed was fixed early in the 20th century and a stud book opened in 1919.

It is a strong, heavy horse, weighing about 1,000 kg (1 ton) – slightly bigger than the Ardennais.

Height about 16 hands. Colours may be bay, chestnut or roan.

Vladimir Heavy Draught This breed was developed in the second half of the 19th century, by using a mixture of Suffolk Punches, Cleveland Bays, Ardennais and Percherons. In 1910 some Shire blood was introduced, but since the First World War no new blood has been added. The breed is now fixed. A strong breed, noted for its energy and competitiveness.

Height is about 16 hands. All solid colours.

Ponies

American Shetland The American Shetland pony has been developed in the United States from specially selected ponies of the British Shetland breed. It is taller than the British version, being up to 11.2 hands, but is lighter in build. Its action is exaggerated – in a similar way to the Hackney pony.

The breed has become very popular in the USA, as shown by the prices paid for top studs. In 1957 a stallion was auctioned for $85,000 and since then $90,000 has been paid for another.

The American Shetland is adaptable. It is used as a family pet, in the show-ring, in trotting races and in pulling contests.

Australian Pony An elegant pony derived from Welsh Mountain and Arab stock. It also has some Timor, Shetland, Exmoor and thoroughbred blood. 'An intelligent and enduring pony', the breeders modestly claim. Unlike the people of that continent it hasn't travelled abroad very much.

Height between 12 and 14 hands.

Avelignese Pony The Avelignese pony comes from Italy, where it is popular as a pack pony in the Alps and Apennines. It is related to the Haflinger pony of Austria. The two breeds look very similar. It is said to contain some Oriental blood, and is descended from the now extinct Avellinum-Haflinger breed. This breed has a gentle character. It is kindly and easy to train.

Its colour is chestnut, with a blonde mane and tail. The height is between 13.3 and 14.3 hands.

Balearic Pony An ancient Mediterranean breed found on the Balearic Islands. It is used on small farms on the islands, where it pulls a wide cart. The main crop of Majorca is almonds, so if you see a pony and cart standing under an almond tree you may fairly assume it's a Balearic pony. Who could prove you wrong?

The Balearic pony has a fine build and a graceful movement. Its mane is upright, which makes the pony look similar to those sculptured on the Parthenon in Greece.

Height is about 14 hands. Colours brown or bay.

Basuto Pony (South Africa) In 1653, the Dutch East India Co. landed four horses in the Cape Province. These horses formed the basis of the Basuto pony breed. Arabs, Barbs, Persians and thoroughbreds were introduced later.

Fearless and enduring ponies, they are able to carry a man up to eighty miles a day. It is thought that this is the result of rigorous natural selection resulting from relatively little care by man in a clime that at most times of the year is inhospitable.

Height about 14.2 hands. Colours grey; also browns, bays, and chestnuts.

Bhutia A more cosmopolitan and slightly larger version of the Spiti. It has obviously evolved from the move to a more salubrious clime and outcrosses to larger stock. It is kept all the way from Punjab to Darjeeling. Some would say that the Spiti is the proof of the survival of the fittest in a more demanding area.

Height up to 13.2 hands. Darker solid colours are seen more commonly than greys.

Bosnian Pony Found all around the Balkan States. It originates from the Bosnia-Herzegovina regions of Yugoslavia, and there are said to be about 400,000 of them in Yugoslavia today. They are used for pack work, in agriculture, and sometimes as riding ponies. The Yugoslavian government controls the breeding of the Bosnian ponies, and will only select a stallion for breeding if it is able to carry a load of about 110 kg (220 lb) for 16 km (10 miles).

The Bosnian ponies are tough and hardy, similar to the Hucul pony. They are affectionate and very intelligent.

Burma (Shan) Pony Bred in the hills of east Burma, in the Shan States. They are related to the Mongolian pony, and are similar in appearance to a small Manipur pony. The Burma ponies were used by British officers in Burma for playing polo, when they couldn't get anything better.

Camarguais Pony (Camargue) These grey-white ponies live in the marshes of the Rhône delta in France. They breed in free-ranging herds in very sparse country, which is bleak in winter and hot and dry in summer. The origin of the Camarguais has not been established, but one French expert, Professor E. Bourdelle, believes that they are descendants of the quaternary horse, *Equus caballus fossilis*. This is based on the fact that Camarguais ponies have seven lumbar vertebrae, whereas most other horses only have six.

The height of the Camarguais is 14 to 15 hands, and its weight is up to 360 kg (800 lb).

Chincoteague and Assateague Ponies These ponies are found on the islands of Chincoteague and Assateague, off the coasts of Virginia and Maryland. It is not known definitely how they came to the islands, but it is claimed that they swam ashore from a wrecked ship which was carrying Moorish ponies to Peru. It is also rumoured that some Welsh stallions have been introduced, improving the breed. The ponies are rounded up every July and the Assateague ponies are swum across a narrow channel of sea to Chincoteague, where they are auctioned with the Chincoteague ponies.

The breed has the appearance of a lightweight horse. It is found in all colours, but the most common is pinto. Its height is about 12 hands.

Connemara Pony In the province of Connaught lies a rugged area which runs into the Atlantic on the west and into Galloway Bay in the south. There, since prehistoric times, a native pony has lived in a wild state.

As they say in Ireland, 'these ponies have been running wild longer than the men.' Certainly the ponies have been there a long time but they've changed more than a bit over the centuries. Some authorities say that the wreck of the Armada in 1588 introduced Spanish blood. But the Galloway merchants were trading regularly with Spain long before that. People may debate the dates of the introduction of Spanish and Arab blood, but no one disputes its presence in the breed.

During the last century both Arab and thoroughbred stallions were used on Connemara mares. The sturdy, dun-coloured Connemara of old, which was used in harness for hauling peat, rapidly evolved into a more stylish riding pony with no mean jumping ability. Fortunately, the breed societies soon recognized that the dilution of the native stock, if followed to its logical conclusion, would result in a completely different type. Since 1928 the policy has been not to recognize any outcrosses. Great attention has been paid to the standards of the stallions particularly, and as a result we have today a pony with stamina, speed, thriftiness and sense. The stud books of the breed society place great emphasis on constitution, staying power, docility, intelligence and soundness.

Although the Connemara was in early years primarily dun, today more than half of those registered are grey. Next come the blacks and then brown and bays. One almost never sees a dun.

Pure Connemara stock is used to produce some of the great Irish hunters and jumpers. One international show-jumper called Dundrum was produced by crossing a thoroughbred stallion called Little Heaven with a pure Connemara mare. It could clear seven feet although it was only 14.3 hands high.

The offspring of all animals transplanted from their harsh home environment to greener pastures tend to get taller and taller. The Connemara is no exception. Before too many horse generations – despite all the efforts of the breed society to retain the hardy, wiry, 13-to-14 hand size – we'll probably have a Connemara *Horse* Society.

Dales Pony In the rugged hills east of the Pennines the Dales pony has been bred and used by farmers for all tasks for hundreds of years. They are powerfully muscled. Although they seldom exceed regulation pony height they are capable of pulling a ton. A Dales pony can effortlessly carry a heavy man all day long. And they are so sure footed and knowing that even the novice rider quickly gains confidence. Every Dales pony registered today can be traced back to a Welsh Cob stallion called Comet who was introduced and used in the 19th century.

In colour they are either black, bay or dark brown. A small white star on the face is acceptable but anything more is considered to be a sign of Clydesdale blood.

Dartmoor Pony Strange that such an inhospitable area as Dartmoor has evolved a pony that *aficionados* describe as the ideal first pony for a child. It is kind, even affectionate, and sensible. Its most striking feature is the head which is classically aristocratic; as you would expect from a pony that has evolved on the exposed moors over a period of many centuries (certainly it was there well before man was able to record his own misdeeds) it has very small ears. There are all sorts of ponies and horses with very small ears who were born with very large ears. 'They got frozen small', would be a cowboy's truthful explanation. The Dartmoor's ears evolved small to save the pain. The conformation of the ideal Dartmoor pony is that of the riding pony as opposed to the bulkier, thicker conformation of the work pony. It combines the strength of its well-muscled back, loin and quarters with the hard, slim (almost refined) limbs one expects to find in what some call 'an easy rider'.

Unhappily, about a century ago, in order to satisfy the apparently insatiable demand for pit ponies, Shetlands were loosened on the moors. The Shetland-Dartmoor crosses proved commercially successful for a period. But during the process the Dartmoor as a breed was almost wiped out. Then, during the Second World War the armed forces took over the moors and the number of wild ponies inevitably declined. However, an enthusiastic breed society has managed to impose strict standards for the breed and it is gradually gaining both in numbers and devotees.

Although skewbalds and piebalds crop up from time to time they are not recognized by the breed society. The colours the breeders try to maintain are the sensible, black, bays and browns without too much white anywhere.

Average height 10 to 12 hands.

Dulmen Pony The Dulmen pony comes from the Westphalia region of West Germany, where it has been bred for six centuries. Today it is a vanishing breed: here are only about a hundred mares in the main herd, living semi-wild on the Meerfelder Bruch. These ponies are owned by the Duke of Cröy, who rounds them up every year to sell unwanted stock.

The Dulmen ponies are found in all colours, but black, brown and dun are the most usual. Their height is about 12.3 hands.

Exmoor Ponies Considered the oldest of the breeds native to Britain, it has survived and propagated on Exmoor without man's help for thousands of years. In actual distance, Exmoor is not all that far from Dartmoor. But the two breeds are quite distinct. This is all the more remarkable when one considers that basically there's not that much difference in the two environments and that over the centuries more than one stallion must have found his way from one moor to the other. As the Exmoor is the older breed, possibly it was the founder or one of the founders of the Dartmoor. This illustrates firstly the remarkable diversity that is to be found within the relatively small boundaries of Britain and secondly the natural process of selection which can occur to produce a distinct type in a closed community – or even one that allows the occasional stranger.

The Exmoors tend to be rather coarser than the Dartmoors. They have good heads with broad foreheads, wide flaring nostrils, and short thick ears – all dominated by prominent eyes which horse people in the area refer to (not disparagingly) as 'frog eyes'. Body conformation is that of a good riding pony – broad chest, well-angled shoulders, powerful loins and well-muscled quarters, combined with trim, hard legs. They carry a peculiar hard, springy coat which has probably evolved to protect them from the merciless winter winds.

Although the Exmoor is a pony and not a big one, it is essentially wild, and requires expert handling in the transition to paddock, stable and riding for pleasure. This can be a patience-racking job, because the Exmoor is both intelligent and strong. It can also be a well rewarded job. Once properly trained they will put their hearts as well as their intelligence and strength into the task in hand.

Although they may be bays, browns or duns all have a cream-coloured muzzle and may have the same colouration on their underbellies.

They average 11 to 12 hands.

Falabella Pony The Falabella pony is the smallest horse in the world, having a height of under 7 hands, i.e. smaller than most Great Danes!

It was developed by the Falabella family in Argentina, on the Recreo de Roca Ranch near Buenos Aires. The family owned a small thoroughbred, which they bred with a small Shetland, giving a miniature pony which has been further inbred with the smallest animals.

The breed is in some demand in North America as a pet and also for harness work. It is said to be a hardy horse, full of character. Any colour may be found in the breed, but Appaloosa markings are favoured.

Some experts would suggest, however, that this tendency towards miniatures is not a forward step in horse development.

Fjord (Westland) Pony It is astonishing that this tough, enduring and willing pony which has remained virtually unchanged since the time of the Vikings is almost unknown outside its native Norway and its Scandinavian neighbours. It is particularly valued for its sure-footedness and its ability to pull loads in terrain too steep for tractors.

It comes in all dun shades – but cream or yellow is most common. It has an upright mane which is traditionally cut short about 10 cm (4 in) high. The body is heavily muscled and very powerful. Height 13 to 14.2 hands.

Galiceno Pony The Galiceno pony is said to have been brought to Mexico from Galicia in Spain. When Cortes invaded Mexico it is thought that he landed sixteen Garrano or Minho ponies on the mainland, which formed the basis of the Galiceno breed. The Galiceno is now found in the USA where it is popular as a family riding pony, because of its good character and great stamina. It is an intelligent pony, easy to handle and very versatile, so is also used for ranch work and light transport.

Its height is between 12 and 13.2 hands and its weight when fully grown is between 270 and 320 kg (600 and 700 lb). Its colouring may be bay, black, sorrel, dun or grey.

Garrano (Minho) Pony The commonest breed of pony in Portugal, its origin is the Garrano do Minho and Tras dos Montes provinces, where it is bred in rich mountain pastures. It is an ancient breed, and has remained unchanged since Palaeolithic times. Cave paintings of the Garrano have been found, showing its association with early man.

The Garrano is a light pony, 10 to 12 hands high, and chestnut in colour. It is well known at the horse-fairs of Vila Real and Famalicao.

Gotland Pony (Gothland) (Skogsruss pony) An ancient breed, believed to be descended from the Tarpan. It originates on Gotland Island in Sweden, and is said to be the oldest Scandinavian breed. It has been running wild on Gotland since the Stone Age, and has been pure-bred since then except for the introduction of some Arab blood in the 19th century. Today the Gotland is also bred on the Swedish mainland in a controlled way. It is used as a children's riding pony and for trotting and jumping. It has a gentle character, although it may be obstinate.

Height is between 12 and 12.2 hands. Practically all colours, including palomino.

Greek Ponies *Peneia Pony* An Oriental type of pony bred in Peneia in the Peloponnese. It is a very hardy pony and a good worker. It is slightly larger than the other Greek ponies.

The most usual colours are brown, bay, chestnut and grey but they may be found in most colours. It may be up to 14 hands high.

Pindos Pony The Pindos pony is thought to have an Oriental origin. Now bred in the foothills and mountains of Thessaly and Epirus. It is strong but light, and may be used as a riding pony or in agriculture.

The colour is dark or grey, and the height is 12 to 13 hands.

Skyros Pony An ancient Greek breed, originating from the island of Skyros. the Greeks use it as a pack pony and also for light agricultural work; and on the mainland it is often used as a small child's riding pony.

Its most common colours are dun, brown and grey. It is a small pony, standing between 9.1 and 11 hands high.

Hackney Pony The word 'hackney' is derived from the Norman French *haquenai*, which was used in the Middle Ages to describe humble horses. The Hackney pony first appeared in the 1860s, probably bred from the Norfolk Roadster trotting horse.

The movement of the Hackney pony is extravagant, the feet flung far forward, and the hocks brought up under the body; in England, this dramatic action is seen mainly in the show-ring, where the Hackney appears usually as a harness-pony, but may also be found in riding and show-jumping, since it has very powerful hindquarters and legs. In the days before the motor car, the Hackney was also used by tradesmen, as a status symbol, to show off their success to customers.

The most usual colours of the breed are brown, black and bay, and the height is between 12.2 and 14.2 hands.

Haflinger Pony From the Tirol region of Austria, where it is bred in the mountain pastures. It is a good mountain pony, as it is very sure-footed, and excellent for pack work. For these reasons the German authorities bred Haflinger ponies during the Second World War, at a stud in Piber, Austria.

The Haflinger is very long-lived. It is said to be able to work until it is forty years old. This is possibly due to the fact that the ponies are left on the mountains until they are four years old, before being broken in.

The colour of the Haflinger is chestnut, and it has a long, flaxen mane and tail. Its height is about 14 hands.

Highland Pony The Highland breed of Scotland is divided into two groups, the Garron or Mainland pony, and the Western Isles pony which is sub-divided according to height into two smaller groups. The Garron is the largest and strongest of the British pony breeds, and one has been seen carrying seven adults at a canter in a circus act.

Traditionally, the Highland pony is known for its association with deer stalking where it is used to carry the deer, as it is very sure-footed in rough country. It has an extremely docile character, and will even allow a hunter to fire a gun from its back.

The Garron has a height of about 14.2 hands, whereas the Western Isles ponies are grouped into two – 12.2 to 13.2, and 13.2 to 14.2 hands. Both types contain some Arab blood and have a powerful body, usually coloured dun, with a dorsal or 'eel' stripe.

Hucul Pony From the Carpathian Mountains of Poland. It is said to be descended from Tarpan stock, so is sometimes called the Forest Tarpan. There were three types of Hucul: Przewalski Hucul, Bystrzec Hucul and Tarpan Hucul, but these have been interbred, so are now almost indistinguishable.

It is a very sure-footed pony, so is ideal for farm work in the high, rough land of southern Poland. It is willing and hardy, and also very strong.

The height is between 12.1 and 13.1 hands. The colour is usually dun or bay, often with dark points.

Iceland Pony Derived from ponies brought to Iceland by Norwegian immigrants in AD 871, and from the ponies of Irish and Scottish settlers who came later. These ponies interbred to form the present breed which is noted for its hardiness and its remarkable homing instinct.

The Iceland Pony was very important for pack work and communications as, until recently, the roads were not very good. It is now used in pack work, riding and draught work. Separate herds are kept for meat, as cattle do not thrive in harsh Icelandic winters.

Most are docile if not downright friendly. Many are controllable by voice alone.

The usual colours are grey and dun, but many other colours may be seen. Height is between 12 and 13 hands.

Indonesian Ponies *Bali Pony* The Bali is a primitive breed of pony. It often shows dark points and a dorsal stripe, and may have an upright mane. It is a strong worker, often used as a pack pony. *Batak* (*Deli*) *Pony* The Batak pony has been specially bred on Sumatra from local mares and Arab stallions. This breeding has been encouraged by the Indonesian government so that Bataks may be used to improve the native ponies of the other islands. Large numbers of Bataks have been exported to Singapore, through the port of Deli.

The Batak is a handsome pony. It may be any colour, although most are brown. The average size is 11.3 hands, but many stretch to 13.

Gayoe Pony The Gayoe pony originates from the Gayoe Hills in northern Sumatra. It is similar to the Batak pony of Sumatra, but has a heavier build and is therefore slower.

Java Pony The Java pony is often seen in Java pulling the Sados, which are two-wheeled traps used as taxis. It is able to pull a full load for a whole day in the tropical heat, and is known for its strength and tirelessness. It is a slightly-built pony, and is about 12.2 hands high.

Sandalwood Pony From the islands of Sumba and Sumbawa. Named after the sandalwood which is exported from the Indonesian Islands.

It is a fast pony, used in bareback racing. It has a fine, burnished coat which may be of various colours.

Sumba Pony A primitive breed from the island of Sumba. It has dark points and a dorsal stripe, which are characteristics often seen in ancient breeds.

The Sumba ponies are ridden bareback and without reins by young boys who take part in dancing competitions on their ponies. The ponies are able to dance to the rhythm of drums, and are judged by their elegance and lightness.

Sumbawa Pony Similar to the Sumba pony. Few people are surprised that it is named after the island on which it is found.

Timor Pony From the Island of Timor. It is the smallest of the Indonesian ponies, being about 11 hands high. In spite of its size it is used on cattle round-ups and for harness work, as it is able to carry heavy loads easily.

The Timor has been exported to Australia and New Zealand, where it is popular as a child's riding pony and may also be seen in the show-ring. It should have a strong back and good girth. The colour is usually dark, but it may be chocolate with cream spots.

Kathiawari and Marwari Two Indian breeds which are difficult to tell apart. Kathiawari ponies come from the Kathiawar Peninsula in the north-west of India. Marwaris come from Rajputana. They are said to be descended from Arab horses, which came ashore from a shipwreck, and native wild ponies – which are generally thin, wretched animals, living on very little but their wits.

The Marwari pony was important as a cavalry pony in the Middle Ages. Records state that the imperial cavalry consisted of over 50,000 ponies.

Kathiawari and Marwari ponies may be any colour. Height between 14 and 15 hands. One characteristic of the breeds is that their ears point inwards, almost touching at the tips. Another is that they kick first and ask questions later.

Konik A generic name referring to several breeds of Polish ponies. Possibly the most important of these 'breeds' is the Biloraj Konik which some authorities claim is a direct descendant of wild horses. They claim the relationship is not remote. There is some evidence that it has been selectively bred from wild horses only since the 18th century.

Polish farmers are pragmatists by necessity. Their ponies are noted for longevity, tractability, fertility and an enthusiasm for work, similar to the qualities the same farmers expect in their wives.

Height about 12 to 13 hands. Almost always dun-coloured with a dorsal stripe. It is said that those more closely related to wild ponies grow white coats in winter.

Landais Pony A semi-wild pony living in the Landes forests in France. The 'Poney Landais' is closely related to the ponies of the Chalosse plains, near the River Adour, and the Barthais pony. The latter are slightly larger, as their pastures are more succulent.

Height is about 12 hands or slightly less. A lightly-built pony, with light bones.

Manipur Pony Bred in Assam for hundreds of years. Records date back to the 7th century when the King of Manipur introduced the game of polo. In the late 19th century the Manipur Cavalry terrorized parts of Burma, but whether they were mounted on pure bred ponies is often disputed. They are thought to be descended from Asiatic wild horses and Arabs.

Height between 11 and 13 hands. All solid colours.

Merens A powerful descendant of Oriental stock, it can and does thrive in the high hills of the Ariège region of France in a semi-wild state. It has a heavy head, lots of bone, and a full-flowing mane.

Height up to 13.3 hands. Almost always black.

Mongolian Pony Bred by nomads in relatively desolate areas for riding, pack and harness. Their milk and meat are considered essential by-products.

There are several variations: Wuchumutsin – a Mongolian type bred on rich grassland; Heilung Kiang – a pony with a large head and slightly convex face; Hailar, Sanho, and Sanpeitze – ponies with some Russian blood standing up to 15 hands; Ili – a Russian-Mongolian pony used as a riding and pack animal.

Black, brown, bay and dun are the usual colours. Aside from those with Russian blood, the usual height is 12.2 to 14 hands.

New Forest Pony This 'breed' is the least distinguishable of the nine breeds of native British ponies. Over the centuries, all sorts of ponies and horses were introduced into the area and it is difficult if not impossible to say which have had the most influence. About a thousand years ago or more, the New Forest covered a much larger area than it does today; it extended almost to the eastern edge of Exmoor. We may fairly assume that at that time the tough ponies of the moors had no small influence on the herds who roamed the New Forest. Certainly there must have been interchange.

In more recent times man has taken a hand at improving the breed. Possibly the most famous stallion introduced was a thoroughbred called Marske. He had done badly on the racetracks, so the owners sold him cheaply. The farmer in Dorset who bought him in 1765 used him on some New Forest mares for four years. Then, in 1769, a horse called Eclipse (sired by Marske before he had been summarily dismissed from the heady heights of the racing world) was raced for the first time. He ran so brilliantly that Marske was quickly located and purchased for the not inconsiderable sum (in those days) of £20. He was moved up to Yorkshire to continue the good work. He never produced another racing prodigy like Eclipse who, in fact, was never beaten during his entire racing career. He was never eclipsed.

From 1852, for some decades, Queen Victoria loaned three Arab stallions to run loose and do their best to help the New Forest pony look more aristocratic. The results are debatable. It may be that the Arab stallions weren't as aggressive as their competitors. When man isn't taking an active hand in the proceedings, speed and good looks are not as important as hardiness and determination. Or it may be that the finer, more classic offspring of the Arabs simply couldn't survive the harsh winters. Whatever the reasons, it takes either a very experienced or a completely non-sceptical mind to pick out the points of today's New Forest pony that are distinctly Arab or thoroughbred. It may be, too, that Lord Arthur Cecil's efforts to improve the breed by introducing Welsh and Galloway blood towards the end of the last century diluted all previous efforts beyond recognition.

Today there are two recognized sorts. Type A is lighter-boned and goes to 12 or 13.2 hands. Type B stands from 13.2 to 14.2 hands. The former is ideal for children. The latter can carry an average-sized adult. Both sorts may be any colour except piebald or skewbald. In appearance they look much of a muchness like any other riding pony. They tend to have rather large heads with intelligent (some owners would say kindly) eyes. The head is carried strongly on a short, powerful neck. The bodily conformation is what you'd expect of a riding pony – powerful back and loins, sloping shoulders, good depth of chest, powerful quarters and clean limbs.

Pony of the Americas In 1956 a Mr L. L. Boomhower of Mason City, Iowa, crossed a Shetland stallion with an Appaloosa mare. The pony produced was a miniature Appaloosa. It was named Black Hand. Black Hand became very popular in shows and a superb children's pony, so was used as the sire of a new breed. This new breed had 12,598 ponies on its register by 1971.

The Pony of the Americas has the characteristics of the Appaloosa horse. It is willing and gentle and is considered ideal for the young rider.

The height must be between 11.2 and 13 hands to qualify for the stud book. The colouring must be a recognized Appaloosa pattern.

Pottok Pony (France) From the Basque region. It has the appearance and endurance of a light Shetland but, like the people of that area, prefers independence. Almost all live wild.

Height up to 13 hands. All colours, piebald and skewbalds are common.

Przewalski's Horse (Mongolian wild horse) Named after the explorer-naturalist who proved the existence of the 'breed', which was thought to be extinct. Truly a wild horse from the Ice Age, it is the precursor of many of our modern horses. However, it doesn't recognize the relationship, and kills domestic intruders with efficient ferocity. There are thought to be less than fifty still living wild. Two or three hundred exist in zoos.

Its dun colour, zebra-striped limbs and crested mane are but the superficial signs that show it to be the only living link in the equine evolutionary chain.

Although its height is only 12.1 to 14.1 hands, even pedantic purists don't call it a pony.

Russian Ponies *Bashirsky Pony* The Bashkirsky ponies are divided into two types: the Mountain pony and the Steppe pony. The Mountain pony is slightly smaller, and is suited to riding. Both types are used to pull sleighs, and are known for their great endurance in snow.

The mares of the breed are often milked to produce a drink known as *Kumiss*, which is said to have medicinal and alcoholic qualities. One mare may produce up to 2000 litres (440 gallons) of milk in seven or eight months.

The colour of the Bashkirsky is usually bay, chestnut or dun. The height averages 13.2 hands.

Caspian Pony Bred on the shores of the Caspian Sea, and also in the Elburtz Mountains of Persia. Although it is thought to be the native wild pony of Iran this has not yet been proved. The Mesopotamians used Caspian ponies in the third millenium BC, but no traces of the Caspian had been found for over 1,000 years until a sober touring scientist in 1965 found them pulling carts by the Caspian Sea. Studies have shown that these 20th-century Caspians are very similar in size and structure to the ancient ponies of Mesopotamia, so it may be possible to trace a connection between them.

A small pony, having a height of between 10 and 12 hands, it is considered ideal for children.

Kazakh Pony The bones of Kazakh ponies have been found in 7th-century tombs of Kazakhstani nomads, who depended on their ponies for food, drink and transport.

The Kazakhs are hardy ponies, able to live in extremes of hot or cold; on the edges of deserts or in deep snow. They are bred for their milk – a mare may yield up to 10 litres ($2\frac{1}{4}$ gallons) a day, and for their meat.

The colour of the Kazakh is usually bay, chestnut, grey or black, but may be odd-coloured or dun. Its height is between 12.2 and 13.3 hands.

Kazanka Pony (Kasanski) Another variety of Viatka, also named after its local province.

Obvinka Pony (Obwinski) A variety of Viatka, named after its province of origin.

Viatka Pony Originates from the Viatsky area of Russia. Descended from the Klepper pony. Now mainly bred in state studs in the Udmurt Republic and the Kirov area.

Used for light agricultural work and to pull *troikas* – sleighs pulled by three ponies.

Colour usually dun, grey or roan; there may be a dorsal stripe and slight zebra-markings on the forelegs. Height is between 13 and 14 hands.

Zemaituka Pony An ancient breed, descended from the Asiatic wild horse. They are found in Lithuania, where the grasslands are good country for the breeding of horses. In pre-war days Lithuanian horses were exported to most European countries.

The Zemaituka ponies are among the toughest ponies to be found; they can survive on the poorest food and in extreme climates, and are still able to travel up to 65 km (40 miles) a day.

The colour of the Zemaituka is usually dun; there may also be a dorsal stripe. The height is between 13 and 14 hands.

Sable Island Pony Sable Island is an exposed Atlantic sandbank off the coast of Nova Scotia, Canada. There are two to three hundred ponies on the island, living wild in very severe weather conditions, with very little shelter. They are strong and extremely hardy, descended from 18th-century New England ponies.

Their height is about 14 hands. Their colour is usually dark chestnut, but may be bay, brown, black or grey.

Senner Pony One of the two pony breeds native to Germany. Now probably becoming extinct. There are some reports that these tough, hardy ponies are still running wild in the forests of the Teutoberger Wald.

Shetland Pony The Shetland is one of the smallest breeds of pony, but is known for its great strength. During the 19th century it was in great demand for work in the coal mines of northern England. A nine-hand pony is said to have carried a 80 kg (170 lb) man 65 km (40 miles) a day.

As its name suggests, the origins of the breed are the Shetland and Orkney Islands, and northern Scotland, where it has been living as a domestic pony since about 500 BC.

There are two theories concerning how the breed came to the Shetlands: one authority claims that it came from further north during the last Ice Age, moving south across frozen seas, while other evidence shows that the ponies may have come from the Biscay areas of France and Spain, travelling north with the early settlers of Britain. Of the two, the latter theory is probably more widely accepted, since a move north to the exposed Scottish islands may have stunted their growth and made them more suited to the climate of northern Britain, rather than a move south from Tundra areas.

Enthusiasts say the Shetland pony is very gentle and docile, and is ideal for children as it is easy to train and found to have great character. A disenchanted minority say they can be nasty and would sooner bite a human hand than eat hay. It has a small head with large eyes, small ears, a thick mane and a long, thick tail. The back is short, but very strong. Similarly, the legs are short but very hard. The feet are small, hard, and effective.

The Shetland is between 9 and 10 hands high, and may be any colour.

Spiti This pony is the equine Sherpa. Bred and traded by the Kanyats, it is noted for its endurance at heights, and its predisposition to irascibility. It's even less happy on the plains.

Height about 12 hands. Most usual colour is grey.

Tibetan (Nanfan) Pony Thought to be related to (if not direct descendants of) Chinese and Mongolian ponies. It is not unlike the Spiti and Bhutia of northern India. Like all mountain ponies, they are deep-chested and sure-footed. A tough all-rounder, used for riding, pack and agricultural work.

Average height up to 12.2 hands. All colours.

Native Turkish Pony This is the native pony of Turkey, originating from the Sivas region. It is a hardy, enduring pony, used in farm work, as a pack pony, in harness, and for riding. Its height is between 14 and 14.2 hands. The colour is bay, brown or grey.

Welsh Mountain Pony *Type a* Records of the Welsh Mountain pony go back to the days of the Romans, when Julius Cæsar founded a stud at Lake Bala and also introduced some Oriental blood. The ponies still roam wild over the mountains and moors of Wales and are rounded up annually when some are sold for breeding.

The legs are fine and hard, giving a quick, free action, and the head is small and tapered, giving an 'Arab' appearance.

The Welsh ponies are quite small, usually being just below 12 hands and, because of their size, were used at one time in the coal mines of South Wales. In 1948 a pony could be bought off the moors for 12/6d. It may be any colour except piebald and skewbald. It is hardy and high-spirited and is very popular as a children's riding pony.

Type b This pony is slightly larger than the a-type, and may be up to 13.2 hands. It is slightly different from the type-a pony because of the influence of the thoroughbred stallion, Merlin, who roamed the hills of Denbighshire in the late 18th or early 19th century.

This type of Welsh pony is described especially as a riding pony, due to its hardy and kind character, and its looks and action.

Welsh Pony (Cob) *Type c* This pony has a strong build and used to be in great demand as a harness pony, before the days of the motor vehicle. Nowadays it is increasingly used by the many visitors to Wales as a trekking pony, being well suited to the rough country and hard work.

It may be up to 13.2 hands high and is hardy and active, always willing to do hard work.

Type d The Welsh Cob is a larger, heavier version of the Welsh Mountain pony. It is very hardy, and has great stamina. At one time it was used by armies, for mounted infantry and pack work, and was much sought after by foreign governments for bringing new blood into their own military horses.

Records of the Welsh cob date back to 1188 when a horse known as the 'Powys horse' was used by English armies. It was derived from the Andalusian and brought to Britain by the Count of Shrewsbury, Robert de Belesme, who bred the horses for their strong character and versatility.

The head of the cob is small, but proudly-carried on strong shoulders. The legs are strong and have a powerful movement, making the pony famous for its speed and ability to jump.

Usually between 14 and 15.1 hands.

Donkeys

Donkeys (so named comparatively recently from their usual dun colour and small size) were, and in many parts of the world still are, more generally known as asses. They differ from horses in their small size – which ranges from 8 to 13 hands at the withers – and in having longer ears, bigger eyes and a shorter neck. They have a wiry mane, no noticeable withers, a broader and deeper girth than horses and a short-haired tail ending in a tuft. They have no chestnuts or ergots, although there is a patch of bare skin inside each foreleg in place of the chestnut: and the males have vestigial teats on the sheath.

A donkey's conformation should, in general, resemble that of a pony, with a light, short head, a short, level back and a shoulder tending to be upright and associated with rather upright pasterns. The feet in foals are remarkably small and narrow and in adults they are narrower than in ponies and have higher heels. These tendencies are exaggerated by neglect. As a guide, the donkey's foot should be encouraged to resemble that of a horse as closely as possible. Donkeys should move freely with a low, straight action.

Common defects in donkey conformation are: a heavy, coarse head; excessively large or long ears; a ewe neck that has a concave upper and a convex lower line instead of both being straight; legs too close together where they join the body; knees bent back; knock-knees; cow hocks with turned-out hind feet; sickle hocks; a roach or arched back; a sloping loin, and a low-set tail.

Donkeys' teeth erupt at the same intervals as those of horses and their age can be estimated in the same way as a horse's age except that the markings on donkeys' teeth are not so clear. In donkeys over eight years old the angle of projection of the lower row of incisors is a good general guide to the animal's age. At eight years old they slope up to meet the upper incisors at about 45 degrees and at thirty years of age the slope of the lower incisors is much flatter at about 15 degrees from the horizontal.

Donkey temperament is usually equable, and most donkeys are well mannered. They are gregarious creatures and need the companionship of other donkeys or horses. Donkeys on their own demand much attention: without it they pine away or become temperamentally difficult. They are, like horses, creatures of habit and, if their routine is disturbed, they become stubborn. Like horses, too, they can be accustomed to almost any routine; familiarizing them with new conditions is most easily achieved by simple repetition. Their stubbornness arises largely from fear of the unknown. Once they have found by experience, helped if necessary by a certain amount of compulsion, that the new conditions are harmless, they will readily co-operate. Stallion donkeys can be aggressive in the presence of mares in season and it is important that they should be accustomed to the simple controls applied by a bit and bridle.

Stallion donkeys bray frequently and deafeningly and this can, like Scottish bagpipes, charm the ear or cause near apoplexy according to the recipient's frame of mind. Mares and geldings bray when they are lonely or in new surroundings in the hope of contacting other donkeys in the neighbourhood. Donkeys also bray or make gentle snuffling noises to express pleasure when greeting familiar people – especially at feeding times.

The small size and weight of donkeys and their lack of ability to move at any speed or to jump obstacles renders them less liable to many of the diseases that are common in horses. They are remarkably free of arthritis and seldom contract many diseases associated with the frequent striking of limbs on hard roads, such as navicular disease, pedal ostitis, ringbone, sidebones, splints and spavins. They do not develop roaring or whistling, which in horses is associated with animals of 15 hands or over.

In temperate or cold climates donkeys are liable to lung diseases. Many of them harbour large infestations of lung worms without showing signs of the disease by coughing or losing condition. Nevertheless, this must weaken the capacity of the lungs to withstand attack by other diseases, and donkeys succumb more readily than horses to respiratory diseases such as influenza, strangles and pneumonia. The fact that many donkeys are carriers of lung worms is a source of infection for horses and the two-monthly routine of worm treatment meted out to all the horses on the premises should also be applied to the stable donkey: lung worm is a very serious disease when it occurs in horses.

Donkeys are economical to keep. They feed on any available herbage, preferring shrubs, hedges and roughage such as thistles to more conventional grass pastures. They are useful for clearing neglected ground, but they soon reduce a well-kept garden to something resembling a desert; and their habit of passing their droppings in one part of the field can be admired as creating a handy manure heap or deplored as yet another of their capacities to make a good field look sick. In countries that have a cold winter, donkeys need supplementary feeding with hay and a pound or so a day of oats or some other horse-corn preparation as long as it is not wheat. Wheat and its product, bread, in significant quantities – that is more than 50 g (2 oz) a day – can lead to serious digestive upsets, colic or laminitis.

Donkeys are used in enormous numbers in tropical and sub-tropical countries for agricultural work and for transport, usually in small groups, but occasionally in large herds, by contractors where the work is not sufficiently urgent to justify using heavy machinery. Donkeys have strong backs and can carry enormous loads as long as they are well distributed. Donkey pack saddles reach from the withers well back over the loins. Donkeys are also capable of carrying a heavy man long distances – provided he sits on the donkey's quarters and not in the middle of the back as is usual with horses. In South Africa, donkeys were used for many years to draw the heavy trekking wagons in teams of twenty-four donkeys, in competition with transport by bullocks (which were used in spans of 6 or 12 animals).

Donkeys play another useful role in fathering that remarkable animal, the mule, which derives its size from the horse mare, its mother, but its characteristics of unwavering endurance and compact strength from the donkey branch of its family tree.

Mules

Mules, the offspring of donkey stallions and horse or pony mares, are probably the hardiest and the most intelligent of all the horse's relatives. Both male and female mules are endowed with the normal organs and behaviour of their sex but they are not capable of reproduction when mated together or with a horse or a donkey. In spite of frequently repeated travellers' tales that mules can produce offspring, there is no authentic record of this event ever having occurred. Dictionaries variously define mules as sterile or usually sterile. The former description is the correct one.

Mules have hybrid vigour demonstrated by remarkable strength for their size – which may vary from 12 to 15 hands according to their parentage, particularly depending on the size of the mare. The mule's desirable conformation closely approaches that of a well-proportioned horse, except that the mule is more upright in the shoulder and foreleg and shorter and stronger in the back, which may even be slightly roached. The feet are narrower and more upright than in the horse. This conformation gives mules a rather stilted action, making them less comfortable than horses as riding animals. Their particular usefulness is for draught and pack work, for which they are extensively used in mountainous country throughout the world. They work well under conditions of considerable hardship as regards climate, terrain, feeding and management. The smaller animals can carry loads of up to 75 kg (150 lb), and the 15-hand mules, provided their limbs are proportionately strong, manage up to twice that weight – and are willing to carry it for long periods over any country. It is generally accepted that a mule can accompany a man anywhere except up a tree.

The mule's intelligence is most noticeable in its capacity to survive, maintaining a cheerful and predictable fortitude against all odds through a working life of twenty years or more, showing none of the nervous reactions to which many horses are prone. Mules respond readily to proper care and treatment but resent violence. This may account for their reputation for being stubborn and vicious; but they only become so if they are bullied or beaten. Mules, like horses, are wary of the unfamiliar; but whereas a frightened horse will lash out instinctively, an aggrieved or surprised mule, apparently incapable of fright, chooses its time and kicks deliberately, very hard and with remarkable accuracy, often without bothering to lay back its ears as a warning signal. However, treated as an equal, any mule is a dependable helpmate when there is troublesome work to be done.

Hinnies The progeny of a she-ass mated by a horse or pony stallion is a hinny. Hinnies are seldom bred deliberately, being less stockily built than the mule and possessing little of that animal's inexhaustible determination. They are more amenable than mules, and their action is less stilted, making them a more comfortable riding animal. Hinnies, like mules, are quite incapable of reproduction.

The horse's family tree

Ordinary horses There is no such thing as an ordinary horse in the same way as there is no such thing as an average man, but the phrase 'ordinary horses' can be taken to refer to horses of no particular breed or, more precisely, to horses of mixed origin. There are tremendous numbers of these horses: riding horses, show-jumpers, hunters, polo ponies, children's ponies, trekking horses, pit ponies and even some high-class show animals – all well suited to their particular work in size, conformation and temperament. Each one has its origins, some more mixed than others; and these can often be deduced by studying the animal's physique and behaviour and other characteristics, all of which are derived from its parents and, through them, from more distant forbears.

Evolution and the inheritance of characteristics The whole process of evolution in horses as in all animals depends on each individual being different from every other individual, even if only slightly different, in height, growth, colour, temperament and in a great many other ways. These variable characteristics are transmitted to the foal by random selection from an ancestral pool, some from the mare's family mixture and some from the stallion's. In a herd of horses where the members reasonably resemble each other their progeny would look alike although each differed slightly from the others. If marked changes in the herd's environment occurred, the changes might favour the slightly taller, faster growing, darker coloured and more aggressive individuals while the smaller, slow developing, light coated and slothful types were eliminated. Over a period of many generations under the new influences that herd would change noticeably. Accumulations of such changes could gradually lead to the development of quite a different animal.

Various types of wild horse survived because there were always some individuals with a mixture of characteristics that could stand up to the new circumstances and live to breed their kind of foal. Survival of a species depends on adaptability, and adaptability depends on the fact that individuals have different characteristics.

It is generally accepted that a large group of animals with a wide choice of breeding partners, making available an infinite variety of mixtures of characteristics, is more vigorous and adaptable than a small group where mating choice is limited so that there will be a close resemblance in the mixtures of characteristics available. Such small groups tend to resemble each other very closely and are not readily adaptable to changes.

Wild horses Wild horses are believed to have evolved from small, 4-toed animals that lived in trees. These changed to 3-toed, tapir-like creatures and later to the one-toed horse. Horses originated in America and spread by land contacts (no longer existing) to Europe and Asia. The horses became extinct in America while those surviving in Euro-Asia developed into several varieties: thick-set, big-boned phlegmatic types in the cold-tundra countries and lighter, more active warm-blooded types in the more southerly woods and plains. It is unlikely that any of them were more than ponies, up to 14.2 hands in height. Man tamed and adopted the horse for various uses, and the wild ones have gone except for a few specimens of Przewalski's wild horse in zoos and perhaps a few in the Asian hinterlands.

Feral horses There may be a few genuine wild horses in Mongolia and Siberia; otherwise any wild groups of horses are feral animals, that is, those which have escaped from man's control and established themselves in a wild state. Herds of these horses existed until recently in parts of western North America but they are now said to have disappeared. There are still such herds in parts of Australia, hardy and intractable animals about 14.2 to 15 hands, known as 'brumbies'. Feral horses are under no control. On the other hand there are herds of horses or ponies living under almost natural conditions in various parts of the world only controlled to the extent that they are periodically rounded up to establish ownership, to pick out suitable horses for work, castrate supernumerary colts and cull obviously diseased or useless animals.

Man's development of breeds For thousands of years man has made use of horses for meat, milk, leather, riding, driving and power. In three ways man's control has helped the marvellous potential of the species to develop into the wide range of horses and ponies now in existence: firstly, by generous feeding and protection from predators and the elements; secondly, by selecting horses with the desired characteristics for breeding together; and thirdly, by cross-breeding the various types which had naturally evolved through thousands of generations in the wild state.

Wild horses had developed into different types because of terrain and weather. Under man's control new types were developed to suit his requirements, though the natural influences of location and climate were still important. Hill peoples found slow, thick-set animals with deep chests worked best for them, while the Tartars and Arabs preferred faster and lighter horses suitable to open country. Under these influences special types of horse became established in different countries until they bred true, and the foals dependably resembled their parents; the outstanding example being the Arab, some of which have pedigrees (recorded by word of mouth but accepted none the less as reliable) dating back to the great flood of 2348 BC.

Breed societies The Arabs started the idea of pure breeds with carefully chosen stock and recorded pedigrees. The English Jockey Club established a stud-book for thoroughbred horses towards the end of the 18th century; and no foals can be entered in the register of thoroughbred horses unless their sires and dams are already in the book. Many other groups have established breed societies for the type of horse or pony that was special to their area or suitable for some particular task. The system helps to maintain the selected type up to a high standard, and it has the outstanding advantage of qualifying any type to be known as a breed, if it produces foals that resemble their parents. The breed societies keep registers and hold or attend shows which encourage good quality and public interest. Through the breed societies anyone wishing to purchase a particular type of horse can be assured, with a little care, that the animal he is buying really is of the kind required and, if bred from, will truly reproduce its kind.

Biologists complain that the breed societies by confining their stud-books to a precisely defined type of horse reduce the range of characteristics available for horse breeding, render their horses less adaptable to any change of circumstances and even increase their susceptibility to disease which may be linked to inherited characteristics: for example, horses over average height are likely to become roarers, while grey horses are subject to black tumour growths.

The breed societies can firmly reply that their horses are specialized animals for particular purposes and that they have no need to be adaptable. They could also claim that hereditary diseases can be eliminated by even further selection. This is true of some diseases but others might defy the most drastic measures. Roaring, for instance, as far as we know at present, could only be eliminated by removing the characteristics for growth so that no horses exceeded 15 hands.

The fact remains that some of the smaller breed societies may have difficulty in improving the conformation of their animals because they do not have enough stock to avoid in-breeding: the mating of related animals. The closer the relationship, the more likely that the parents' conformation, good or bad, will be repeated in their offspring. The desirable course is usually to out-breed – that is, to mate unrelated stock. As suggested already, in a small group it may be difficult to find a mate that is not a cousin of some sort.

Cross-bred horses A great advantage of having numerous established breeds of known characteristics is that horses from different breeds may be mated together with a fairly clear idea of what the progeny will turn out to be. While the established breeds consist of highly specialized animals, the result of cross-breeding may be a foal suitable for quite other occupations, with desirable characteristics from both parents. For example, a Cleveland Bay mare mated to a thoroughbred stallion would produce a fast-moving animal up to considerable weight; while a good quality child's pony can be bred from a New Forest mare put to a thoroughbred horse; and the opposite cross would produce an animal of similar quality and rather more height, since it is the mare that controls the size of the progeny. This last point is important and renders it safe to cross-breed animals of very varying size. The physical problems of actually mating animals of different sizes can be overcome by standing the mare on a hump of ground or in a hollow. In extreme cases, artificial insemination would be required. If colts and mares are run together it is never safe to assume that mating will not take place because of marked discrepancy in size. If the mare is in season, love laughs at a small matter of hands and inches!

An added advantage of cross-breeding is a phenomenon known as hybrid vigour. While true-bred horses closely resemble the mare and stallion because they inherit well established groups of similar characteristics from each of their parents, the cross-bred animal inherits characteristics from the mare that are quite unrelated to those from the stallion, and the new combination is likely to be invigorating. The outcross of a thoroughbred horse and a coarser type of mare which is used for hunter production owes some of its success at least to hybrid vigour. The Hunters Improvement Society make available thoroughbred stallions in various parts of the country at a reasonable and subsidised fee for the express purpose of improving the quality of the foals produced.

Breeding from mares of mixed origin A great many countries now have horse-breeding regulations that prevent indiscriminate breeding. In the British Isles a permit is required to keep a colt after it is two years old; thus, stallions for breeding are approved animals, though not necessarily of a recognized breed. Permits are only issued after inspection to check that colts are of good conformation and not likely to transmit hampering diseases. Animals that do not reach the required standard must be castrated. Apart from being well proportioned, approved colts must not be affected by cataract, roaring, whistling, ringbone, sidebone, bone spavin, navicular disease, shivering, stringhalt or defective genital organs. The effect is that there are no poor quality stallions available for mating. Mares are not inspected. Most breeders are sensible enough not to waste time and money breeding from unsuitable mares. Thoroughbred colts and some pony breeds are exempted from inspection because it has been found that the people concerned adopt rigid controls without legislation.

The owners of mares of mixed origin can never produce pedigree stock from these animals. However, they have a wide range of stallions to choose from to mate with their mares, though there will be no certainty that the resulting foals will be quite what they hoped for. This is because, while the laws of inheritance work very consistently with pedigree stock, their effects cannot be anticipated when dealing with mixed origins. If the mare's antecedents are unknown and she is put to a well-bred stallion, any foal she conceives is likely to benefit from his influence; but if she is sent to a stallion, duly approved, which is also of mixed origin, it is quite a gamble as to which of the variety of ancestors will contribute their characteristics to the foal. It must be borne in mind that each conception results from a fresh shuffle of the ancestors' characteristics, so that a cross-bred mare mated with the same cross-bred stallion year after year would not produce a series of similar foals. Their foals could be as widely varied as the brothers and sisters in a human family. The resulting foals are once again of mixed origin but they have a father of certified quality and a mother almost certainly bred from a good stallion, and herself obviously well known to the breeder. These young animals form the great majority of riding, jumping and driving horses and ponies; and they have all the advantages of a rich mixture of characteristics inherited from their outcrossed ancestry, which can hardly fail to instil them with hybrid vigour.

3 Locomotion

Lameness

An exercise in detection Lameness is the most frequent cause of trouble with horses. A lame horse – that is, one which is limping or has departed from its normal gait – is in pain and should not be worked until the cause of lameness has been found and suitable treatment given. The causes of lameness are legion (a Roman Legion was 3,000 to 6,000 men), varying from a stone under a shoe which can be hooked out with the nearest boy-scout's knife to an obscure arthritis that may puzzle the veterinary specialist. Nevertheless, the cause of lameness can be discovered in the vast majority of cases. Until the cause is known no proper decisions can be made about treatment, when to return to work and how to prevent re-occurrence. Nothing is more unsatisfactory than treating lameness blindly with pain-killing drugs in the hope that it will go away.

The routine examination As lameness can nearly always be traced to an observed and demonstrable item of disease or injury, vets have evolved a routine of examination which will uncover the majority of possible causes. The horse is seen at rest and under controlled movement, being led at a walk and then at a trot. The limbs and the feet are each carefully examined. This examination may be halted at any point if the cause of lameness has been confidently established. Short cuts may save time but caution is needed as an obvious injury may not be responsible for the lameness. With practice and experience a full examination can be conducted fairly quickly; and it may be worth completing even though the probable cause of lameness has already been detected. Going through the whole process makes sure that all the likely causes have been considered. After that the signs that have aroused interest can be investigated further and, if the cause of lameness is clear, treatment can be arranged. If this preliminary examination has met with no success the assistance of nerve-blocks, radiography, faradism, laboratory examinations or a second opinion may have to be called upon.

History It is likely to be of help in deciding the cause of lameness to know something of the horse's history: what work it usually does, what it has been doing recently and whether it has been ill or lame before. The attendant's knowledge of the animal and its habits and peculiarities are always interesting and may be invaluable.

Examination in the stable The horse should first be looked at in the stable or loose-box. If the animal has difficulty in moving or cannot move at all the cause might be an injured back, laminitis, tetanus, azoturia or some other acutely painful condition. If it moves awkwardly or staggers one should consider brain and spinal injuries or disease, spinal arthritis, fractures, pelvic injuries, thrombosis, wobbling and stringhalt. While in the stable, the body and limbs should be looked over and the hand run over them to detect deformities, swellings, wounds, scars or wasting muscles. One fore foot rested on the ground in advance of the other suggests navicular disease; any foot rested on the toe suggests pain in that limb, though that is often a normal resting position for a hind foot.

Examination outside the stable The horse is to be watched for faults of action as it leaves the stable. The animal is then held still while it is looked at carefully from all sides for any unusual signs. Unless the cause of lameness is already obvious or the horse is crippled, it may now be led away in a straight line for about twenty metres at a walk and walked back, then trotted a little further and trotted back. If the horse is lame it is at this trotting stage that it may be confirmed which limb is at fault. From the side, the horse appears to take a shorter stride with the affected leg. The foot of the injured limb is always put down less firmly than the sound foot and this may be detected by ear. Viewed from the front, the horse drops its head as the good foreleg strikes the ground and raises its head to relieve the limb of weight as the painful leg comes down. From the back, if a hind leg is affected, the point of the hock of the good leg makes a greater up and down excursion than the point of the hock of the painful limb.

Examination of the limbs If a particular limb is suspected it should be further examined in the stable or outside, as convenient. Even though lameness is most frequently traced to the foot it is advisable to survey the limb first, to detect heat or swellings, and then to extend and flex each of the joints for signs of pain. At this stage or later, when the foot is being examined, the pedal joint in the hoof may be flexed by pressing the toe towards the back of the fetlock, and extended by placing a wedge of wood under the toe to raise it 2.5 cm (1 in) above the heel. If this appears to cause pain when the other foot is picked up it may be a sign of some arthritic condition in the foot. As well as wounds, bruises and abscesses, the fore limb inspection may reveal any of the following signs of disease: ringbone, sidebones, quittor, mud-fever and cracked heels; strains, dislocation, immobilization, bursitis and arthritis of any of the joints; rickets, split pastern and cannon bones, splints, fractured splint bones, sore shins, filled legs and strains of the tendons and ligaments; skin changes from firing, blister and charges; broken knee bones, strain, paralysis and atrophy of the shoulder muscles; girth galls and fistulous withers.

In the hind limb there could be, as well as most of the above list, bruised shins, curb, spavin, capped hocks, strained hock ligaments, a slipped perforatus tendon, strained or wasted muscles in the quarter, or swellings affecting the sheath, scrotum or mammary glands.

Aids to lameness examinations It may be obvious that lameness arises from a particular leg but uncertain if the trouble is in the foot or from higher up the limb. This may be decided by using a local anaesthetic injected over the nerves which lead to the foot. This deprives the foot of all sensation. If the nerve block enables the horse to walk and trot without the signs of lameness seen earlier, then the lameness was almost certainly from the foot. With this knowledge it is worth while using x-rays to produce radiographs which may show arthritis, sidebones, fractures or such things as nails or gravel embedded in the hoof or frog. Nerve blocks are very dependable when used on the fore limbs. They are more difficult to apply and interpret in the hind legs.

If the nerve block does not relieve the horse's lameness the pain must be from higher up the limb. A further careful examination may suggest the use of x-rays on a higher part of the leg, but if nothing significant is noted the trouble may lie in the muscles that cover the upper part of the body, most of which are directly involved in limb movements or are affected by them. These muscles can be activated singly or in groups by using a faradic current; and injured muscles may be detected by noting the horse's reactions to this stimulus.

The spinal column

Brain injury and disease A horse whose brain is injured by accident or disease may indicate its condition by losing interest, becoming lethargic, appearing to be blind, and leaning its body or pressing its head against the wall. Alternatively, the signs may be excitement, uncontrolled head-tossing or box-walking, lack of balance, sudden collapse with galloping movements, convulsions, and coma. Some cases are rapid and dramatic, others creep on insidiously but, when the condition is diagnosed, these allow time to plan remedial measures.

As well as rabies, anthrax, tetanus and other diseases that produce septicaemia or toxaemia and end fatally by poisoning all the tissues, there is a wide variety of causes of brain disease. Shortage of oxygen is one of the more usual reasons and this may sometimes be traced to lung, heart, or blood-vessel trouble interfering with the supply of oxygen to the brain. Other causes of brain injury are larvae of the warble fly or of various species of worm which have penetrated to the brain by chance, destroying brain cells directly or causing haemorrhages which damage the nerve tissue by pressure. Accidents to the skull similarly cause injury from the pressure of fractured bones or from haemorrhage, while brain tumours destroy nerve tissue simply by the pressure of their growth. Another cause is a virus – encephalitis – which occurs in epidemic form in various parts of the world from time to time, fatally affecting the brain.

Many cases of brain damage cannot be treated, but pressure from a fracture or an obstruction to the circulating blood can sometimes be relieved, and the administration of oxygen may help. The animal should be kept quietly in a darkened box under sedation. Some cases of minor brain damage may recover gradually. Damage persisting for any length of time is likely to be fatal, as nerve tissue under pressure or seriously deprived of oxygen for more than a few hours is incapable of recovery.

The spinal column There are fifty-four bones – the vertebrae – in the horse's spine. They form a column that reaches from just behind the skull, down the neck and along the back into the tail. There are seven large bones in the neck, eighteen smaller thoracic ones to which the eighteen pairs of ribs are attached, six wide lumbar bones behind the saddle, five sacral bones fused together forming part of the pelvis, and the remaining eighteen becoming smaller and smaller extending to the fleshy part of the tail. Each of the vertebrae consists of a solid body of bone, surmounted by a bony archway, except for the last eight or ten in the tail which are simply small rods of bone.

When the bones of the spine are in place, the row of archways forms a tube, the spinal canal, wide in the neck and narrowing all the way to the tail. The spinal cord, which is nerve tissue extending from the brain, fills the whole length of this canal. Nerves branch off from the spinal cord, emerging from the canal between the vertebrae or through holes in the bony archways to reach all parts of the body and deliver messages to and from the brain.

Many of the vertebrae have bony processes or extensions: some reach forward and some back, and these overlap with similar projections from the next bone ahead or behind in the column and help to link the bones together in a flexible chain, except for the solid wedge of sacral bones. Each of the thoracic vertebrae has a bony extension, flat from side to side, rather like a thick knife-blade, straight up from the top of the arch. These extensions increase in height from the first to the seventh of the thoracic bones, making the rising curve of the withers, and they then decrease to the last, the eighteenth. The other important processes are on the lumbar bones, all of which have a blade-like projection on each side. All the vertebrae are held together by numerous ligaments of flexible fibrous tissue and the whole column of bones is buried in masses of muscle.

Examining a horse's back Some neck and back injuries are the result of spectacular falls but the majority of spinal troubles are insidious in onset. Often the first sign is loss of flexibility, detected as a reluctance to carry out some ordinary movement. The unwillingness may be conveyed to the rider by a feeling that the horse is being awkward, or that it is using more ground than usual to turn on. If these indications only apply to one particular manoeuvre there is almost certainly some pain involved. Such behaviour is often put down to obstinacy. It is worth remembering that changes in a horse's behaviour nearly always have a physical cause.

To examine a horse suspected of neck or back trouble it should be looked over in its box and the hand run over both sides of the neck and body for obvious signs of injury: wounds, swellings, galls or warbles that might be causing discomfort. If the animal moves over both ways easily and turns round without difficulty it should be led out, inspected again in the better light and then seen in action; led away and back at a walk and then at a trot. The horse should then be turned right round each way, pulled with one hand close up by the head collar or bridle and pushed by the other just behind its elbow. Turned steadily in this way the animal should turn easily in its own length and the inside hind leg should reach across the front of the outer leg at each step. The horse should then be backed a few paces.

With the horse standing still, another minute or so should be spent making a careful inspection by hand pressure and by eye of all parts to note enlargement or wastage of muscles or any difference of appearance between the left and right sides. Running the finger and thumb along either side of the spine, from the withers to the loins, with some pressure from the fingernails causes most horses to dip their backs freely and, if the same pressure is continued over the croup to the tail, the back swings boldly up again. Horses whose spines can be moved in this way are flexible in that part of the spine. Those that resist do so for some reason. They may be stubborn or frightened but they may be resisting because of pain.

Back in the stable, or outside if more convenient, each leg should be picked up, the shoe inspected for unusual wear, the joints flexed to confirm their mobility, and each limb, with the joints flexed, drawn away from the body and then pushed as far as convenient under the body. Most trained horses will permit this manipulation without serious resentment, although there is bound to be some reaction. The objective is to discover if any movement produces particular resistance when applied to one leg.

It may be thought unnecessary to manipulate the limbs when no lameness has been detected and suspicion is directed to the back; but slow-motion photography shows clearly that horses in action consist of four legs whose musculature meets somewhere under the saddle and, while back troubles often occur without apparent limb lameness, there is frequent involvement of one or more limbs which can be revealed by limitation of stride or pain caused by applying unusual traction to the muscles.

The simple examination will have eliminated the more obvious troubles: cases of major spinal fractures are unable to rise from the ground; set-fast and azoturia cases have a high temperature and a history of sudden onset; wobblers reel as they are turned and have difficulty in remaining on their feet when they are backed; shiverers show their defect clearly when backed or pushed from side to side; croup paralysis presents a flaccid tail and difficulty in manoeuvring the hind legs; stringhalt shows itself clearly at a steady walk and pelvic displacement and fractures of the point of the hip or the buttock are seen as marked changes in the horse's outline.

This leaves the more frequent causes of neck and back troubles: muscle injuries, minor fractures and arthritis.

The general examination is likely to have confined the search to a fairly small area. Minor fractures are likely to be acutely painful to pressure or to movements involving the affected bones. Muscle and ligament injuries become more painful if the horse is exercised, while cases of arthritis improve with exercise but are later in a worse state than before and require a day or two to recover to their previous condition.

If a diagnosis has not been reached the muscles of the suspected area should be stimulated by using faradism. Healthy muscles contract painlessly, injured ones are painful. If it is clear that muscle injury exists, a carefully graded course of faradic massage is likely to bring about a cure. Care must be taken in differentiating arthritis from muscle injury as muscles contracting near arthritic bones may produce a painful reaction which is arthritic and not muscular. Arthritis may be diagnosed with certainty by using powerful x-ray machines.

Muscle injuries Muscle injuries may result from falls or other obvious accidents but a great many are insidious in onset, resulting from slipping up at work, from the wrench of regaining balance from an awkward movement, or from tired muscles required to produce some quite ordinary effort too frequently. The signs of such injuries may be stiffness (often shown as a reduction in normal flexibility, especially when turning sharply), poor performance, a reluctance to carry out some movement, or bucking, jibbing or refusal. Difficulties in turning left are likely to be due to muscle pain on the right side and vice-versa, as muscles show more pain when stretched than when compressed. By contrast, arthritis pains are exaggerated by compression.

The location of muscle pain can often be assumed from the horse's alteration in gait or difficulty in making some movement. A shuffling action of the forelegs is obviously from the fore-end of the horse and may be traced to any area from the base of the neck, over the withers and down to the pectoral muscles. Turning all in one piece is likely to derive from the loins or under the saddle. Awkward action in the hind quarters may be traced to muscles in that area, but may derive from spinal troubles much further forward – bearing in mind the example of wobblers whose signs mostly affect the hind legs while the cause lies in the spinal cord of the neck.

The activation of muscles by faradism causing them to contract rhythmically is essential in locating muscle injuries other than superficial ones. The whole area of the muscle masses on the neck, back and quarters can be examined in about twenty minutes, though a much shorter time than that is likely to be needed as only a particular part of the horse usually requires searching for the injury. Normal muscles contract and relax painlessly while injured ones are painful. This causes the horse to fidget, turn its head round, or move away from the operator. Only a very few horses show any resentment against the activation of their normal muscles; most thoroughly enjoy the massaging effect.

Early diagnosis of injury is important. Day by day reduction of the signs of the trouble indicates rapid recovery and no treatment is likely to be required other than rest from vigorous work. Gentle exercise should be given several times a day, to keep the blood circulating adequately. Complete idleness is liable to lead to accumulations of blood and discharges in the injured part, with the formation of adhesions and deep seated scars which can end up as a permanently painful fibrositis.

If recovery is not obviously progressing satisfactorily, the best treatment is a course of faradic massage which exercises the injured muscles and the adjoining ones, keeps the circulation active and helps to reduce any discharges. Recovery is hastened, swellings reduced and the risk of adhesions almost certainly eliminated. The main advantage of faradic treatment is that the horse can be returned to full work in considerably less time than if left without treatment which is the only other option. Pain-relieving drugs are useful on humane grounds in cases of severe injury, but they have no curative effect.

Major spinal fractures Major fractures of the spine are usually the result of steeplechasing, hunting falls, or road accidents. Any fracture that involves the spinal canal, the tube of bone through which the spinal cord runs, is certain to be fatal because subsequent damage to the spinal cord causes paralysis. Horses that get off-balance and land on their noses over a jump are liable to break their necks just behind the poll. The neck bends so sharply that a projection of bone on the second neck vertebra cuts cleanly through the spinal cord and death is instantaneous. Fractures across the back paralyse the horse's hind quarters so that it is unable to rise and it has to be destroyed. There is a problem for those responsible to decide if a horse that lies collapsed and still after falling over a jump has a broken back or is only winded. It is necessary to wait until the horse attempts to get up. A horse with a broken back tries to get up using only its fore legs. The winded horse, exhausted but comfortable on the ground, may take as long as a quarter of an hour before it will make any effort to rise and will then calmly get up using all four legs and walk back to the stable. The inevitable delay can be exasperating but there seems no quicker way of avoiding making an irrevocable mistake.

Some spinal fractures do not have an immediate effect. The bone breaks but the parts are held together by the surrounding muscles. The horse may travel home in apparent good health and lie down in its stable. When it gets up again the thrusts and strains necessary to lift its enormous weight off the ground displace the bones and the back is broken, sometimes as much as twenty-four hours after the fall occurred. It is interesting to speculate that if such cases could be foreseen, the horse might have recovered by being kept in slings until the bone parts healed together, though it is more likely that eventual pressure on the spinal cord would cause a hopeless paralysis.

Pelvic fractures Fractures of the pelvis may occur from falls or other accidents or, in the case of the point of the hip, from unbalanced muscle activity causing a spontaneous fracture while galloping. This particular fracture is plain to see but the muscles often accustom themselves to the new bone alignment and the horse may return to normal work after 4 or 5 months' rest. If lameness continues the broken piece of bone may have to be removed. Fractures of parts of the pelvic girdle may cause any degree of trouble from slight inconvenience to complete paralysis. They may be diagnosed by finding various parts of the pelvis unnaturally moveable on each other, in some cases by a manual examination through the wall of the rectum. A pelvic fracture involving the hip joint is almost certainly hopeless. Other fractures may heal satisfactorily if there has not been marked displacement of the bones or injury to the internal organs adjacent to the pelvis.

Pelvic displacement The sacrum is a solid portion of the spine which is made up from the sacral vertebrae which are fused together and form the roof of the pelvis. In older animals the sacrum and the pelvic bones are solidly locked together where they lie flat against each other on either side. In young horses the opposing surfaces, while not forming a moveable joint, are slightly adjustable on each other. If a severe wrench in a fall overdoes this adjustment the pelvis may be seen from behind to be slightly misaligned and from the side to be more than usually angled or goose-rumped, one or both points of the croup projecting well above the spine. Although replacement is not possible many horses affected in this way are able to continue satisfactorily in work.

Spinal arthritis A number of painful backs are due to arthritis of the blade-like vertical processes that form the withers or the horizontal ones that project laterally from the vertebrae in the loins.

Growth of inflamed arthritic bone extends so that the blades of bone impinge on each other and their grinding together gives rise to such pain that the horse cannot face up to work. A surgical approach is to remove alternate blades leaving large gaps between the remainder which cannot possibly touch each other and so the pain is relieved.

Arthritis may also arise from small processes on adjoining vertebrae rubbing against each other. The general area involved may be defined by watching the horse's difficulties of action or by its refusal to move in certain ways. The painful part may sometimes be located by finger pressure and this can be confirmed if the pain disappears when local anaesthetic is injected near to the diseased bones, enabling the horse to move freely for a short time. It is important to differentiate between arthritis and injured muscles because muscle trouble can often be treated successfully, while arthritis cannot be eliminated, though many cases may be rendered painless or much less painful. Pain from injured muscles is persistent while they are being used and usually becomes steadily worse if the horse is worked. By contrast, pain from arthritis is variable and is often reduced or disappears completely during exercise but returns, after a short rest, more fiercely than before. A slightly arthritic horse ridden gently is likely to move quite freely after the first ten minutes or so and continues comfortably for a long period even through some pressure of work; but if there is occasion to stop on the way, even for a few minutes, the rider has a crippled horse on his hands requiring twenty-four hours to recover to its previous condition.

The use of faradism may help to locate an arthritic area because the horse gives indications of pain as the contracting muscles move the arthritic joints, but faradism is of no value in the treatment of this disease. Radiography can establish the presence of arthritis with certainty by revealing changes in the outline of joints but, while standard machines are useful for confirming arthritis in the feet and lower limbs, very powerful x-ray equipment, usually only available at veterinary schools or equine veterinary hospitals, is necessary to produce radiographs of any part of a horse's spine because of the bulk of muscle that surrounds it. Phenyl butazone is a most useful drug for horses that are suffering from minor arthritic ailments, allowing them to continue in work. The use of this preparation to enable horses to compete is forbidden by many of the organizations that control equine events.

Cold backs Horses with cold backs dip their spines excessively when being girthed up or mounted. Many of them settle down quite quickly and work well in spite of the complaint but it seems likely that there is a slight degree of arthritis involved in some of these cases.

Jinked back Horses are jink-backed when the hind limbs appear to follow a course slightly to one side of that set by the front end of the animal. There are several conditions that may be responsible: small fractures of bony processes on the vertebrae, spinal arthritis, and chronic muscle injuries such as adhesions or fibrositis. Treatment depends on the basic cause but in most cases the condition is permanent. Many jink-backed horses work quite satisfactorily in spite of the peculiarity of action. Those that present signs of pain may sometimes be relieved by the use of phenyl butazone.

Slipped discs Horses do not suffer from slipped discs in the way that human beings and dogs are affected. The successes claimed by back manipulators in treating horses' vertebral injuries are probably due to slight adjustment of spinal processes giving pain relief, at least for some time.

Wobblers Wobblers reel as they walk, stagger if they are asked to turn, and collapse if attempts are made to rein them back. The condition is a partial paralysis, mostly affecting the hind legs, due to damage to the spinal cord in the lower part of the neck; many cases have been found on post-mortem examination to be the result of pressure on the spinal cord from a congenitally narrowed spinal canal. Wobbling can show itself at any age but is more frequent in colts than in fillies, and it usually occurs at around two years of age. This may be a result of boxing matches and other rough play indulged in by young horses whose immature and possibly mis-shapen bones are exposed to unusual stresses by their exuberant activity. Affected animals cannot be used and there is no known treatment that is of any help.

Shivering Shiverers show the signs of their complaint if they are startled when shouted at, or if they are backed or turned sharply. The muscles of the hind quarters tremble and twitch, accompanied by an up and down pumping action of the tail. The cause is degeneration of some of the nerve tracts in the spinal cord. Shiverers do not recover but the condition may remain static for many years, the affected horses continuing in steady work. There is no satisfactory treatment.

Stringhalt Horses with stringhalt develop a snatching action when they lift their hind feet as they walk: in some cases the action is so exaggerated that they strike the belly with the foot at each step. The peculiar action is most marked in the walk. Some stringhalt cases trot normally, and many can canter with complete freedom of action. The cause, like shivering, is traced to degeneration of spinal nerve tissue the cause of which is unknown.

Croup paralysis This disease, also known as *Neuritis cauda equina* develops in young horses as a paralysis of the muscles for some distance around the tail. The cause is some defect in the terminal branches of the spinal cord and it is apparently an hereditary condition. Affected animals are quite useless and there is no treatment. Animals whose offspring have developed this disease should not be used for further breeding.

Azoturia Azoturia, also called myo-haemoglobinaemia, has now, unfortunately, been given the name rhabdomyolysis but the shorter name is established and is a great deal easier to pronounce. This is a disease of management. It occurs almost exclusively in fit horses, well fed for hard work, which have not had their rations reduced during a spell of idleness and are then ridden or driven at speed. An affected horse begins to move unevenly and with increasing difficulty and soon comes to an unsteady standstill. Severe cases collapse completely and these may be rapidly fatal. Less seriously affected horses show signs of distress and pain, breathing hard, sweating freely and biting at any objects within reach. The temperature is raised to 39° or 40°C (103° or 104°F). The most characteristic sign is the passing of very dark brown urine. The muscles of the back are violently contracted, very painful and as hard as a board.

Azoturia is due to chemical changes associated with the violent activity of muscles overloaded with starch stored for energy. The starch changes to sugar faster than it can be used up and the excess sugar changes to damaging amounts of poisonous acetic acid. The disease used to be a common market-day complaint when young farmers tried to beat their neighbour's time record for the weekly journey into town. Weekend polo ponies whose owners are lavish with heating foods but have no time to exercise their animals during the week are other likely victims of this disease.

Azoturia cases should be transported home by horse-box. Even walking short distances may alter the condition from bad to hopeless. The horse should be sedated and rugged up to keep it warm and to prevent self-damage. Hot packs or fomentations on the back may help to relieve the muscle tension. Medication should include cortisone and bicarbonate intravenous injections. Convalescence must not be hurried as the affected muscles are severely and sometimes permanently damaged. Azoturia may be avoided by ensuring that feeding is reduced if exercise has to be curtailed.

Set-fast Set-fast appears to be a mild form of azoturia, occurring most usually in yearlings or two-year-olds in racing stables which are being pushed rather too hard in their work. The horse stiffens up across the back after exercise and the temperature is raised. Most cases respond to a light laxative, slightly reduced feeding and a course of sodium salicylate medication with a very gradual return to increased exercise.

The limbs

Fractures *Broken bones* A broken bone in a horse's leg usually results in its destruction. There are sound reasons why this should be done, but every case must be carefully assessed because some may be suitable for treatment, though persistent lameness is likely.

The damage caused by a fracture is frequently so extensive that there is no possibility that the leg could be used again. Attempts at treatment in these cases are pointless.

In the treatment of less serious fractures there are two facts to be considered; first, that a horse with a broken leg must not be allowed to lie down and get up because the leverages created – in spite of all possible support from plating, splints and casts – would cause further injury: and secondly, that a horse cannot be treated on the ground for long periods because of the development of hypostatic pneumonia and paralysis due to pressure. The animal, in consequence, must be treated standing up. However, even this creates difficulties because a horse standing on three legs for any length of time is liable to develop acute laminitis which, in these circumstances, would be fatal. To avoid this the horse needs to be put into slings to take the extra weight. Very few horses have the stamina and temperament to survive the 4 to 6 months in slings necessary for the fracture to heal. Even with devoted attention and no restriction on costs such a task could defeat the most efficient veterinary hospital.

The cases that qualify for treatment are the splint bones which hardly bear any weight, some of the knee bones, which share the weight between them, and the bones of the fetlock and pastern region which, in simple fractures, can have the pieces of bone screwed together and their weight-bearing temporarily transferred by padding and casts to a higher part of the limb. Since fractures of these bones, except the splint bones, are bound to roughen the previously smooth joint surfaces, the horse is likely to be lame for the rest of its life and of no value except as a companion animal or, in the case of colts and mares, for breeding purposes.

Cracked bones When a horse has been kicked or involved in some other violent accident resulting in a painful bone injury without obvious displacement, there is always the possibility and the hope that the bone has not been broken but only cracked. Cracked bones are often more painful than broken ones because with a crack a swelling occurs under the periosteum putting extremely painful tension on this sensitive membrane. With a break the periosteum is torn and the parts are separated, so there is no tension. It can be observed that horses with broken legs are not feeling any pain while those with bones that are only cracked resent the slightest pressure.

It is advisable to x-ray the bone to determine the extent of the injury. There is often the risk that pressure or leverage on a cracked bone may extend it to a break. For this reason it may be inadvisable to allow the horse to lie down and slings can be used to prevent this. Cracks heal very much more rapidly than any break, but the decision to allow the animal to lie down and get up depends on the extent and position of the injury and the progress of the case monitored by x-rays. When this time does come the horse should be given plenty of room in a large box with a soft bed of straw or peat to avoid the risk of slipping.

Time is the most necessary factor in the healing of cracks, though there are some cases where creating an inflammation by using a stimulating ointment or giving support by a bandage or a hot plaster, known as a charge, may be helpful.

Broken splint bones Fracture of a splint bone is usually caused by the horse striking the bone with the shoe of the opposite foot. The fracture is difficult to differentiate from a developing splint but the suspicion may be confirmed by x-rays. Limb movements keep the fractured ends rubbing against each other preventing healing and causing lameness. The only satisfactory treatment is surgical removal of the lower segment of bone.

Bone chips – joint mice Small pieces of bone can be chipped off in minor accidents or are pulled off by the wrench of a ligament. They cause trouble by acting as foreign bodies, giving rise to discharging sinuses that require surgery.

Loose fragments of bone in a joint may move about causing intermittent lameness. These are known as 'mice', presumably because they are erratic in their movements, small in size and of considerable nuisance value. They are detected by x-ray examinations of the troublesome joint and are removed by surgery.

Spontaneous fractures Fractures are called spontaneous when it is the horse's own tissues that cause the break.

Hip down If a galloping horse becomes unbalanced it can happen that the uncoordinated muscles of the quarter break off the point of the hip with a loud crack. The piece of bone, measuring about $3\times3\times6$ cm ($1\frac{1}{4}\times1\frac{1}{4}\times2\frac{1}{2}$ in), buries itself in the muscle mass leaving that hip rounded while the other hip retains its point. The horse is acutely lame but usually recovers its action after resting at grass for four or five months and can then return to full work. No treatment is usually necessary, but if lameness persists the broken portion of bone should be extracted by surgery.

Split pastern This fracture usually occurs in soft going. The horse gets off balance and puts a foreleg slightly to one side to recover. The foot drives into the soft ground with the small joints at the lower end of the limb exactly straight so that they cannot bend in either direction, mechanically known as a dead end. The whole weight of the horse is momentarily thrust down the column of bones in the foreleg and one of the pastern bones cracks, or it breaks in two, or it explodes into 30 or 40 pieces. It is not always a pastern bone; it may be the cannon bone that gives way. X-rays reveal the extent of the damage. Cracked bones recover with little treatment; split bones may be repaired by screwing the pieces together; the exploded bone cases are usually destroyed unless the animal has very high breeding value when there is the possibility that the leg may be supported until the mass of fragments fuse together leaving a very stiff lower leg.

Bone dislocation Bones are held together by ligaments to form joints. When some mishap occurs and the bones are completely separated or dislocated, the ligaments are stretched or torn. As the ligaments are anchored in the thin membrane, the periosteum, covering the bones, this stress is likely to set up periostitis and arthritis. In short, a dislocated joint, even if the bones can be correctly re-aligned, is likely to become arthritic with the horse chronically lame.

Any joints may be dislocated. Spinal dislocations often lead to sudden death from pressure on the spinal cord or nerve roots. Dislocated limb joints, other than the shoulder or the fetlock, are usually accompanied by so much tearing of ligaments and other tissues that destruction is usually the only course, though isolated examples of remarkable recoveries are reported from time to time.

Dislocated shoulder The shoulder joint may be dislocated in a fall or collision with very obvious displacement of the bones. This joint is almost devoid of ligaments so that, if the bones can be re-aligned under a general anaesthetic, there is a good chance of recovery without arthritis following. The chief problem is re-occurrence. To avoid this, the area should be treated with a stimulating ointment to produce an inflammatory reaction and exercise should be carefully controlled for several weeks.

Dislocated fetlock The fetlock may be dislocated dramatically in a fall leaving the pastern and foot projecting laterally at a right angle. The proper alignment is easily restored, usually without an anaesthetic, and it requires supporting bandages to keep the parts normally in place. The accident causes severe tearing of ligaments so that arthritis and persisting lameness are almost certain to follow.

Dislocated patella – stifle slip The horse's patella slides up and down on the lower extremity of the femur in front of the stifle joint as it extends and flexes. In the resting horse the patella lodges at the top of its range of movement on a ridge of bone on the femur. Owing to a lack of tension in the tissues of a young or unfit horse the patella may move too high and become locked over the ridge. This prevents the stifle joint from flexing and the horse remains unable to move, with the affected leg extended backwards. The condition may occur at intervals in one or both hind legs. The dislocated patella frees itself if the horse extends its stifle by giving a plunge or is encouraged to make a sudden forward movement by being struck with a whip.

There are usually no after-effects, but the dislocation may be repeated frequently, upsetting the horse and interfering with its work. Most horses grow out of this complaint if they are built up with more and regular work. Some, successfully treated in this way, start slipping their stifles again as soon as they are eased off in their work, losing muscle size and tension. Persistent cases may be cured by surgical section of the internal patella ligament which is partly responsible for retaining the bone in fixation. Cutting the ligament does not appear to interfere with the horse's normal activities.

Slipped flexor tendon The superficial flexor tendon of the hind leg passes over the point of the hock, being held in place by lateral ligaments. By accident or the horse's unbalanced action, the holding ligaments may be torn and the tendon slips to the outside of the hock. The mishap may cause a temporary lameness but the tendon soon accommodates itself to its new alignment and the horse's galloping and jumping activities are not usually affected. With the horse standing and the leg picked up, the tendon can be moved under the skin by finger pressure and restored to its original position; but as there is nothing to retain it there, it immediately slips again to the side of the hock. Surgical interference is not helpful.

Subluxation of joints (jumping bumps and knuckled-over fetlocks) Joints are subluxated when the bones forming them are shifted out of their normal relationship without actual dislocation. Subluxation may be sudden and accidental or it may develop gradually.

The sacro-iliac joint, formed between the spine and the pelvis on either side just below the point of the hip, is liable to be wrenched suddenly in a fall or to be gradually shifted by constant jumping activities. In either case the front of the pelvis moves upwards so that the points of the croup show on either side above the mid-line of the spine creating what is known as a jumping bump. The cases that result from a dramatic fall may cripple the horse's action for a while but in most cases a return to normal work can be expected after a few months. The cases that develop the jumping bump gradually do not appear to be affected by the altering angulation of the bones. There is no treatment other than rest when required.

Gradual subluxations occur affecting the joints from the fetlock to the foot where attempts to avoid the discomforts of jarred joints, strained ligaments or chronic laminitis cause the horse to hold these joints more and more upright until in some cases, the fetlock joint is knuckled over in advance of the foot. Radiographs may show quite dramatic alterations of the alignment of the bones. Every effort should be made to enable these horses to move more comfortably by careful farriery or other means of reducing the jarring impact of this development.

Bone diseases *Rickets* Rickets is not a common disease in horses but it may appear in foals and yearlings, being recognized by enlarged and tender swellings at the lower end of the ribs and just above the knees. The forelegs may be bowed. X-rays of the bones show them to be unusually transparent with obvious irregularities at the youthful growth junctions.

Rickets is due to a deficiency of calcium, phosphorus, and Vitamin D in the food, and to the young animals being short of exercise and sunshine. Treatment consists of adjusting the diet to less corn and adding ground limestone to the ration. Vitamins may be added in the form of cod-liver or halibut-liver oil. Sunshine helps the natural production of Vitamin D and reasonable exercise is needed to enable the limbs to recover.

Osteomalacia and osteodystrophy These two conditions occur when adult horses are fed on a grain diet that supplies too much phosphorus and too little calcium. In osteomalacia, which may occur in mares that are suckling one foal and are pregnant with another, the bones on the face lose calcium and become soft. The limb bones are also affected and lameness occurs. In osteodystrophy the facial bones become swollen, sometimes to such an extent that the nasal passages are narrowed and snoring beathing is heard. Affected horses move very stiffly and their joints creak.

Treatment of both conditions is to balance the diet: the corn feed is reduced to lessen the intake of phosphorus, and calcium is increased by feeding clover, lucerne or alfalfa and adding ground limestone to the manger food. Recovery is usual except in very advanced cases.

Arthritis and periostitis The chief cause of arthritis in horses' limbs is the sudden impact of their heavy weight on hard ground, and the next most likely contribution is poor quality bone from rapid growth. Ponies suffer little from arthritis: their weight is less and they are usually allowed to mature slowly, an essential condition for the production of hard bone.

The fine membrane covering horses' bones, the peri osteum, produces new bone growth when it is jarred, irritated or inflamed. This is periostitis. When joints are involved it is known as arthritis. For general purposes it is convenient, if not scientifically correct, to use the more familiar word arthritis for all these new bone growths.

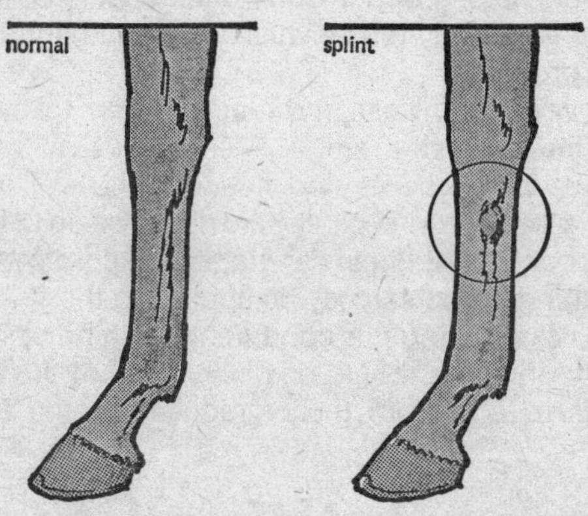

Splints The splint bones are attached on either side of the back of the cannon bone, actually lending support to the lower row of knee bones. They are bound closely to the cannon bone for one third of the way to the fetlock joint, then each continues as a shaft that runs unattached to the cannon bone and ends in a knob that can be clearly felt above the fetlock joint.

Splints are growths of bone usually developing from the ligaments binding the splint bone to the cannon bone; consequently they occur most frequently on the upper third of the splint bone. A great many horses develop small splints in this area. They are painful for a while but become painless after a few weeks and do no harm. Splints high up on a splint bone are known as knee-splints. They can cause persisting lameness if they interfere with the normal movement of the knee bones. Splints that project into the groove where the tendons lie at the back of the cannon bone are called peg-splints. They may cause lameness by pressing against the tendons or the suspensory ligament.

Splints cause lameness by putting tensions on the sensitive periosteum covering the bones. Pain and lameness disappear when the new bone stops growing and the inflammation has subsided. In some cases the process can be hastened by applying stimulant dressings. Splints developing in mature horses frequently cause a persistent lameness. Some of these cases respond most satisfactorily to electro-cautery. Knee-splints and peg-splints may require bone surgery for their removal but success is not assured.

Sore shins Sore shins can be recognized by the horse's reluctance to put its feet down firmly and by finding the front of the cannon bones extremely tender, usually only on the forelegs. The condition is a diffuse inflammation of the periosteum on the cannon bone caused by working on hard ground. Sore shins occur most frequently in young horses, especially those which are fat and unfit and have been fed for rapid growth.

Treatment consists of rest, and recovery may take several weeks. As horses that are rested are inclined to put on weight, feeding should be restricted and limited freedom allowed, such as being turned out in a well-bedded cattle yard. Exercise on soft going should be given as soon as the horse can manage it comfortably. Calamine or other soothing dressings may be applied to the shins.

As a means of avoiding this condition young horses that may have to be put to work early should be given some of their slow exercise on the roads to accustom them gradually to the effects of hard ground.

Bucked shins Bucked shins are usually seen on the hind cannons. The front line of the cannon bone, instead of being perfectly straight, is convex to some degree from below the hock to the fetlock joint. The condition occurs in jumping horses from bruising on the top of obstacles. The injury usually involves the periosteum over the cannon bone and the extensor tendon and its sheath that run down the front of the cannon may also be inflamed. The injuries seldom cause more than temporary lameness. Calamine, lead lotion, or iodine ointment may be used on recent injuries. Protective boots or bandaging are a help in preventing the recurrence of this bruising.

High ringbones (Low ringbones are referred to in the section on foot injuries.) The only difference between high and low ringbones is that high ringbones can be felt around the fetlock or on the front of the pastern while low ringbones are hidden in the feet. Both are new growths of arthritic bone that occur on the front and sides of the bones from the fetlock to the foot, being seen more commonly on the fore limbs. They may not be prominent when they first occur but are painful to pressure. At this stage they show on x-ray plates as a hazy line in place of a clear cut edge of bone. Ringbones may grow to be very obvious and can spread to such an extent that they overwhelm the fetlock and pastern joints, completely immobilizing them. Small ringbones not affecting the joints may settle down after a period of rest. Horses with ringbones that interfere with joint action and cause lameness can sometimes be restored to years of activity by un-nerving. Whether un-nerved horses are safe to put to work depends on the particular circumstances of each case, but the animal certainly feels no pain.

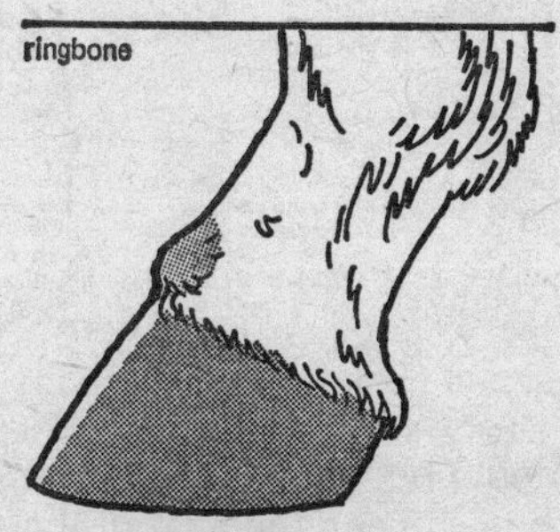

Osselets (*ankle bones*) Young horses in work sometimes develop round bony swellings on the sides of the cannon bones where they form part of the fetlock joint. These are known as osselets or ankle bones. They may be associated with a slightly stilted action for a while but they usually settle down without treatment after a period of rest and relief from working on hard ground. They often reduce in size as the horse matures.

Carpitis (*knee arthritis*) Arthritis of the knee bones can be a serious problem in young horses required for fast work. Rest and iodine dressings may encourage recovery but the pain and lameness recur when fast work is started again and permanent damage may be done. Some success has followed the use of radium implants or applications to the knees. Conservative treatment is to put the horse back for a year in its competitive programme.

Spavin (*bone spavin*) The most important arthritic condition affecting the hind limb is bone spavin. It affects the small bones at the front of the hock, low down on the inner side of the joint. The spavin can be seen as a rounded projection of bone which may be very small or as large as a walnut. Lameness is caused by the movement of the inflamed bones of the hock against each other. Horses affected with spavin put weight on the toe and it may be noticeable that the toe of the shoe shows more than usual wear.

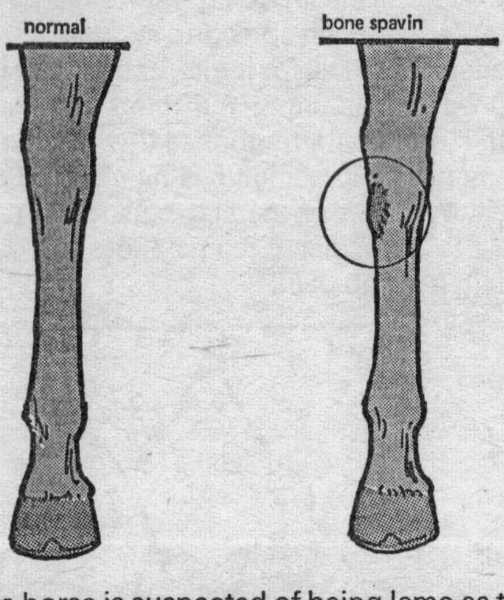

The spavin test If a horse is suspected of being lame as the result of a spavin, the animal should be trotted away from the observer and its degree of lameness noted. Then the foot of the affected leg should be picked up and held for one minute at about hock height under the stifle so that the hock joint is tightly flexed. At the end of the minute the attendant holding the horse must be ready to trot the horse away as soon as the foot is put down. If the horse trots away distinctly more lame than at the previous trot the spavin is probably to blame for the lameness. If there is not a marked difference in the trotting the lameness should be sought elsewhere.

The treatment of spavin A number of spavins cure themselves by ankylosis, which indicates that the arthritis has filled up the space between the bones and locked them together so that they can no longer move one upon the other. As there is no movement, so there is no pain and the horse trots without lameness. It is a fortunate chance that the movement of these bones does not appear to be necessary to the horse's activities.

It follows from the above that horses with bone spavin enlargements need not be lame. No doubt each of them has been lame for a time but recovered when the bones ankylosed. A horse with a big spavin and no lameness is not likely to suffer further from that condition.

Horses with spavins causing lameness require treatment. Waiting hopefully for ankylosis to occur spontaneously may be fruitless and condemn the horse to years of painful progress. Ankylosis is produced surgically by deep thermo-cautery or by drilling between the affected bones so that their smooth opposing surfaces are inflamed and heal solidly together.

Bursitis An oily fluid, synovia, lubricates the joints and tendons to enable them to move without friction. The synovia is secreted by a membrane which encloses the joint or forms a sheath for the tendon, the enclosure being known as a bursa. Synovia also occurs in small bursas on prominent bony points so that the skin can slide over them easily. Any bruise or injury stimulates the bursa to produce more synovia, causing a swelling – a condition of bursitis.

Examples of bursitis on the limbs are capped elbow, tendon sheath swelling over the front of the knee, windgalls above and below the fetlock, capped hock, bog spavin and thoroughpin on the hock joint, and swelling in front of the stifle.

Capped elbow This swelling is due to bruising of what is normally a small bursa on the point of the elbow. The bruising is caused by a heel of the shoe while the horse is lying down with the leg folded underneath it. The shoe heel may be shortened and further bruising prevented by strapping a padded leather roll, known as a sausage-boot, around the pastern when the horse is not working. This prevents the shoe from contacting the point of the elbow.

Tendon sheath bursitis The tendon that runs over the front of the knee in a bursal sheath is subject to bruising from the horse hitting an obstacle when jumping or striking its knee under the manger as a sign of impatience at feeding time. A sausage-like swelling develops down the front of the knee. The hunting or jumping accidents cannot always be avoided but boarding-in the front of the manger will prevent recurrences from that cause.

Windgalls Windgalls are small swellings that appear at the side of any or all of the fetlock joints. Some are caused by tendon sheath bursitis, others are from the fetlock joint bursa. In young horses they are a sign of faulty action or of excessive work. In older horses they are often looked upon as wear and tear, honourable signs of a long hard-working life.

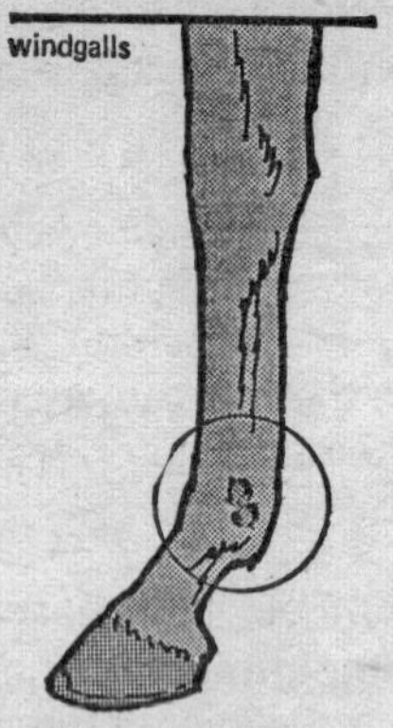

Capped hock A bursa on the point of the hock may be bruised on a hard stable floor or by kicking against a partition, causing a capped hock which may be as large as a tennis ball. When first bruised the

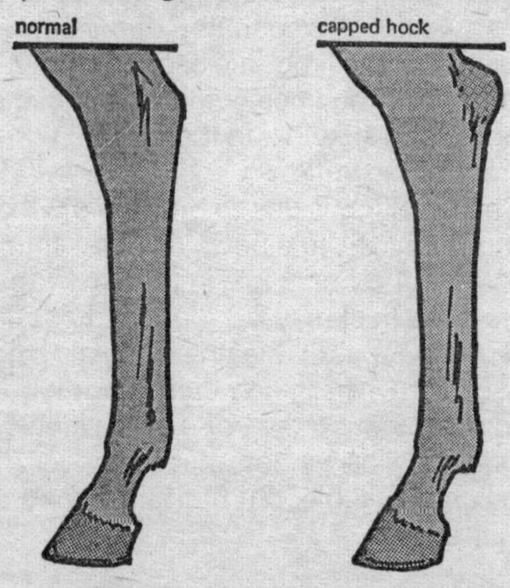

capped hock is extremely painful making the horse lame. The lameness does not usually persist but the bursa remains swollen and resists treatment. It is very unsightly but does not affect the horse's performance.

Thoroughpin There is usually a distinct hollow between the point of the hock and the back of the joint. When some strain or injury causes a bursitis at this site the hollow alters to a swelling that bulges out on both sides and may reach the size of a large grapefruit. It is usually quite painless.

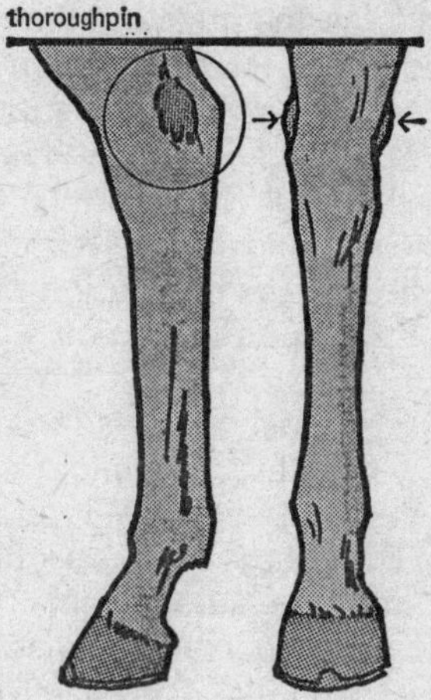

Bog spavin On the front of the hock and towards the inside a bursal swelling occurs, usually rather soft, fluctuating and painless. This is

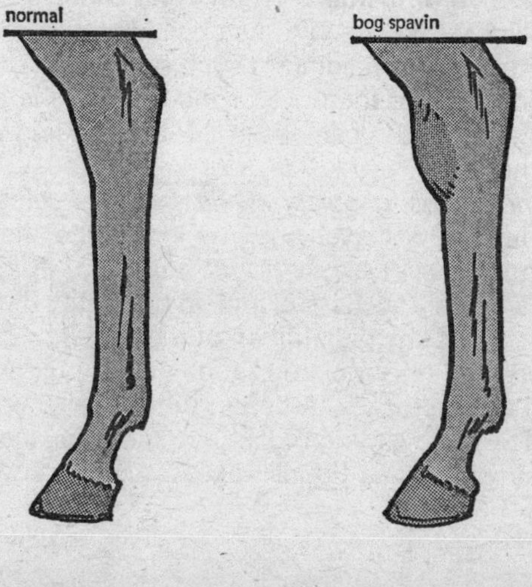

a bog spavin, being only slightly higher on the joint than the site of bone spavin.

Treatment of bursitis Most bursitis swellings are offensive to the eye but have little effect on the horse's performance. Windgalls, thoroughpins and bog spavins are likely to be due to faulty action. A better alignment of the joints can sometimes be brought about by careful shoeing. Thoroughpins and bog spavins are eased by thickening the shoe heels to lessen tension on the hock joint. Work may be reduced but complete rest, that is confining the horse in a stable, is not advisable, as the result of the slowing down of the blood circulation encourages fluids to accumulate in the limbs. An active circulation is needed if swellings are to be reduced. Pressure over bursal swellings is helpful. This may be applied by bandaging as far as the knee or the hock for swellings below that level. The knee and hock joints do not lend themselves to bandaging but steady pressure may be applied to them by using charges. Padded hock boots are sometimes used but it is extremely difficult to keep them functional.

Charges These are chemical plasters, resembling sealing-wax, which are melted and then brushed into the hair over the bursal swelling and around the joint in several layers alternating with thin layers of cotton wool. The charge shrinks slightly as it cools and acts as a pressure and supporting bandage, remaining firmly in place for a month or more over parts, such as the knee or hock joints, which cannot be bandaged satisfactorily. The charge can be removed when hair growth has separated it from the underlying skin.

Blisters Various stimulating paints or ointments containing mustard, iodine, biniodide of mercury, tar, or cantharides are used to reduce bursal swellings. They need to be applied with care to avoid any of the irritant dressing spreading to such sensitive areas as the back of the knee, the front of the hock or the heels at the pastern because inflamed skin in these positions may crack causing wounds that are difficult to heal.

Tapping and injecting bursal swellings It is seldom advisable to draw fluid from bursal swellings. The immediate effect is striking but the swelling refills in a few hours. Injections to suppress further secretions are rarely successful and do not justify the risk of infection that accompanies any penetration of a bursa.

Infected bursas Infected bursas, of which poll-evil and fistulous withers are examples, are abscesses which may have serious consequences. The synovia is an ideal nutriment for the organisms that cause disease. Bacteria flourish exceedingly in any bursa and may spread from there to cause a generalized blood poisoning. Even if they do not spread, local damage done to joints or tendon sheaths may so injure a horse as to make it permanently lame and, in consequence, useless.

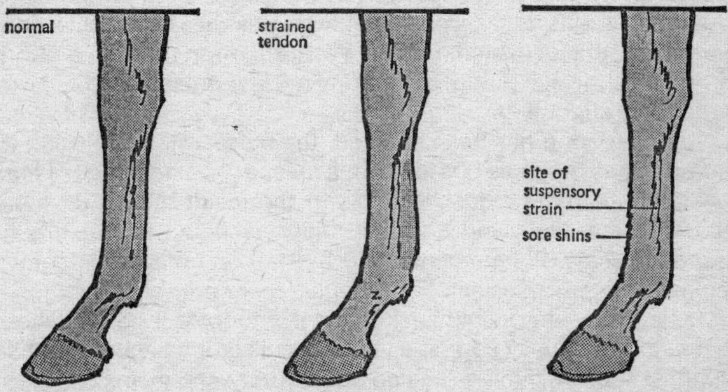

Strained tendons and ligaments Strain of the flexor tendons at the back of the foreleg between the knee and the fetlock occurs most frequently in horses that are doing fast work, especially when jumping is involved. Strains are more liable to occur in unfit horses than in those that are fit, in tired horses than in fresh animals and on hard going than when the ground is soft. When the tension in a galloping horse's tendon becomes too great the tissues give way. Fluids leak into the tear causing a soft swelling and the part becomes painful and hot. The strain may be in the superficial tendon, the deep tendon, the suspensory ligament or the check ligament. A tendon strain is recognized by noting that the tendon area is swollen and feeling the injury by running the hand down the back of the horse's leg. Lameness is sometimes present but in small injuries there is often no lameness. Horse trainers know from experience that if a horse showing these signs of strain is allowed to continue in work much more serious injuries will occur.

Tendon healing takes place by the natural process of inflammation. When blood vessels and fibrous tissue have penetrated the whole swelling, the blood supply diminishes and the fibres shrink, forming scar tissue which contracts the swelling and gives firm support. Eventually the leg becomes hard and cold again with a lump at the site of the tear and this may throw the back line of the leg out of true causing a 'bowed tendon'. In some cases the whole length of the tendons may be involved so that there is a diffuse thickening.

Treatment is only necessary if the horse is to return to the same type of strenuous and fast work as before. When the natural healing process has occurred stimulant dressings, blistering ointments or electric cautery are applied to repeat the inflammatory process in an exaggerated form so that the leg is eventually strongly supported by additional fibrous tissue. Considerable success has been achieved by reinforcing the damaged tendon with an inserted strip of fibro-carbon mesh which guides the natural healing process into a correct and strong alignment.

When a tendon has been strained, the horse will avoid using the injured leg as much as possible. This means that the opposite leg is constantly carrying extra weight with the result that, if the horse returns to fast work and a further injury occurs, it is probably the sound leg that will be strained and not the one that was originally damaged. Every consideration should, therefore, be given to the sound leg and, when stimulant treatment is adopted, both legs should be dealt with equally so that as the horse is gradually brought back to fitness the work will be shared equally between them.

Curbs Tendon and ligament strains occur less frequently in the hind limbs. Treatment is the same as may be applied to the fore limbs. A common ligament strain in the hock is known as a curb. It occurs at the lower part of the back of the joint where it meets the top of the cannon bone. The ligament joining the hock and the cannon bone is normally embedded in the bones and does not disturb the perfectly straight line from the point of the hock down the back of the leg. When the ligament is strained it shows as a bulge clearly seen from

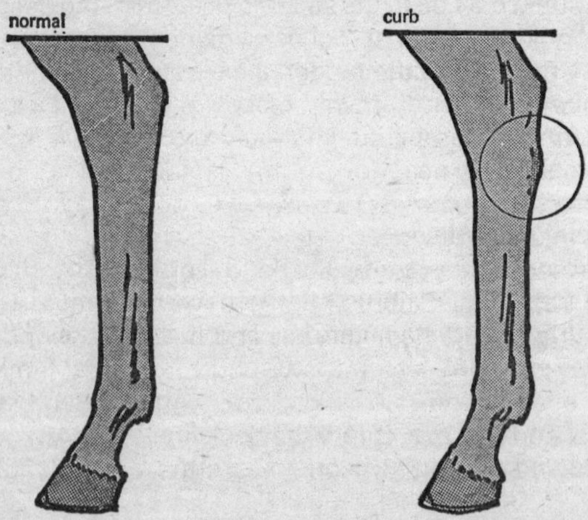

the side. Harness horses starting a heavy load or jumping horses taking off unbalanced at a jump, or some other mishap throwing stress on the hock may cause this strain. Rest is the most essential treatment. Most cases return to normal work but the swelling persists. If lameness continues stimulant dressings or electric cautery may be needed to establish a strong fibrous support.

Curby hocks Legs, on which the back line from the point of the hock angles forward at the junction with the cannon bone, are not suffering from a strained curb ligament. The conformation is congenital and is considered to be a weakness and a fault. Such horses are said to have curby hocks.

Firing Firing is the application of heat therapy to the skin and underlying tendons, ligaments or bones, so that the parts are acutely inflamed.

Horses normally heal their injured tissues by inflammation. Sometimes the blood supply cannot produce sufficient inflammation to effect a cure. In such cases the extra stimulus of firing, which repeats the inflammatory process in an exaggerated form, often brings about a recovery and enables the horse to return to work.

The operation of firing, accurately carried out under anaesthesia with electrically heated instruments, is applied to strained tendons and ligaments, splints, curbs, ringbones and spavins. In line-firing, the heat is applied in lines to the skin. This inflames the skin and the tissues below it. In addition to the healing effect, the lines of skin become less elastic than before, acting as a supporting bandage. In point-firing, metal pins penetrate the skin to various depths into injured or diseased tissues. The resulting scars in the skin are insignificant. It is interesting that even when tendon sheaths are pierced no persisting adhesions result. Spavins are fired even more deeply into the arthritic condition between the small hock bones so that they fuse together and eliminate the painful movement that is the cause of spavin lameness.

Firing has been practised for thousands of years; it was a painful process before anaesthesia became available and is criticized as unnecessary because, it is stated, most cases treated by firing would recover with the lapse of more time. The reply is that under modern systems of surgery and after-care these operations need cause the horse no distress, and experience has shown that without the stimulus of firing to the inflammatory healing processes many horses would have to be retired on account of chronic lameness when they might have many years of successful work ahead of them.

Other operations have been devised for the treatment of strained tendons of which carbon fibre implants appear to be the most promising.

Firing as a cure for strains has acquired such a reputation over the centuries that it has, probably mistakenly, been used to prevent strains occurring. Firing to strengthen the curb ligament was at one time a prevalent practice in Ireland; in the Indian sub-continent, Swat Valley mules are readily recognized by firing marks on the shoulders and quarters applied in patterns considered suitable to improve muscle power in these important areas.

The fetlock area The fetlock is in constant action and is designed to eliminate the concussion created by placing the foot on the ground under the heavy thrust of the horse's weight. The flexor muscles at the back of the limb gently relax to lower the joint and then reverse the process and contract to raise the joint up and thrust against the ground to drive the horse forward. The necessary leverage around the back of the fetlock joint is helped by the presence of the two sesamoid bones and the fetlock joint is prevented from sinking to the ground by the powerful suspensory ligament.

The design is well suited to normal progress on a grass surface. Troubles arise from progressing for considerable periods of time at the unnatural work of trotting, on a hard surface, carrying the weight of a rider. An uneven surface makes matters even worse; while tired horses, weary from working too long or too fast, become unbalanced in action. The uneven surface and the unbalanced action both cause stresses and strains.

Jarred joints The ligaments holding the bones together suffer from many small strains and become thickened. These enlarge the fetlock joint and limit its activity often without causing lameness.

Ringbone The ligaments are variously attached to the periosteum covering the bones. Strains on the ligaments irritate the periosteum and new growths of bone develop around, usually below, the fetlock joint as periostitis, arthritis or ringbone.

Windgalls The bursal membrane of the fetlock joint or the bursal sheath of the flexor tendons are likely to be involved in the stresses and produce more lubricant fluid which bulges at the side of the joint as windgalls, not usually causing lameness. They may be due to faults of conformation, working young horses too hard or, in aged horses, to the wear and tear of years of work.

Sesamoiditis The sesamoid bones can be affected by strained ligaments, arthritis or tendon strain. The bones are so well covered at the back of the joint that their injuries or diseases are difficult to assess and often impossible to treat. Lameness attributable to sesamoiditis can only be treated by long periods of rest, without any certainty of success.

Suspensory strain or injury The suspensory ligament may be involved in tendon strain or injured by external blows and may be a cause of lameness. Treatment is on the same lines as suggested for strained tendons.

Brushing Brushing wounds or scars are caused by the shoe of the opposite foot cutting the inside of the limb, usually on the side of the fetlock joint. These may cause acute lameness which usually disappears when the bruising effect has resolved. Brushing results from improper shoeing or faulty action from tiredness. Horses that turn their toes out from bad conformation are very liable to injure themselves in this way and they should be carefully shod.

Knuckling over The gentle slope of the leg below the fetlock joint, 50 degrees from the horizontal, is important to smooth and comfortable action. In some horses the fetlock joint lies more forward, an upright conformation. Age and wear and tear tend to have this same effect and in some cases the joint lies even further forward than the front of the hoof. This condition is known as knuckling over and such horses are very liable to stumble, injuring the front of the fetlock joint which may carry scars from this cause. Horses which never lie down are particularly liable to develop this condition.

Filled joints Horses suffering from some slight interference with their circulation, which may be due to lack of exercise or overfeeding, are liable to develop soft, painless swellings in various parts. The hind fetlock joints are often the first to fill. Treatment is to remove the cause of the trouble if it can be discovered.

The knee Considering the complication of the knee joint's arrangement of eleven bones and its constant activity, the knee usually keeps remarkably free of troubles.

Knee wounds The most frequent injury is from stumbling on to the front of the knee on a hard road surface. Lively horses at exercise are frequently fitted with knee boots to protect them from this damage. In these wounds a whole area of skin may be torn off. Deceptively, the underlying tissues appear clean. If the knee is bent to the angle at which it struck the road the mobile skin slides down the leg and the severe damage to the deeper parts may then be seen through the hole in the skin. Some surgery may be needed to drain these wounds satisfactorily. Numerous scars on the front of the knees indicate that the horse stumbles frequently, probably because of some arthritic condition in or near the feet.

Knee arthritis Arthritis of the knee bones is not common but it may occur in horses that are put into fast work too young. They can recover if stopped immediately and given a year's rest. Some cases have done well after treatment by radiotherapy.

Kneebone fractures Fracture of any of the knee bones usually has a crippling effect on the horse from the resulting arthritis, although small pieces of broken bone may often be removed surgically with success. A flexor muscle is attached to the upper part of the accessory carpal bone at the back of the knee. Extreme tension placed on this muscle in some fall or awkward landing is liable to break this bone, usually into two almost equal parts by a vertical fracture. Six months of idleness in a limited area to prevent any movement beyond a walk usually permits healing and some cases can return to fast work. Surgery is not helpful because removing the loose piece of the bone would prevent proper knee action and the parts cannot be screwed together or plated because the bone is shell-shaped and has not sufficient substance to retain the screws.

Tendon sheath bursitis A bursitis may affect the sheath of the extensor tendon which runs vertically over the front of the knee. In that situation it is easily bruised and becomes distended as a sausage-like swelling. It is usually painless and does not interfere with the horse's activity.

Popped knees The bursal capsule of the knee may become inflamed following minor frictions within the joint, often without causing lameness. The resulting bursitis appears as one or more small bulges on the front of the knee, a condition known as a popped knee. Either of these conditions of bursitis, if painful or causing lameness, may be treated with stimulant dressings or the joint can be enclosed in a charge.

The elbow joint The most serious injury to the elbow joint is a fracture of the point of the elbow which is formed by the head of the ulna bone. In some minor fractures the joint can be repaired by plating and screwing but the necessary immobilization for recovery is difficult to arrange. That particular bone's only function is to act as part of such a powerful lever that further displacement is almost inevitable.

Dropped elbow In cases where pressure on muscles or nerves has interfered with the shoulder's activity the elbow joint is let down and lies several inches lower than its fellow on the other foreleg. The horse is unable to move, or else progresses on the other three legs, dragging the affected limb and allowing it to swing forward passively at each step.

Such cases frequently recover if massage and stimulant treatment to the shoulder muscles are able to restore them to activity.

The shoulder The shoulder area takes the brunt of a good many falls and collisions. Fractures of the blade bone are not common, but as that bone is only partly covered by a muscular layer there is not enough muscle to hold the parts in place against the powerful leverages of movement and any major fracture is hopeless. A small point of the blade bone that projects over the shoulder joint is sometimes broken and while the injured horse can get around, permanent lameness is almost inevitable.

Fracture of the humerus which runs from the point of the shoulder to the elbow, though well surrounded by muscles, is hopeless to treat for the same reason, the tremendously powerful muscles that are anchored to this bone preventing the broken parts being held together during a long healing process.

The shoulder joint is a shallow cup and ball with weak surrounding ligaments. A sideways thrust on this joint is unusual, but may occur in a fall or other accident, dislocating the joint. This dislocation may be successfully reduced under a general anaesthetic though a long period of rest is required to allow the strained ligaments to re-establish themselves and the horse's activity should be limited by the use of slings and later by a blister over the joint.

Bruising of the shoulder joint by accident or from ill-fitting harness may give rise to bursitis, showing as a soft swelling over the point of the shoulder. The size of the swelling may interfere with the horse's usefulness, though the animal may not be lame. Treatment consists of ensuring that further damage does not occur. The swelling should be reduced with the help of stimulant paints or absorbent ointments.

The foot and shoeing

The hoof The hoof is constructed to withstand contact with the ground. Constant use wears it down and this is balanced by steady growth of about 8 mm ($\frac{1}{3}$ in) a month. The hoof is also designed to diminish concussion to which the horse is particularly susceptible because its limbs have only one toe. Apart from the horse and its

Bones of the lower limb

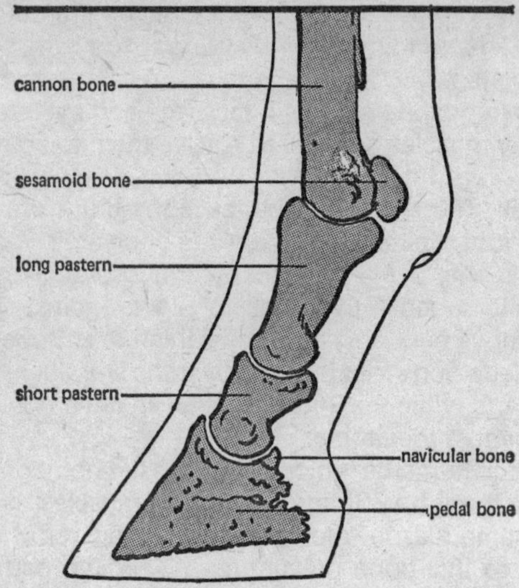

immediate relatives all large and fast-moving animals have several toes to share the shock of impact with the ground.

In action the weight of the horse is thrust into the hoof by the single column of bones which, from the fetlock down, are the long pastern, the short pastern and the pedal bone and, tucked in horizontally behind the pedal bone, the boat-shaped navicular bone.

The pedal bone (coffin bone or the 3rd phalanx) is shaped like a small hoof. It is extended back on each side by plates of gristle, the lateral cartilages. Its sloping front and sides are covered by vertical strips of flesh which interlock with strips of horn that line the wall of the hoof. The wall grows down from the coronet which surmounts the hoof. Each side of the wall is divided arbitrarily into toe, quarter and heel. At the heel the wall turns sharply forward forming an acute

Normal

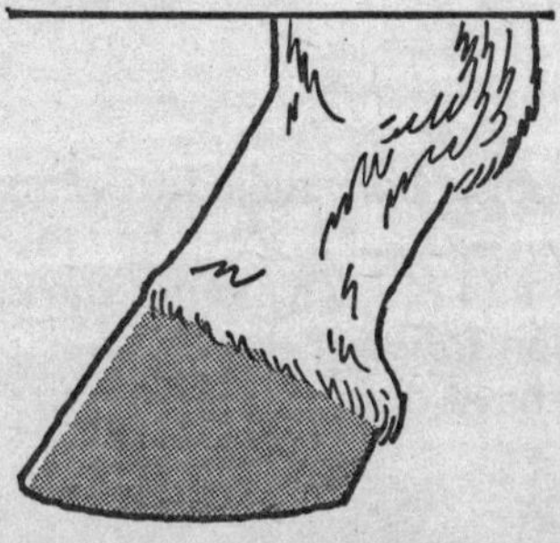

The sole

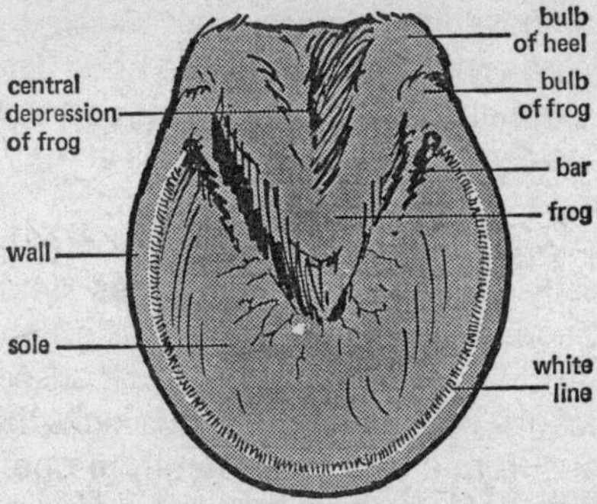

angle known as the buttress. The part of the wall that runs forward inside the angle is the bar. The pedal bone's lower surface carries a fleshy layer that secretes the sole. The sole is slightly arched and its perimeter is attached to the inside of the wall forming a junction of rather powdery horn known as the white line. Behind the sole is the frog, a wedge of rubbery tissue, its point at the centre of the foot and its broad end gripped between the bars on either side. Above the frog, inside the hoof and lying between the lateral cartilages, is a mass of firm but spongy tissue, the plantar cushion. All these parts are involved in reducing concussion.

A horse puts its foot down so that the heel reaches the ground first. The frog and the plantar cushion, compressed between the horse's weight and the ground, bulge sideways. The lateral cartilages and the walls at the heels are pressed outwards by the bulging plantar cushion and the frog. As the horse's weight pivots forwards, the arched sole flattens and extends slightly at its circumference, allowed to do so by the soft horn of the white line and some elasticity in the sloping hoof wall. When the foot is relieved of the horse's weight during the next stride all these tissues spring back to their resting position.

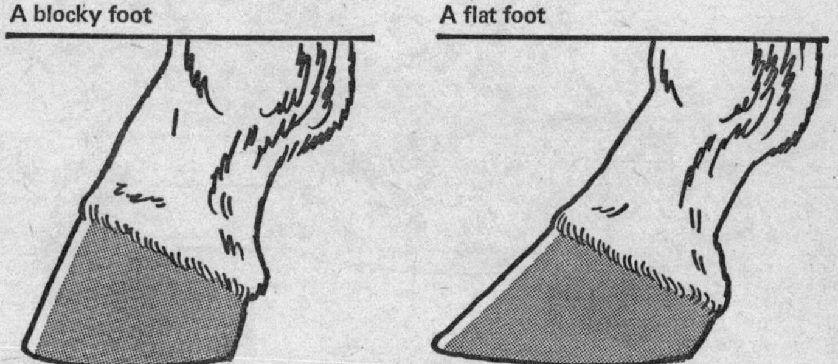

This repeated expansion and contraction of the hoof is essential to the horse's comfortable progress. It also assists in the process of pumping blood through the vessels in the hoof. The most important requirement for normal hoof activity is a broad contact of the frog with the ground to force the heels outwards at each step.

Shoeing Shoeing is necessary because normal growth of the foot cannot keep up with the wearing effect of regular work on hard surfaces, especially in wet weather. Horses whose activities are limited may manage very well without shoes if they are kept off the roads. Horses at grass are better unshod because their feet remain healthier and because the playful or jealous kicks that they exchange are less dangerous from a bare foot than from one shod with metal. All the same, the feet of horses at grass should be inspected regularly because they may not be getting enough wear. Feet that grow too long throw the joints out of balance and subject the limbs to strains. Unshod feet need to be pared and rasped regularly to keep them short and the sharp edge well rounded off. Wide, flat feet are particularly liable to split or break off pieces of horn at the quarters

The shod hoof

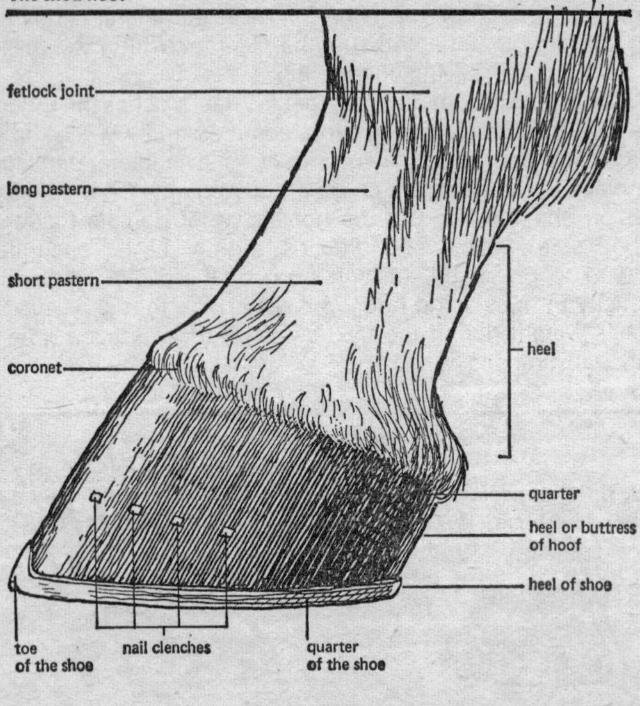

if they are allowed to grow too long, and if this has occurred they are difficult to treat unless they are shod.

Shoes are made from bars of mild steel which are shaped to the foot and nailed on through the hoof wall. Holes are sunk in the shoe to accommodate the tapered heads of the shoeing nails. When the shoe is nailed on, the long shank of the nail comes out at about one third of the height of the wall and is turned over to form a clench to keep the shoe tightly in place. Nails are held tight in the shoe by the accuracy of their fit in the nail hole. Shoes are made of various weights according to the horse's work, the aim being to provide a shoe that will resist wear to the best advantage of the horse. Shod horses wear down the shoe but the hoof continues to grow. In a month the hoof has grown about 8 mm ($\frac{1}{3}$ in) and needs to be rasped back to its proper proportions. This requires removal of the shoes. In most horses on regular work a new set of shoes will be needed at this time.

Growth of the shod foot The hoof wall always grows faster at the toe than at the heels. This is a provision of nature to balance the extra wear that results from the foot pivoting on the toe at each step. In shod feet the toe is completely protected from wear by the firmly fixed shoe, but the heels expand on the upper surface of the shoe each time the foot bears weight and contract each time the foot is lifted. This repeated movement, even if the heels are moving on a perfectly smooth shoe, wears the heels down slightly. The result is that the toes need considerably more reduction than the heels, when the horse is re-shod. The toes grow forward and if the shoe is left on much longer than a month this growth not only throws the foot out of balance, putting some strain on the joints, but it draws the heels of the shoe forward so that they may reach a position where they are likely to bruise that portion of the sole that lies between the wall and the bars, causing corns. If the shoe is not excessively worn down during the month's use it may be replaced after the foot has been trimmed back.

Calkins Heavy horses used to have the shoe heels turned down at right angles by as much as 2.5 cm (1 in) to improve their grip on hills and rough going. These heel grips are known as calkins. An equally thick bar was welded across the toe to keep the shoe level and add further purchase. This practice removed the frog from any ground contact and led to contracted heels. It is now discontinued but there are still steep streets in some towns paved with square stones set with gaps of about 2 or 3 cm (1 in) to supply a good grip for calkins and toe pieces. Small calkins are used on the hind shoes of riding

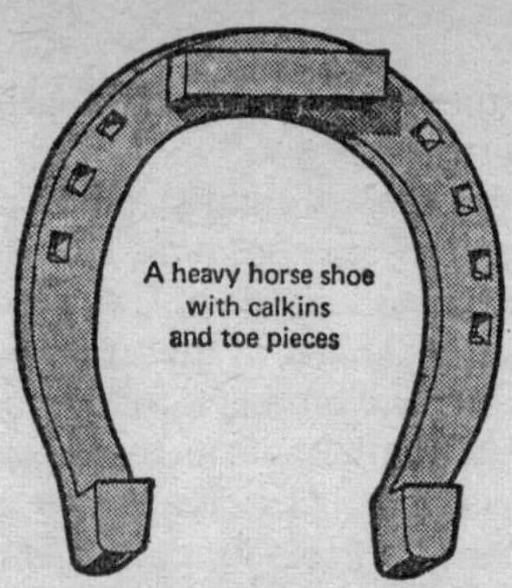
A heavy horse shoe with calkins and toe pieces

horses to prevent slipping and especially to help polo ponies in their quick changes of pace and direction. Care must be taken that calkins do not unbalance the foot on the limb. They are unsuitable for road work for light horses. For general use flat shoes are preferable as they allow the frog to come into contact with the ground. Frost cogs, which are calkins that can be screwed into the shoe when needed, are useful for horses working on snow or ice.

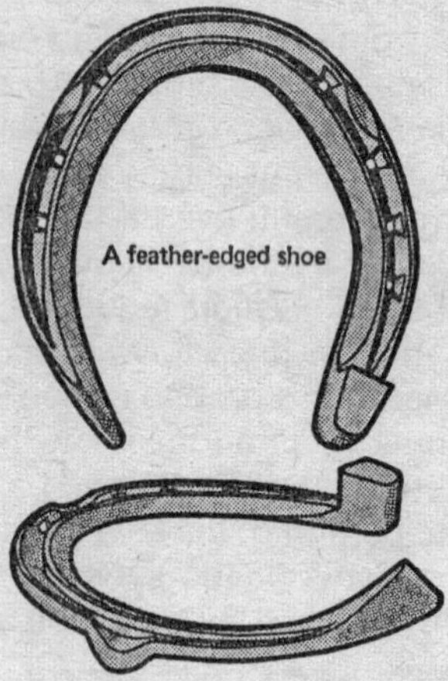
A feather-edged shoe

Fullering the shoe The ground surface of the shoe is often grooved for its full length. This is fullering. The groove fills with earth and grit which gives an anti-slipping area on the shoe, useful on smooth surfaces. The contact of the shoe with the ground is important. On turf, sand or other soft going, the shoe digs in and the impact is gradual. On hard ground or on road surfaces the impact is more sudden and it is a great advantage if it can be a sliding stop. Plain metal on smooth roads may cause slipping. Adding rough spots of hardened steel to the ground surface of the shoe causes an immediate stop on impact which jars right through the horse. The grit-filled groove in a fullered shoe gives the required happy medium of a shoe that grips without either slipping or jarring.

Clips Shoes are often made with clips which are 1.25-cm ($\frac{1}{2}$-in) rounded projections forced from the outer edge of the shoe. They may be placed at the toe or one on each side of it. They slope back against the hoof wall and help to retain the shoe in position.

Shoeing nails Shoes are attached to the feet by as many nails as the farrier finds necessary to keep them in position. In the United Kingdom seven nails are usual, four on the thicker outside of the foot and three on the slightly weaker inner side. This is traditional and satisfactory though, in America, four nails are used on each side with equal satisfaction and clips are usually dispensed with. The nails are spaced out equally on either side of the toe to reach back only slightly beyond the widest part of the hoof. The rest of the hoof is left free of nails to allow for the necessary expansion at the heels and the foot surface of the shoe should be very smooth to minimize friction. The heels of the shoe should be sufficiently wide to accommodate this expansion without the hoof overlapping the edge of the shoe.

Shoes for hunters For hunters and other riding horses likely to be sinking their feet into soft wet ground, the inner edge of the shoe is usually sloped from a normal width at the foot surface to a narrow fullered ground surface. This is a concave shoe. The narrower ground surface creates less suction and the horse can pick up its feet or drag them out of the mud more quickly in preparation for the next stride.

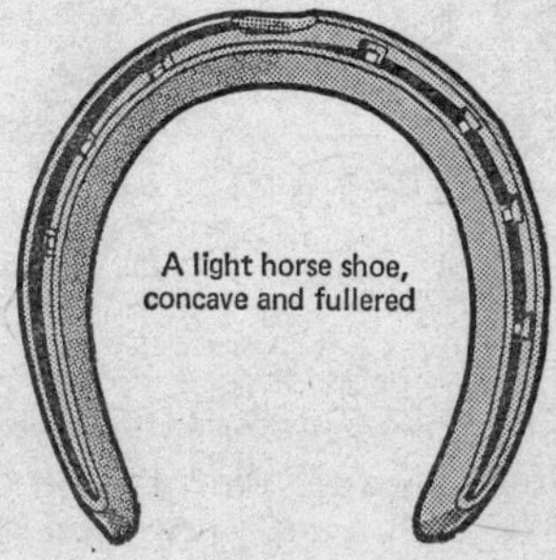
A light horse shoe, concave and fullered

Points of good shoeing

With the foot on the ground:

1 The nail clenches should be flat and broad and in a sloping line about one third of the height of the wall.

2 The shoe should fit the foot, neither overlapping the other except at the heels where the shoe should be 4 mm ($\frac{1}{6}$ in) wider on a hind shoe and 2 mm ($\frac{1}{12}$ in) wider on a fore shoe.
3 The walls should not have been rasped to make the foot the right shape for the shoe.
4 Any clips should be rounded, low and broad.

With the foot picked up:
1 The nail heads should be well driven home.
2 The hoof and the shoe should touch all the way round.
3 The shoe heels should be shaped to the angle formed by the wall, buttress and bar and sloped to the line of the buttress, rounded and smooth like a hazel nut, except the outside heel on each hind shoe, which should be round and upright.
4 The frog should be able to reach the ground.

These points of good shoeing apply to normal healthy feet. Farriers have to use their experience and discretion in shoeing damaged or neglected feet, or feet of poor conformation, and their expertise in improving the action and usefulness of these horses is invaluable to owners and their veterinary surgeons when problems involving the feet are presented.

Variations in shoes With the advent of synthetic materials and modern technology many different methods of shoeing horses have been suggested and some of them are useful for special purposes. Racehorses run in aluminium shoes, known as plates, for lightness.

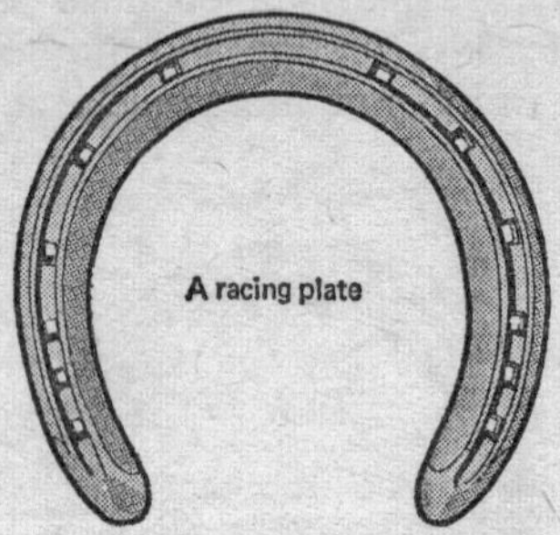

It is considered that any extra weight on the foot is a handicap equivalent to twenty times as much in the saddle. The racing plate weighs 50 g (2 oz) compared with 300 g (12 oz) for a hunter's shoe and 1 or 1.5 kg (2 or 3 lb) for a shoe for a heavy horse. As heavy shoes cause horses to lift their feet higher and this shortens the stride, it is logical to use light shoes for racing and heavy shoes for Hackneys. Shoes can be fitted with a rubber pad between the heels as a non-slip device. This acts as an artificial frog and may be useful with a heavy shoe that prevents the frog contacting the ground. But, whenever possible, using thinner metal for the shoe and encouraging natural frog pressure is preferable. Shoes of hardened rubber or hard wearing synthetic material do not adapt to varying ground surfaces as well as metal. They are liable to grip so firmly that the horse is jarred, or not to grip at all on wet surfaces, causing dangerous slipping. Their slight compressibility drags at the nail clinches at every step and loosens the nails. Nailed-on plastic shoes are usually lost because the nails break between the foot and the shoe or the nails tear off the pieces of hoof to which they are clinched.

With modern adhesives synthetic shoes can be glued to the feet, but if the adhesive is adequate to hold the shoe on for a month the farrier cannot remove it when the foot needs to be trimmed and the walls have to be broken. There is a fortune waiting for the inventor of a simplified method of protecting horses' feet against wear but, up to the present, nothing has been found to be more satisfactory than nailing on steel bars.

Hoof growth: 1 Grass rings The wall of the hoof grows down from the coronet and faint or distinct rings or ridges parallel with the coronet often develop on it. These are growth rings or grass rings and they may be irregularly spaced but the spacing is the same on all four feet. They indicate variations in the horse's food supply. Horses at grass all the year round are likely to produce thicker hoof horn when they are on summer grazing than on their less palatable winter food and they may show broad bands of differing horn around their hooves, indicating variable food supplies over past seasons. Horses not being worked for long or short periods for any reason carry a diary of these holidays in the growth rings on their feet. Grass rings or growth rings are quite harmless, merely indicating the different planes of nutrition properly fed to horses which may be in strenuous work over some periods and, at others, not getting so much exercise. Laminitis rings occur on the feet of horses with chronic laminitis. They differ from grass rings in that they are not parallel to the coronet and to each other but are closer together at the toe and wider apart towards the heels.

2 Slow hoof growth In starved or debilitated horses the hoof may grow very slowly and this corrects itself if the animal's feeding and management are satisfactorily adjusted but, occasionally, hoof growth slows down in horses that are in good condition and appear to be properly fed. The cause may be some mineral or vitamin deficiency which a summer at grass would almost certainly correct but, failing such a break, hoof growth can usually be restored by

An overgrown foot

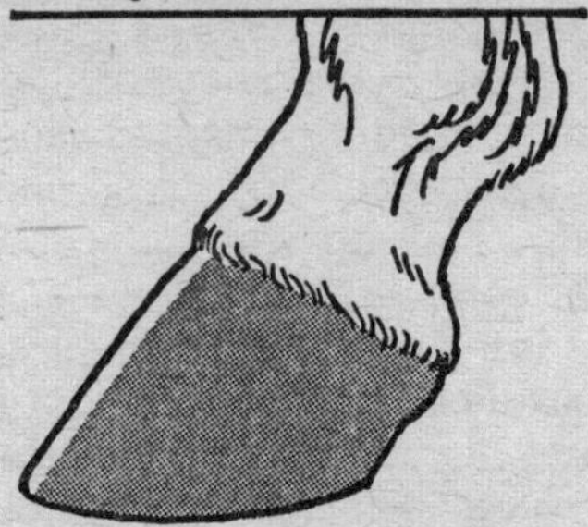

stirring up the local circulation with a creamy paste of mustard and water rubbed around the coronet for a few minutes once a week.

3 Hoof over-growth Feet that are not kept trimmed by natural wear or by monthly foot rasping grow too long, especially at the toe and this puts extra leverage and strain on the joints and tendons. The heels grow down and turn in over the frog putting it out of action as far as expanding the heels is concerned. The farrier can trim these feet back but he may have to do it in several stages to avoid damaging sensitive parts before normal proportions can be restored.

A grossly overgrown foot

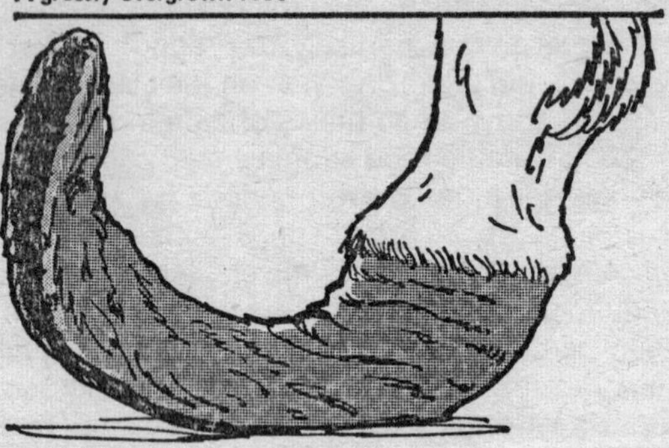

Horses' feet that have grown untrimmed for years become tubular and curl up in front like a ram's horns. They are sometimes seen in neglected horses on marshy land.

Pain in the foot Most diseases and injuries of the feet are accompanied by some inflammation which increases pressure inside the nearly inflexible hoof. This extra pressure causes pain and even a slightly inflamed foot may be acutely painful.

Apart from dealing with the actual cause of the trouble in the foot, steps must be taken to relieve the pain. This makes the horse more comfortable and enables the examination and treatment to be carried out more satisfactorily. Relief from pain in the foot may be obtained by soothing the horse with tranquillizers such as acetylpromazine, reducing the inflammation with cold water or with anti-inflammatory drugs such as phenyl-butazone, softening the hoof by tubbing (see below), relieving pressure by grooving the walls or deadening sensation by using local anaesthetics or by un-nerving. Very often operations on the foot can be dealt with by using a local anaesthetic but for long or complicated operations a general anaesthetic is more satisfactory both for the surgeon and the horse.

Grooving the hoof Some alterations in the feet, such as ringbones, side-bones, pedal ostitis and keratoma, cause continuing pressure in the hoof. This may be relieved temporarily by tubbing the foot but a more lasting effect may be obtained by grooving the hoof. This consists of cutting grooves in line with the growth of the horn, two or three spaced out on either side of the foot, 3 or 4 mm ($\frac{1}{8}$ in) wide, from the coronet to the ground surface through nearly the whole thickness of the horn of the wall without drawing blood. Care should be taken to avoid damaging the newly forming horn just below the hair line at the coronet. The segments so formed can separate slightly from each other and so increase the accommodation inside the hoof and also enable the new horn to grow as a larger hoof. The horn cuts more readily if there has been an opportunity to soften it by tubbing the foot for a day or two but the farrier may choose to burn the outer layers of horn which cut more easily when they are hot. The grooves grow out with the hoof and may need extending upwards from time to time.

Tubbing the hoof Inflammation of any sort is extremely painful in the hoof because of its inflexibility which does not allow it to swell or expand, as other parts of the body do, to accommodate the fluid secretions that accompany inflammation. The hoof can be made slightly flexible and more accommodating by tubbing; that is, standing it in a tub or a hard rubber bucket in 5 litres (1 gal) of hot water to which has been added 0.5 kg (1 lb) of Epsom salts and 0.5 kg (1 lb) of washing soda, for about 20 minutes. This may be repeated twice a day for several days, but the effect is cumulative and the foot becomes so soft that shoe nails cannot get a grip in the spongy horn. The water should not be hotter than one can hold one's hand in comfortably. Softening the hoof in this way as well as reducing some of the pressure building up in an inflamed hoof is also useful when cutting or grooving the hoof becomes necessary for dealing with abscesses, false quarter, seedy toe and other foot troubles.

Poultices The most satisfactory poultice for a horse's foot is a poultice pad of cotton wool on a fabric backing which is impregnated with an antiseptic paste. These are readily obtainable from chemists and saddlers. Dipped in hot water, not too hot to hold the hand in, and wrung out, the poultice is wrapped around the hoof, covered with a thin sheet of plastic and held in place with 3 or 4 metres (yards) of 8-cm (3-in) adhesive tape. The hollow of the heel needs to be well padded, either with the poultice if its activity is needed there, or with a pad of cotton wool, as, without such padding, there is the risk of bandaging too tightly above the hoof and interfering with the circulation of blood to the foot.

The poultice softens the hoof and skin and absorbs discharges from wounds. A poultice may need changing frequently or at long intervals according to the injury being treated. Properly applied the poultice will stay in position for 2 or 3 days even if the horse is at grass, though it will wear through much sooner on a hard floor.

When the poultice is removed the bulbs of the heel may appear to be separating from the skin, but the separation is superficial and harmless. Repeated poulticing is cumulative in its effects and the tender skin in the heels may be scalded if the poultices are applied at a greater heat than that suggested (comfortable to hold in the hand). It is advisable to check this personally. Dairy workers' idea of hot water involves superheated steam that would nearly melt the shoe let alone the horse's hoof.

Foot injuries and diseases

Loss of the hoof The whole horny box of the hoof, covering the pedal bone and the end of the limb, may be wrenched off by accident. When horses were used for shunting railway wagons they sometimes caught a hoof in the points and the oncoming wagons pushed the horse forward leaving the hoof wedged in the rails. The hoof may also be shed because inflammatory fluids from laminitis or an abscess in the hoof have completely separated the horny layer from the fleshy underlying tissues.

In theory the hoof could grow again in about a year, but the injuries associated with its loss are usually too severe to allow normal replacement. Although the horse is not usually noticeably in pain, immediate destruction is the only humane course to take in the majority of such cases. In the event of a hoof being shed under what appear to be hopeful conditions, the foot should be covered with a mild antiseptic paste of medicinal liquid paraffin and sulphanilamide powder under a generous cotton wool and gauze dressing. Slings may be needed until the horse has learned to bear some weight on the injured limb. Even in favourable cases it is unlikely that the result will be better than a misshapen horny stump. The smaller the animal the better the chance of success. Large and heavy animals are unable to support themselves even for a short time on three legs and usually develop a painful and incurable laminitis in the uninjured leg which is carrying the extra weight.

Acute laminitis Laminitis is an inflammation of the fleshy tissue on the front of the pedal bone, the parts that interlock with the strips of horn that line the wall of the hoof. Laminitis usually results from poisons – produced by bacterial diseases – circulating in the blood stream or by some form of food poisoning or indigestion. Why the fleshy parts on the front of the pedal bone should be the only tissues to swell up and secrete inflammatory fluid in these cases is not understood. The fact remains that horses suffering from severe feverish diseases such as pneumonia or inflammation of the womb and horses given a surfeit of grain or other unsuitable food may suddenly show acute pain in the feet from the pressure of inflammatory fluids.

A horse with acute laminitis stands fixed, unwilling to move because shifting its weight increases the pain and, for the same reason, it will not allow a foot to be picked up. The horse puts the fore feet as far forwards as possible and brings the hind feet under the body to take weight off the toes and on to the heels. The feet are hot, and tapping them lightly with a hammer causes flinching. Acute laminitis cases run a temperature up to 41 °C (104°F), which can be attributed partly to the poisoning disease and partly to the painful feet.

Acute laminitis may also result from excessive galloping on hard ground. Some versions of Dick Turpin's ride to York suggest that he rode one or more horses to death on the way and, if that was so, they probably died of foot founder, the name given to acute laminitis caused in that way. Horses travelling long distances by sea, unable to lie down or take exercise for weeks on end, frequently developed acute laminitis during the passage or after their first walk on land, the predisposing causes being strain on the feet from long standing and digestive disturbances associated with feeding problems under sea-going conditions. A frequent cause of laminitis is an injury that prevents the horse from putting any weight on one leg for a long time. The uninjured, opposite leg, having to carry twice its usual burden without remittance, is likely to develop acute laminitis suddenly. This may be avoided by giving a seriously injured horse the support of slings.

During the first twenty-four hours of a laminitis attack it is vitally important to relieve the horse from the acute pain which can become unbearable and contribute to the animal's collapse and death. After that time, medicinal and other treatments, which will vary according to the cause of the disease, should be taking effect and the pain is likely to be lessening.

A good soft bed should be put down and the horse may get relief from slings or even from being pulled down with ropes when it will often lie for a considerable time. It is sometimes suggested that the shoes should be removed and the feet poulticed. Poultices are certainly to be recommended but removing the shoes is impossible in many cases because the horse cannot bear the pain of standing when one foot is lifted. Cortisone injections and local anaesthetics give remarkable relief for some hours and may be repeated to allow the horse to be given exercise so that circulation is restored to the feet. The sensitivity to pain may be reduced by acetyl-promazine or phenyl-butazone. Saline laxatives are needed and antibiotics are indicated as a guard against the development of a complicating infection.

Careful nursing is important. The patient needs to be kept warm and encouraged to eat sloppy mashes and to drink freely. The horse should not be disturbed if it is lying down but exercise is important and when it is standing it should be encouraged to move about as every step improves the sluggish circulation. In convalescence care of the feet resembles that described for chronic laminitis cases.

Chronic laminitis Chronic laminitis is as insidious as acute laminitis is dramatic. Chronic laminitis results from an imbalance between feeding and exercise in the form of persistent overfeeding. The most usual victims are ponies on ordinary pasture. Ponies are naturally adapted to derive their nourishment from heaths and moorlands where the grazing for most of the year is sparse and of poor quality and they have to take a great deal of exercise to find enough to eat. Good pasture and little work over indulge them so that they put on weight and suffer from a mild chronic indigestion which poisons the blood stream. The poisons inflame the fleshy tissues under the hoof walls and fluid accumulates in front of the pedal bone. Horses that are overfed in relation to their work become similarly affected.

Normal foot in section

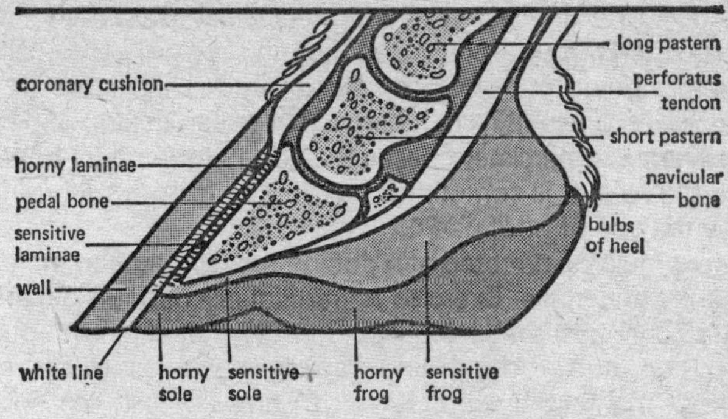

Laminitis foot in section

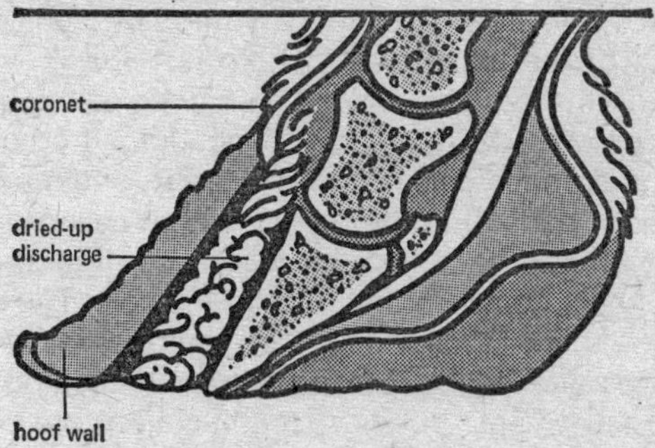

Changes in the feet occur gradually, over months or years. The fluids on the front of the pedal bone gradually force the toe back and down in the hoof. The toe grows long and low and the front of the wall becomes concave. The heels may be upright and narrow. Growth rings appear around the hoof horn, close together at the toe and wider apart towards the heels. The lower edge of the pedal bone

A chronic laminitis foot

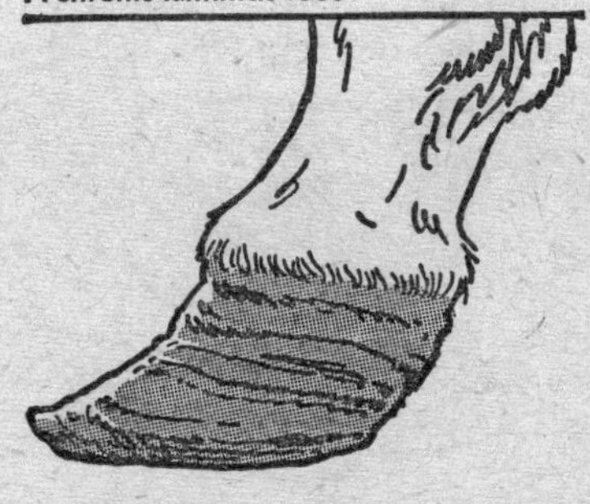

is pressed against the sole which becomes convex, instead of being arched, and bruises easily, causing lameness. When walking the feet are often thrown forward as though they were loose on their hinges before being put down on the ground. This is due to some disturbance of the usually exact balance between flexion and extension. In severe and persistent cases the edge of the pedal bone may penetrate the sole. It is sometimes possible to restore such a foot to normal by the use of hoof pads.

Treatment must be directed at reducing the feeding and increasing the amount of exercise. Exercise is particularly difficult because of the painful changes that have occurred in the feet. It should be conducted on soft ground and rapidly becomes much easier. Attention to the feet by farriery is of prime importance. The toe should be rasped back to restore a normal shape to the foot, as far as possible. This is likely to expose a dry mass of crumbling horn at the toe instead of the usual wall of horn but it will eventually be replaced by growth from the coronet. The walls at the quarters and heels should be lowered sufficiently to encourage frog contact with the ground. The dropped sole is thin and tender and may need to be protected by hoof pads or by a layer of leather nailed on under the shoe. The shoe should be seated out (see illustration on page 196), except at the heels, to avoid pressure on the sole. The shoe suited to most cases is thick at its widest part, the quarters, and thinned towards the toes and heels. If frog pressure is lacking a bar may be added across the heels. All these modifications are combined in what is known as a rocker-bar shoe, but a simpler shoe should be used as soon as the horse's action improves. Exercise is important

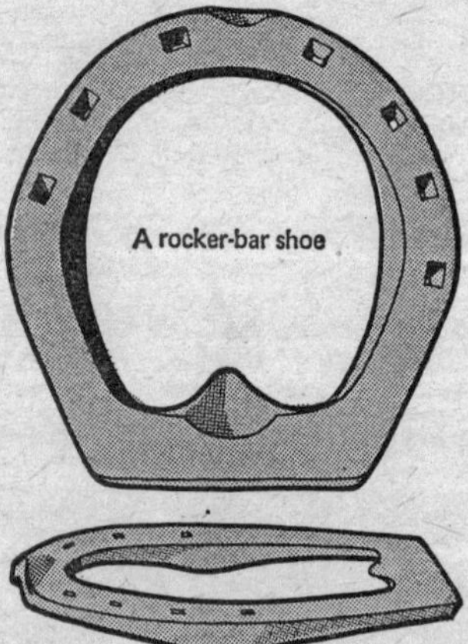

and should be given on soft going several times a day, increasing the distance each day as progress permits.

Horses with chronic laminitis should be put on to a laxative and reducing diet. It may be necessary to stable a laminitis case for long periods each day without any food because some horses can eat more than enough grass for their maintenance requirements in a couple of hours. A yard is useful in which the patients can take some exercise on their own. Later, as their action improves, they may be allowed more food to counterbalance the work they are doing, but reducing the weight of an overfat horse or pony with tender feet requires determination of an exceptional degree.

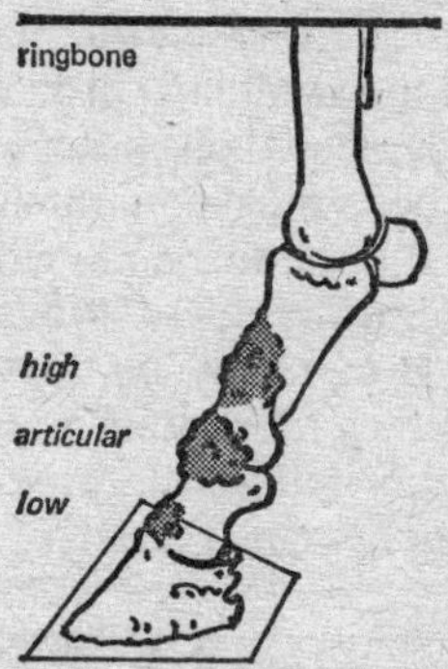

Bone injuries and diseases *Ringbones* Ringbones are an extra growth of bone on the long or short pastern bones. They are caused by strains, injuries or by concussion. If large enough they may be felt as prominences, most commonly on the front of the bone just above the hoof. Small ringbone formations and those below the edge of the hoof may only be detected by x-ray.

Ringbones are sensitive to pressure when they are forming and

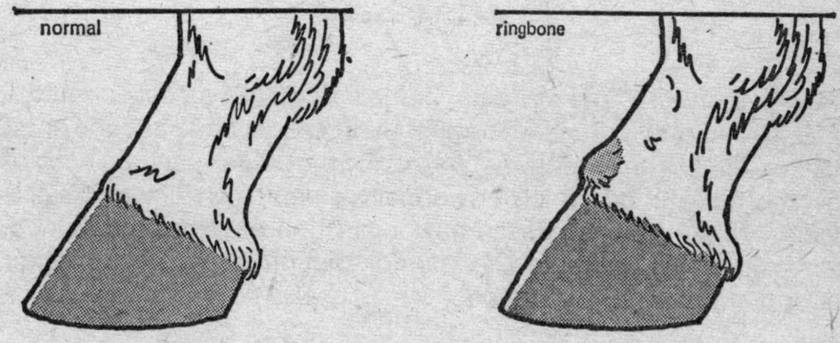

cause lameness. Later they become insensitive but may still cause lameness if they extend to the joints, above or below the short pastern, causing interference with the movement of the bones or the related ligaments and tendons or, if they are below the level of the hoof, by causing pain from pressure.

Ringbones may be treated by resting the horse until the inflamed bones become insensitive. This may be hastened by using a blistering dressing. Phenyl-butazone helps to relieve the pain. Grooving the hoof may be required to accommodate low ringbones. Un-nerving may be the only remedy in cases where joint action is affected.

Pedal ostitis Pedal ostitis occurs as extra growth or defective growth of any part of the pedal bone. It always causes lameness because of increased pressure within the hoof. The highest point of the pedal bone is called the pyramidal process and when this part is affected it is known as pyramidal disease. This site is just below that part of the short pastern bone most commonly affected with ringbone and the two conditions, ringbone and pyramidal disease may be present together, interfering with the movement of the bones on each other. Pedal ostitis can only be detected by x-ray. Phenyl-butazone usually gives some relief. Rest and tubbing the hoof alone or with grooving the hoof should be tried. Some cases are considerably helped by a hoof pad. Persistent cases may have to be relieved by un-nerving.

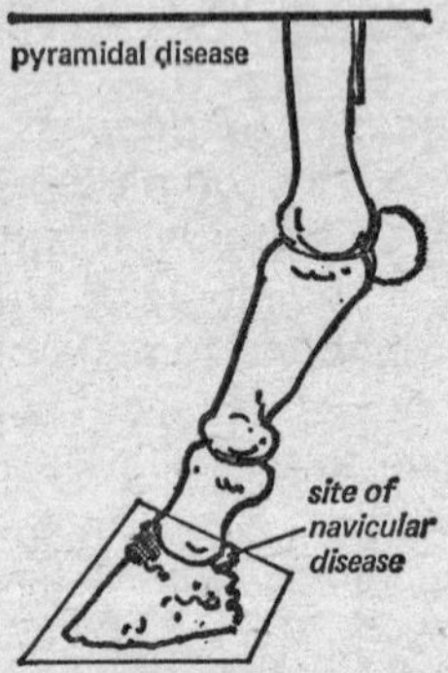

Navicular disease The navicular bone, shaped like a boat, lies at the back of the joint in the hoof formed by the pedal bone and the short pastern bone. The tendon that flexes the foot slides over the back of the navicular bone which is normally smooth. Navicular disease occurs when the back of the navicular bone becomes roughened, lameness being attributed to painful friction between the flexor tendon and the rough surface.

Navicular bone, showing navicular disease

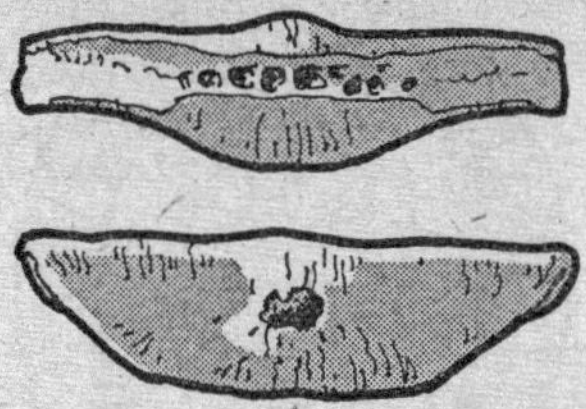

Navicular disease nearly always develops insidiously. The horse loses freedom of action and length of stride and is inclined to stumble. These signs are most noticeable as work starts but fade away as the horse warms up. After a period of rest they become obvious again. In the stable the horse often 'points' a toe, placing the affected foot flat on the ground a little in front of the other. If both feet are involved first one and then the other is 'pointed'. A wooden wedge placed under one fore foot so that the toe is raised an inch above the heels and left there while the other foot is held off the ground for a minute, puts considerable pressure on the flexor tendon where it runs over the navicular bone and, in affected horses, causes increased and marked lameness for a short while. The existence of navicular disease can usually be confirmed by radiographs which show areas where the bone has been thinned and eroded and that the channels through which the blood vessels enter the bone are considerably enlarged.

The cause of navicular disease has recently been shown by the Equine Research Station at Newmarket to involve blood clots obstructing the vessels supplying the bone so that it degenerates from lack of nutrition. It is suggested that this degeneration is painful and is the cause of lameness. Why clots should form in the blood vessels in this particular area has yet to be explained.

Navicular disease has been looked upon as an incurable condition which could be alleviated by judicious management and the use of such drugs as phenyl-butazone and cortico-steroids, and careful shoeing. The most useful shoe is thin at the toe which is 'rolled' or turned up slightly (see page 186) to overcome the tendency to stumble, and is gradually thickened to the heels. Un-nerving has been used and has kept many navicular disease cases going for years. Work at the Equine Research Station suggests that treatment with warfarin may so improve the circulation to the navicular bone that degeneration of the bone may be arrested and normal action restored.

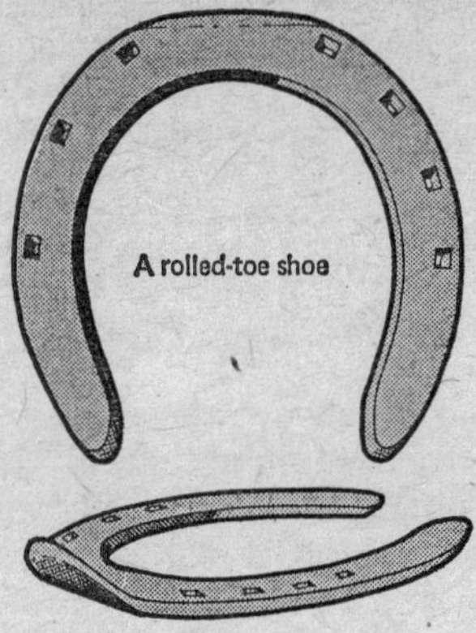
A rolled-toe shoe

Sidebones The lateral cartilages, extensions of gristle on either side of the back of the pedal bone, gradually change from cartilage to bone with advancing years, usually causing no trouble, though they reduce the expansion of the hoof. Sometimes, following some injury, large sidebones form, greatly exceeding the size of the original cartilages, and they appear as hard ridges on either side above the heels. They show very clearly on x-ray plates.

Horses with sidebones may go lame but a careful search for some other cause of the lameness should be made as sidebones, unless associated with a recent injury, are not often responsible for lameness. Their restriction of hoof expansion increases the effect of concussion and so they may in that way be an indirect cause of arthritic changes in the foot. They may be associated with corns since the sole is readily bruised between the heel of the shoe below and the inflexible sidebones above. Sidebones that are causing lameness can be made more comfortable by grooving the hoof and phenyl-butazone may ease the pain.

Fractures of bones in the hoof Any of the three bones in the hoof, the pedal, navicular and short pastern bones, may be fractured. As with

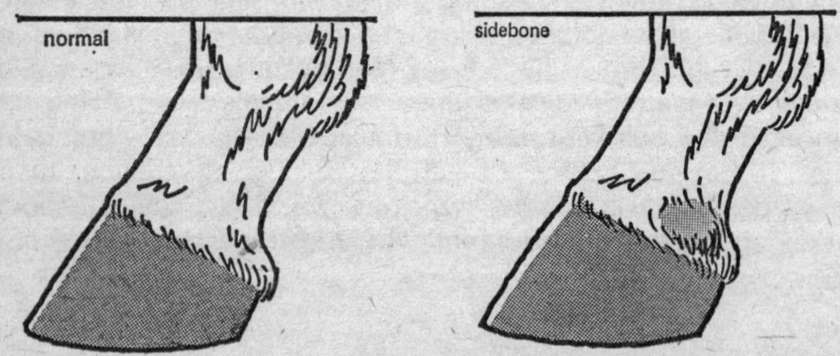

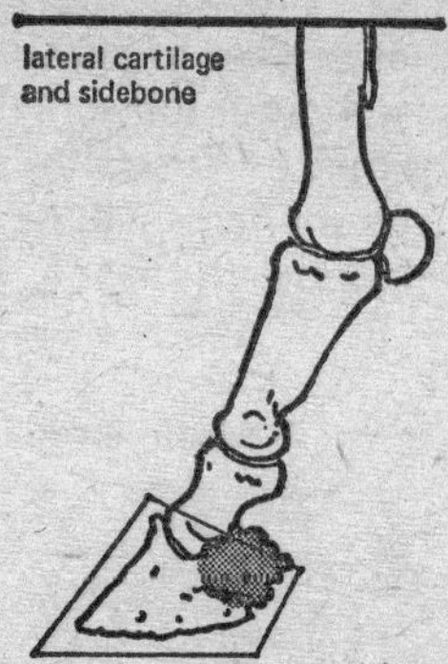

all cases of broken bones in the horse, a decision must be taken as to whether it is sensible to treat the animal or destroy it because of continued pain or the likelihood of treatment being unsuccessful. Broken bones in the foot can often be justifiably treated. Pieces of the pedal bone may be broken off when the horse, in action, strikes its foot suddenly against a solid object. Nails, glass or pieces of metal that puncture the sole may penetrate so far that they break either the pedal bone or the navicular bone. Navicular disease may so weaken that bone that it fractures at work. Fracture of the short pastern bone is usually caused by violent compression from above, when the weight of the galloping horse, off balance, is thrust violently down the rigid limb. This may break the bone vertically into two pieces, a condition known as a split pastern; sometimes the bone disintegrates into 30 or 40 pieces with a noise like a pistol shot. In any fracture small pieces of bone moving against each other are extremely painful. The horse goes lame or refuses to move and flinches with acute pain if the foot is picked up and twisted in the hand.

Suspected fractures of bones in the hoof should be well supported by bandaging over cotton wool, moved as little as possible and with great care, and x-rayed. Small breaks of the pedal bone are held in place by surrounding tissues and they usually heal in six months or so. Fractures resulting from sharp objects penetrating the sole are complicated by the wound which is likely to be infected. A split pastern, without displacement, may recover completely after a few month's rest with no more support than bandaging, though in many cases the two pieces of bone may require to be screwed together. If one piece of bone is quite small it may be best to operate and remove it. Multiple fractures of the short pastern bone usually lead to a decision to destroy the horse but they can sometimes be sufficiently supported by a plaster cast to allow the pieces to bind together in a confused mass, though this will never allow freedom of action. Any of these cases may end up with bony enlargements and lameness, but some horses injured in this way may be helped to reasonable activity with phenyl-butazone, hoof-grooving or unnerving.

The sole, showing keratoma

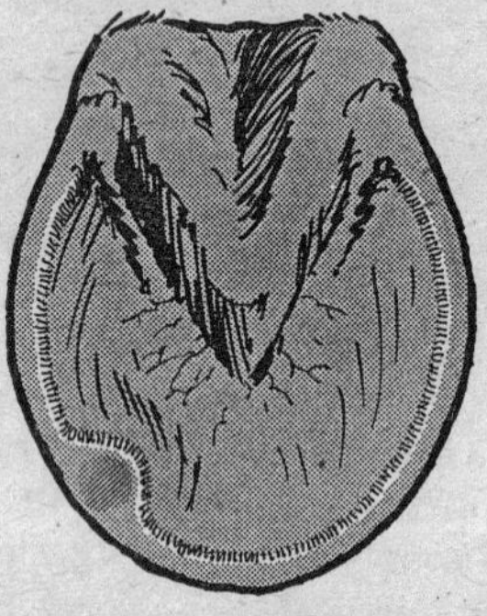

The coronet and walls *Keratoma* A keratoma is a horny tumour of the foot, an extra growth of horn that occasionally develops from the coronet and grows down inside the wall. The cause of such growths is unknown. The increased pressure causes lameness and may deform the shape of the pedal bone. The keratoma can usually only be seen when it has reached to the ground surface of the wall and appears as a rounded segment of horn causing the white line to make a detour around the front of it. Its effect, a deep groove on the front of the pedal bone, may be seen on x-ray plates. Treatment is directed at relieving the pressure and may involve removing a segment of the wall including the keratoma, though it is likely to recur with new hoof growth. Tubbing the foot and grooving the hoof on

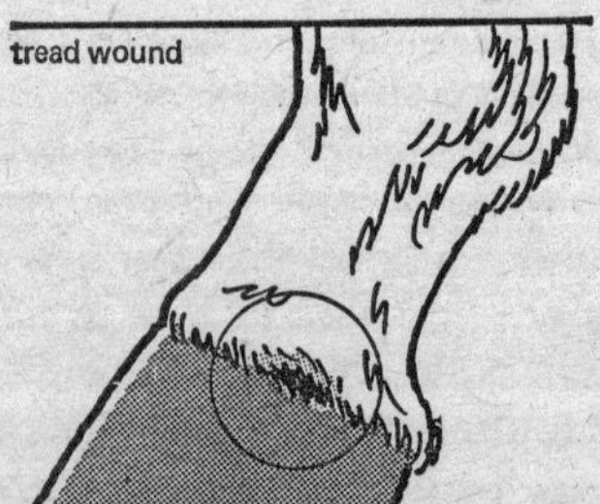

either side of the growth may allow sufficient expansion to accommodate the keratoma and allow the horse to continue work without lameness.

Tread wounds A tread is a wound on the coronet caused by the horse putting one foot on top of the other when turning sharply, the cut being caused by the sharp edge of the shoe or by a calkin. A tread wound may equally be caused by another horse. The wound should be carefully treated, the chief danger being that this damage to the coronet interrupts horn secretion causing the development of a false quarter. (See illustration opposite, below.)

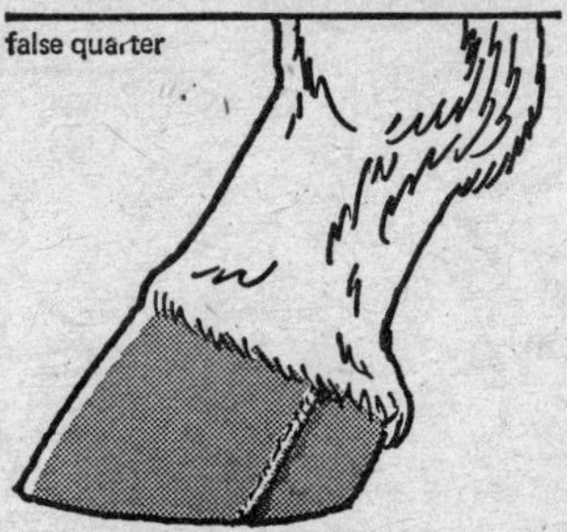

False quarter If the coronet has been injured by a tread from above or an abscess from below it may not be able to secrete horn for wall formation at that point. As a result, a break in the wall appears just below the injury and, as the wall continues to grow down, a line of defective horn develops. This is known as a false quarter, because, though it may appear at any part of the wall, the most common site is at the wall's quarter. Small false quarter lines are harmless apart from spoiling the smooth appearance of the surface of the hoof wall. Larger ones may develop a deep groove exposing the fleshy tissue below to the risk of infection or to be pinched between the sides of the groove, causing lameness. Paring the edges of the groove may prevent pinching and allow access to the deeper parts for antiseptic dressings. Pain may be lessened if the heel on the affected side of the foot is immobilized by fitting a bar shoe, nailing back towards the heel and drawing a clip on the other branch of the shoe, exactly opposite the false quarter. False quarters that cause serious trouble may be improved by surgical excision of part of the wall as described under Sand crack.

Sand crack – quarter crack Sand cracks are vertical splits in the hoof wall that develop suddenly just below the coronet as a result of some major effort. Heavy horses starting a load are liable to develop a sand crack at the front of the hind foot; light horses racing on hard ground

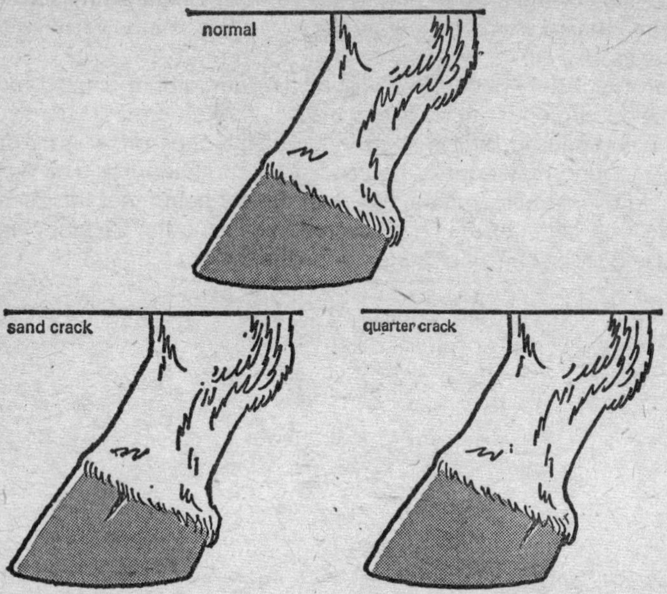

are more likely to develop one towards the heel where it may be called a quarter crack. A crack may develop at any point around the hoof head if a horse, plunging about, strikes a foot suddenly on hard ground. If a crack is not treated the normal stresses of hoof activity will keep it opening and closing and prevent the coronet from secreting sound horn at that point so that a false quarter follows. The sand crack is often acutely painful causing lameness. It may not be visible under the hair overhanging the hoof but is readily detected by pressing a finger around the coronet.

To prevent sensitive parts being pinched between the edges of the crack or to avoid the formation of a false quarter, a triangular piece of the whole thickness of the wall should be taken out. The 2.5-cm (1-in) base of the triangle lies just below the coronet and the apex 2.5 cm (1 in) lower. This removes all stress from the coronet and enables it to secrete a continuous strip of wall while the triangular gap is growing down the hoof. The hoof should be softened by tubbing before the operation which is carried out under anaesthetic. In about a month, when the hoof horn has begun to form from the coronary band the gap will have coated over with a thin layer of horn and can be filled up with acrylic resin to the level of the rest of the wall and the horse returned to normal activities. In

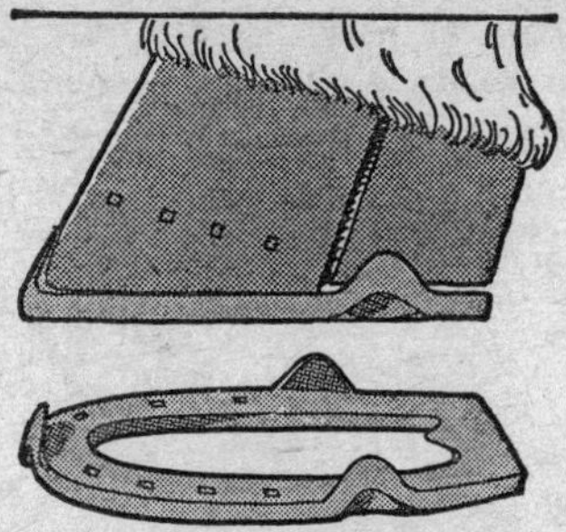

A bar shoe with three clips
for a quarter crack

quarter cracks that occur close to the heel, a wedge of horn reaching to the back of the foot may have to be taken out, though expert farriery may be able to keep a horse working, in spite of a quarter crack, using a bar shoe with several clips.

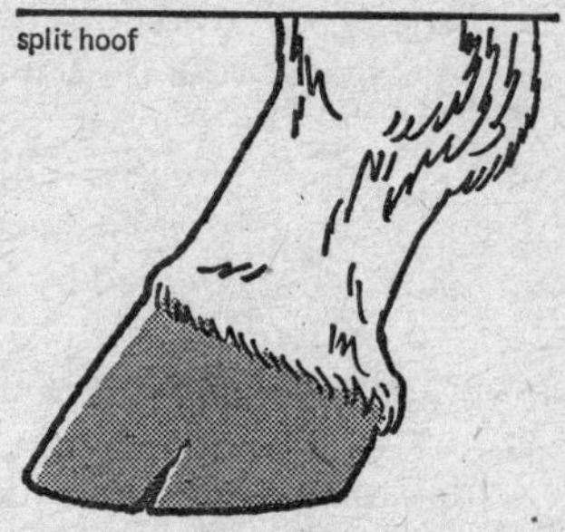

Broken hoof walls Large pieces of hoof wall may be pulled off if a horse loses a shoe; bare-footed horses, especially those with shallow, shelly feet, may split the lower rim of the wall or break pieces off. The broken edges of wall should be trimmed so that the injuries do not extend up the wall when weight is put on the foot after it has been shod. Shoeing prevents further damage. If fleshy sensitive tissues are exposed, an antiseptic dressing held in place by adhesive tape should be applied immediately and again after the shoe is put on. Any raw areas soon cover themselves with a thin protective layer of horn, after which the cavity can be filled up with acrylic resin level with the undamaged wall.

Gravel abscess Gravel is a stable name given to trouble arising from grit or gravel being driven up into the white line and developing painful pressure or an abscess under the wall. Tapping the wall over the affected part with a hammer causes flinching. The foot should be tubbed or poulticed and the foreign matter extracted from the white line. A piece of the wall may have to be removed. If not relieved gravel may develop into a seedy toe or it may form an abscess which discharges through the coronet resembling a quittor.

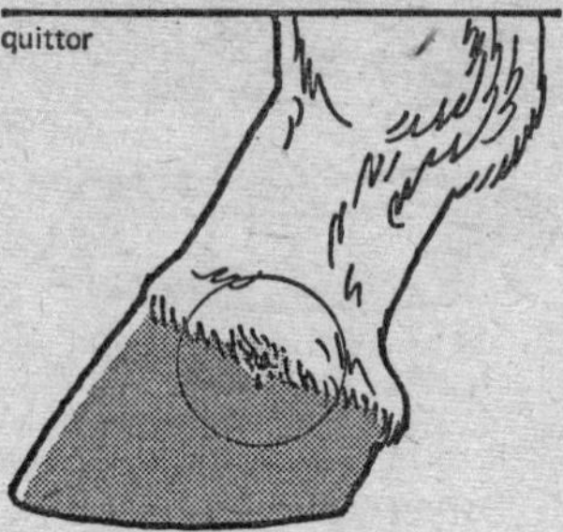

quittor

Quittor A quittor is a discharging wound on the coronet usually at the quarters. It is the opening of a channel leading down to an area of diseased lateral cartilage. This condition follows damage to the lateral cartilage following a tread wound from above or an infected corn from below. Opening up the corn to encourage downward drainage from the part, combined with antibiotic treatment may bring about a cure. In cases where there is extensive disease of the lateral cartilage it may have to be removed by a major development of the operation described under Sand crack. The object is to cut out the diseased portion of the cartilage without interfering with the coronet's secretion of horn for the wall of the hoof. It is important to arrange downward drainage from the operation wound.

Seedy toe In seedy toe a hollow develops in the white line and extends upwards under the wall of the hoof. It is usually filled with dry, crumbly horn and is quite painless. The cause of the separation of the horn of the wall from the fleshy tissue beneath is not usually

The sole, showing seedy toe

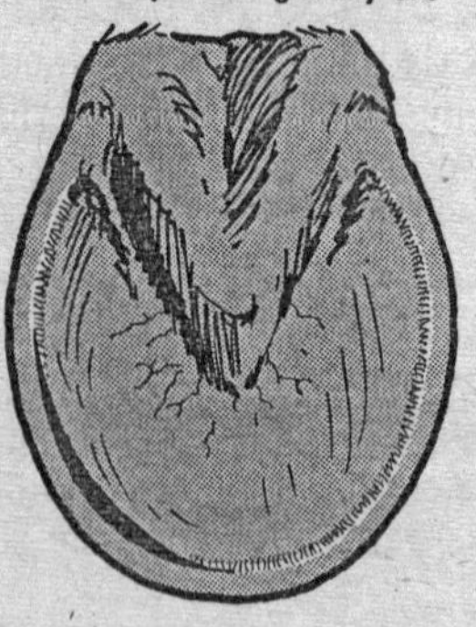

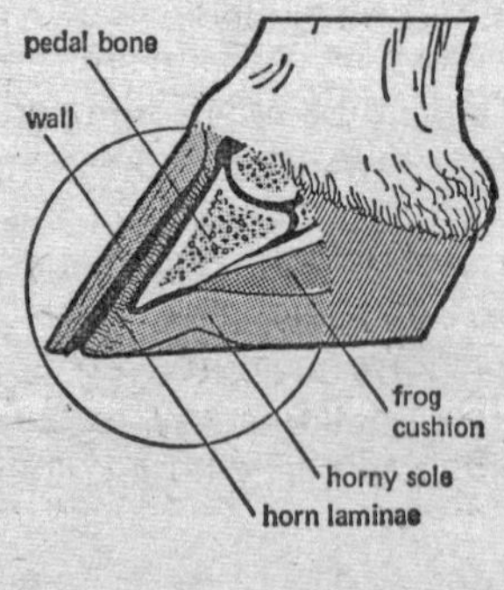

discovered. It may have been due to grit or gravel forcing its way into the white line or to pressure from a shoe clip or to some simple injury. Once established a seedy toe is liable to persist and to extend upwards and eventually cause pain and lameness from the pressure of material wedged in the space under the wall. Treatment consists of removing the whole of the outer covering of the cavity. This is quite painless and leaves a hollow on the face of the hoof which grows down with the natural hoof growth. The underlying fleshy tissues are not exposed, as they cover themselves with a thin layer of horn as the seedy toe develops. The unsightly depression on the front of the hoof may be filled in with acrylic resin to the normal shape of the hoof. This condition is very common in donkeys.

Nail bind If, when shoeing a horse, the farrier drives a nail too deeply in the hoof wall so that it presses on the underlying fleshy tissues, pain is caused and the horse flinches. The farrier draws out the nail and replaces it less deeply. If the nail were to be left in, the horse would go lame from a nail bind or press. A farrier always trots a horse after he has shod it to make sure that the shoes are comfortable. If the horse trots lame the farrier puts slight pressure with pincers over each nail to see if one of them is too deep and needs altering.

Pricks In shoeing a horse the farrier may direct a nail too deeply into the wall of the hoof and injure the sensitive tissues below. This is a prick, an accident which must be classed as an occupational hazard for both the horse and the farrier. It is liable to occur from time to time even in the most expert hands and can be attributed to variations in foot growth, the impetuous fidgetting of mettlesome horses or an error of judgement. A prick is a wound and the horse's foot is a dirty object giving rise to the possibility of infection. The usual treatment is for the farrier to open up the wound sufficiently to apply an antiseptic dressing and continue with the shoeing. If lameness does not develop and the horse is protected against tetanus no further attention is necessary. If the horse goes lame as a result of the prick the case must be treated as a wound in the sole.

The sole *Picked-up stones* One of the most widespread items of knowledge about horses is that they can pick up stones in their feet. Stones and other objects become jammed between the frog and the heel of the shoe and they can cause acute and immediate lameness which is cured as quickly by hooking them out with a hoof-pick, an essential item in every grooming kit, chiefly used for regularly cleaning out the feet before and after work. Small stones can sometimes get in between the hoof and the shoe and the shoe may have to be removed to reach the stone. Picked-up stones can cause severe bruising on the sole.

Bruised sole The sole is often bruised or cut by hard or sharp objects which are trodden on. Bruising causes lameness and the bruise may sometimes show as a blood stained mark when the sole is washed clean; others may only be detected by the horse flinching when the foot is examined with hoof testing pincers. Bruises usually clear up with a few days' rest unless they are so severe that they have damaged the pedal bone. They may be helped by tubbing the foot or by poulticing and are helped by hoof pads. Corns are a bruising of the sole at the heel.

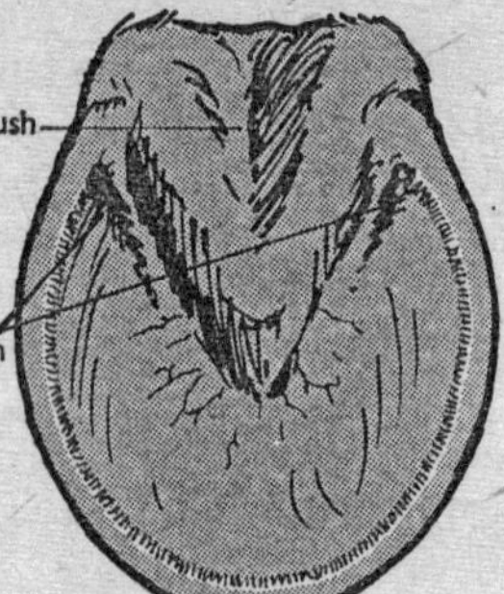

Corns A corn is a bruise of that part of the wall that is enclosed in the angle formed by the wall and the bar. The sole in this area is comparatively thin and the 'heel' of the pedal bone lies closely above it. The bruise is almost always caused by pressure from the shoe, sometimes because the heels of the foot have been lowered too much or because the shoe, left on too long, has been dragged forward by the growth at the toe and the shoe-heel presses directly on to the seat of corn. When the shoe is taken off, the horn at the site of the corn is seen to be discoloured from blood stains and the horse flinches if that part is compressed with hoof testers. The treatment of corns consists of cutting out enough of the bruised sole to ensure that there is no pressure on that part when the horse is re-shod with a properly fitting shoe. The cavity formed should be filled with a pad of antiseptic dressing as a protection against dirt packing in under the shoe. A corn may be infected so that an abscess has formed. The pus can be discharged through an opening made by cutting down on to the corn. If not released in this way the pus is likely to take the line of least resistance and break out at the coronet, possibly resulting in a false quarter or a quittor.

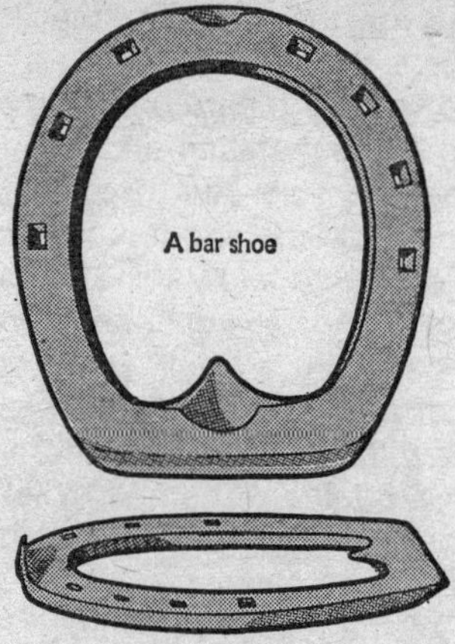

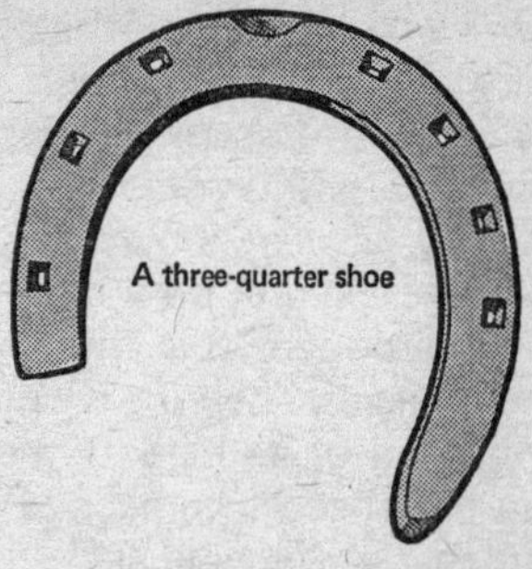

Special shoeing may be needed temporarily for feet badly affected by corns. A bar shoe takes pressure off the heels and transfers it to the frog. A three-quarter-bar shoe takes all the pressure off a bad corn and leaves the part available for attention but is not a suitable shoe to work in as there is no direct protection over the corn. A set-heeled shoe is suitable for a slight corn that is not preventing a horse from being worked. This shoe has the heel on the side of the corn only half the thickness of the rest of the shoe so that that part has little contact with the ground and impact and jarring are reduced.

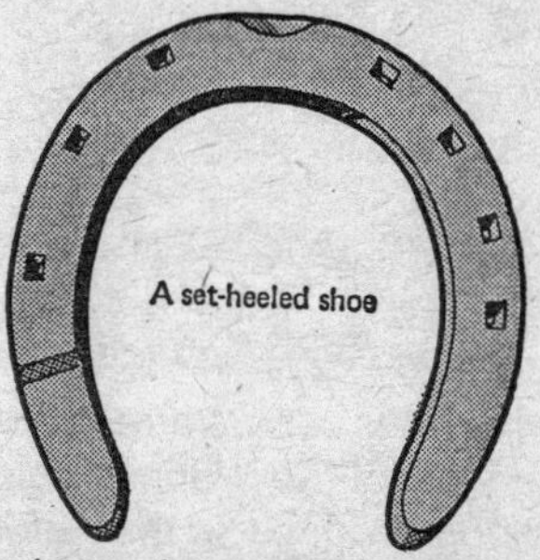

Prevention of corns depends on regular and careful shoeing. When fitting a shoe the farrier, as a preventive measure, ensures that the shoe does not press on the sole at this point and he may remove a little horn to ensure this. Horses with contracted heels, sidebones or shallow feet are especially liable to develop corns and the farrier should be consulted as to the best type of shoeing for each case.

Punctured sole – under-run sole Cuts in the sole from sharp stones or nails can let dirt and bacteria through the horn into the fleshy tissues below and an abscess may develop. The wound in the horn is likely to close up so that there is no way for the accumulating pus to escape and this spreads under the sole separating the horn from the fleshy tissues, known as an under-run sole. An abscess in the foot is very painful from the pressure of the pus and it is necessary to make an opening in the insensitive horn to allow the abscess to evacuate itself. The sole is cut through with a searcher knife which has the end of its blade turned back to form a small, sharp hook. When the abscess is reached it will often discharge itself violently. A suitably large hole is left to allow further drainage from the abscess and the foot is covered with a poultice. The hollow left by the emptied abscess in the fleshy tissues is soon lined with new horn. Antibiotics and protection against tetanus are needed.

Dropped sole Dropped sole is one of the results of laminitis. The inflammatory discharges that are produced in front of the pedal bone in laminitis cases press the toe of the bone down against the sole which loses its arch, flattens and then becomes convex or 'dropped'.

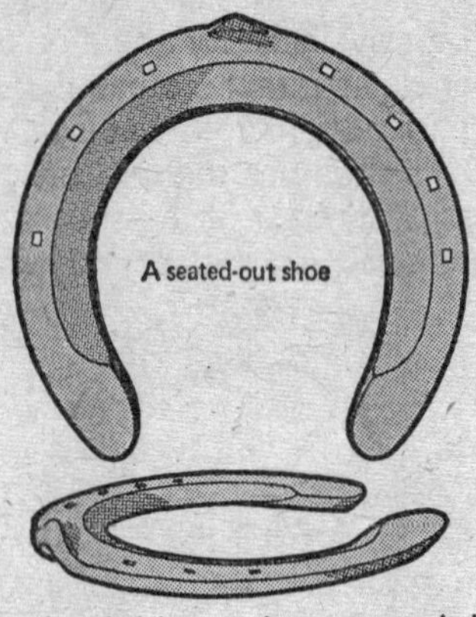

If the progress of the laminitis can be arrested the horse may be able to continue in work in spite of the dropped sole. The inner rim of the foot surface of the shoe requires to be sloped inwards to avoid putting pressure on the sole. This is a seated-out shoe.

A dropped sole is thin and tender and bruises easily. It is often protected by fitting a piece of leather across the foot, nailed on with the shoe, or by a hoof pad.

The frog *Contracted heels* The cross-section of the hoof wall resembles a powerful C-spring and it is inclined to close unless its

A contracted foot, sole view

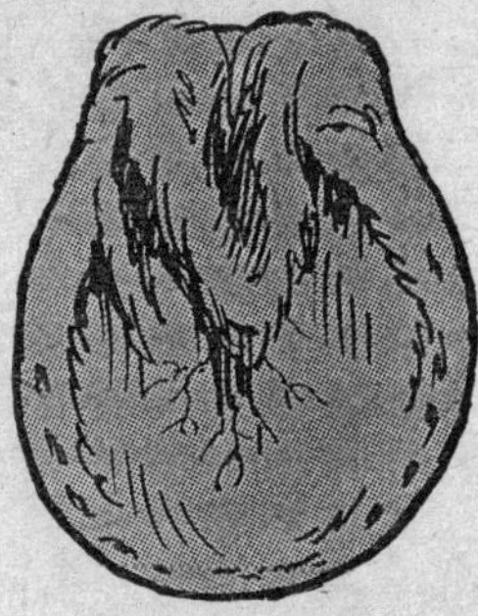

sides are kept apart by a well developed frog. If the frog is allowed to wither from lack of active contact with the ground because of a thick shoe or overgrown hoof walls, the heels close in on each other, the condition of contracted heels. This tendency can develop to such an extent that the heels meet together and the hoof becomes a tube. Contracted heels are objectionable because they interfere with the health and efficiency of the foot and affect the horse's action. When contracted heels occur their proper separation should be restored by encouraging development and activity of the frog. This may be brought about by lowering the heels and allowing the horse to run barefoot or with bare heels, the toe being shod with a short shoe that tapers away at the quarters. This shoe is called a tip. If the horse is to be worked, a thin shoe may allow the frog to reach the ground or, in some cases, a bar shoe may be needed which carries the shoeing iron across the back of the foot for the frog to press upon. In addition to frog pressure, contracted heels may be encouraged to spread by sloping the upper surface of the shoe gently outwards for the last 5 cm (2 in) of the heels, and placing the shoe nails nearer the toe than usual to allow more freedom for the heels to expand. Contracted heels are often associated with a condition of thrush of the frog.

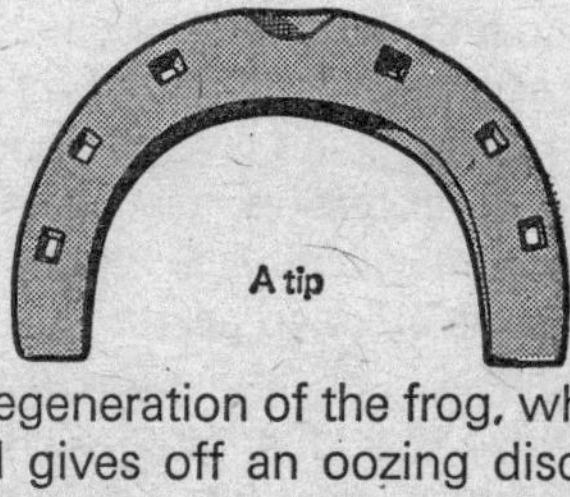

A tip

Thrush Thrush is a degeneration of the frog, which becomes moist, black and pitted and gives off an oozing discharge which has a musty, unpleasant smell. The central depression of the frog extends

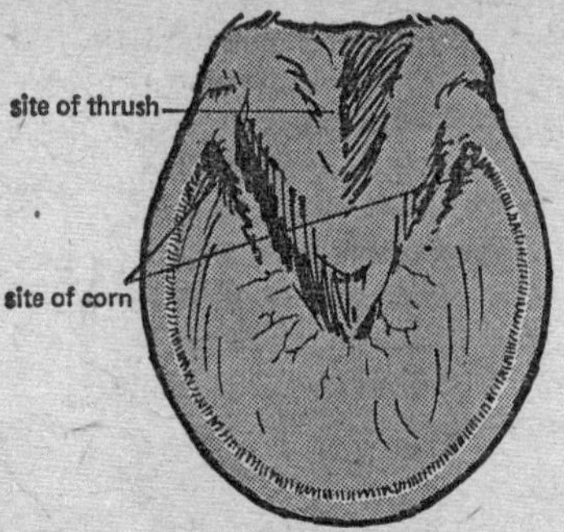

to become a deep cleft. The cause of thrush is not clearly understood but contributing factors are moist and filthy stable conditions and failure to clean out the feet regularly. High heels, contracted heels and lack of frog pressure often accompany the disease. The hind feet are more usually affected than the fore feet.

Treatment consists of cutting away as much as possible of the moist, pitted frog tissue without damaging the fleshy parts beneath. The heels should be lowered reasonably and shoeing arranged to restore frog pressure. A mild antiseptic powder should be dusted over the frog and clean, dry bedding supplied. Maggots occasionally develop in the depths of a thrushy frog. They are easily sluiced out with an antiseptic solution or a little hydrogen peroxide.

A thrushy frog gives poor protection to the sensitive tissues below, which may be bruised and cause lameness. The horse will rapidly improve if turned out to grass. If exercise has to be given on hard or rough ground the feet may be protected temporarily with a piece of leather or linoleum strapped on with sticky tape. These covers should be removed on returning to the stable because thrush cases recover best if exposed to the air. The disease usually clears up satisfactorily under conditions of improved hygiene and persistence in attempts to restore frog pressure.

Canker Canker is a wet eczema of the sole and frog whose cause is not known, though, like thrush, it is usually associated with damp and filthy conditions of stabling. The affected parts are wet under a thin scab which easily rubs off and reveals a peculiar smelling cheesy layer in which fern-like fronds of tissue are developing. Canker spreads slowly in some cases, rapidly in others. Treatment consists of exposing the whole of the affected area and applying antiseptic and caustic dressings under considerable pressure. A useful method of obtaining pressure is by placing strips of hoop-iron across the foot with the ends tucked under the shoe. The centres of the metal strips are then hammered down flat. Antibiotics should be used locally as well as by injection. The disease is stubborn to treat and liable to recur. Fortunately it is now rarely encountered.

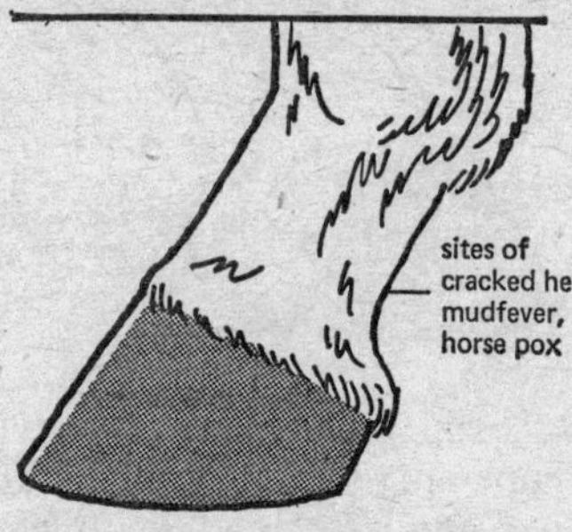

The heels *Heel wounds – cracked heels – mud fever* The skin at the back of the pastern is especially liable to injury and disease because it is thin and soft and very close to the ground. Wounds in this area are likely to be caused if the horse tramples over large stones, broken bottles, discarded tins or stubs of brushwood. Horses may also injure this part by putting a foot over a low fence wire. If they pull back suddenly the bulbs of the heel can be trapped by the wire and, especially if it is barbed, an ugly wound may result.

Cracked heels may develop when the heels are irritated by dirt, wet and cold. The inflamed skin cracks into a series of horizontal sores that keep breaking open because of hinge-like action of this part every time the foot is moved.

Mud fever is an inflammation of the skin in the heels associated with muddy conditions. Most horses are not affected by standing in mud or by carrying it around to dry on their legs. Washing the mud off for the sake of appearances, leaving the heels wet and raw in cold weather makes matters worse. If they require washing they should be dried off and bandaged. The colour of the horse's hair and the type of soil make some difference to the likelihood of trouble from mud fever. The pink skin of horses with white hair in their heels is much more sensitive than dark, pigmented skin and clay soil is worse than any other for giving rise to irritation. The inflamed skin of mud fever can rapidly develop into a condition of cracked heels.

All these breaks in the skin can become infected with dirt and bacteria, causing wet discharges, a high temperature and lameness. Most wounds in horses heal up satisfactorily under a dry scab but wounds in the heels that scab over crack open again constantly. They heal well if kept soft and moist with an antiseptic ointment or paste.

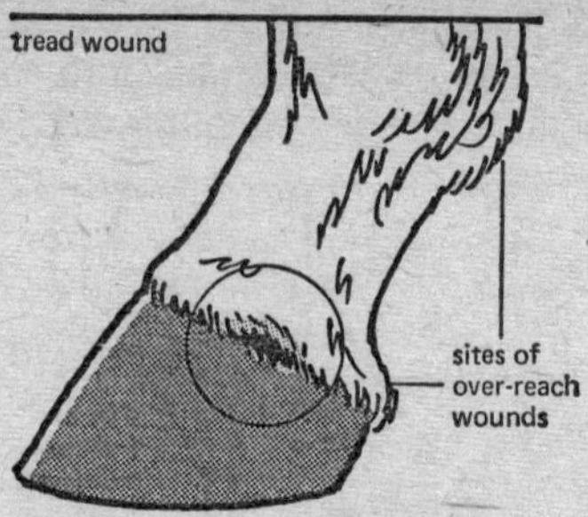

Sulphonilamide and medicinal liquid paraffin as a paste, or zinc and castor oil as an ointment, are useful and they should be covered with cotton wool and gauze and bandaged. Even large wounds do well under this treatment. In very severe cases a plaster cast may be needed to limit movement but this makes any change of dressings difficult. Stitching of any wounds in the heels should be avoided as drainage from them is essential to recovery.

Over-reach wounds Over-reach wounds are caused by the shoe on a hind foot cutting down on the back of a fore limb as it is leaving the ground when galloping. The bulb of the heel is the common site of an over-reach although it may occur at the back of the fetlock or even as high as the flexor tendons. They are serious wounds because they are made by a dirty shoe, at speed and from above downwards. The dirty shoe leaves infection in the wound, the speed of the blow causes serious bruising and the downward drive leaves a flap of skin hinged at the bottom making drainage from the wound difficult. Over-reach wounds usually heal better if the hinged flap is cut away solving the problem of drainage. Otherwise they need to be treated like other wounds.

While most over-reach wounds are isolated incidents resulting from the horse being thrown off balance while galloping or jumping there are some horses that repeatedly injure themselves in this way. This tendency to over-reach may be corrected by altering the timing of the foot movements. This is done by rolling the toes of the fore shoes to speed the take up action of the fore feet and by leaving the hind feet slightly longer at the toe so that their forward flight is somewhat delayed. The inner edge of the hind shoes' ground surface should be rounded off at the toe as this is the edge that actually does the cutting of the wound. The fore legs may also be bandaged or put into protective boots if it is thought that the horse's action or the state of the ground might be conducive to over-reach injuries occurring. Untrained and tired horses are particularly susceptible.

Grease Grease is an inflammatory infection of the skin at the back of the pastern first noticed as a waxy discharge with a very offensive smell. The hairs stand up gummed together in tufts. The skin thickens in ridges and, later, warty growths appear in groups which has led to the condition being known sometimes as 'grapes'. Grease is seen on the hind limbs more usually than on the forelegs, and occurs more commonly in heavy horses than in light horses or ponies.

Grease in the early stages affects the horse very little. As the skin thickens and growths appear the disease causes irritation and sometimes lameness. The affected part should be soaked in a solution of 100 g (4 oz) of washing soda in a gallon of warm water to clean the area and then dressed with a paste of medicinal liquid paraffin and sulphanilamide powder. Such treatment is only palliative.

Grease is stubborn and very difficult to cure. Caustic dressings or surgery may be needed to remove growths interfering with proper activity. When antiseptic dressings or a natural self limitation finally settle the disease, considerable permanent and ugly scarring often remains. Prevention consists of ensuring that any injuries in the heels are treated properly.

Heel-bug Heel-bug is a name given to a number of conditions that may affect horses' heels and has no specific meaning. It may refer to horse-pox, cracked heels, mud fever or grease. It is a very useful diagnosis for the indefatigable know-all.

Horse-pox Horse-pox commonly occurs in tropical countries and occasionally spreads to temperate lands. It occurred widely in England in 1938 and 1939.

This disease is an infection due to a pox virus. It usually breaks out in the skin of the heels and may confine itself to that area or may spread on to the limbs and appear around the mouth, by the girth and on the genital organs. Like cow-pox, small-pox and chicken-pox it produces spots which go through a series of stages from watery blisters to little abscesses and, finally, to dry scabs. It is impossible to observe these stages in horses' hairy heels. All that can be seen is a wet discharge in the folds of skin at the back of the pastern with matted hair and, in horses on nutritious feeding, a swelling that extends up the legs to the knees or hocks. The heels dry up in 4 or 5 days and the swellings subside. There is no unpleasant smell as there is with grease.

Horse-pox is highly infectious. Animals that contract the disease may run a temperature of 38° or 39°C (102° or 103°F) and go off their food for a day or two before the heel eruption occurs Others may show no sign of illness before the spots occur. The disease is self-limiting and lasts for about three weeks from the first rise in temperature to the stage when the dry scabs are flaking off the healed skin.

Treatment consists of resting the affected animals, reducing the rations and avoiding grooming over the affected parts. It is almost impossible to prevent horse-pox spreading and attempts to do so are only likely to extend the time it remains in a stable. Any discharges are infectious and it may be reasonable in some circumstances to spread the disease right through a stable by using a swab of cotton wool soaked in saliva from an infected horse to wipe around all the horses' mouths. Horse-pox does not affect human beings or any animals except horses, mules and donkeys.

4 The heart and circulation

Blood circulates from the heart to every part of the body, absorbing oxygen from the lungs and digested foodstuffs from the intestines and delivering them where they are required. The heart keeps the blood circulating by driving it forcibly into large arteries. The arteries branch repeatedly into smaller ones with thinner walls until they become fine capillaries, so thin that the blood is able to exchange substances with the body cells. The blood in the capillaries then flows on into small veins which join other larger ones and these finally deliver the blood back to the heart.

The heart consists of two simple pumps that lie side by side. The right side of the heart pumps blood to the lungs and this returns to the left side of the heart which then pumps it round the rest of the body. The blood returns from the body to the right side of the heart and the process is repeated.

Each side of the heart resembles the rubber bulb of an old-fashioned motor horn that can be squeezed to empty it and springs back to fill itself. The muscles of both sides of the heart contract together to drive the blood into the arteries and relax together to allow the cavities to refill from the veins. In horses at rest the heart muscles contract and relax, which together constitute one heart beat, about thirty-eight times a minute. The speed of the beats is controlled from the brain and by the heart's own pacemaker and it is varied to meet the horse's needs. The flow of blood is directed by valves: two inlet valves and two outlet valves on each side of the heart.

The heart lies in the chest between and slightly above the elbows. By listening just behind either elbow with a stethoscope the heart of a horse at rest can be heard beating regularly at 35 to 40 times a

Diagram of the heart and circulation

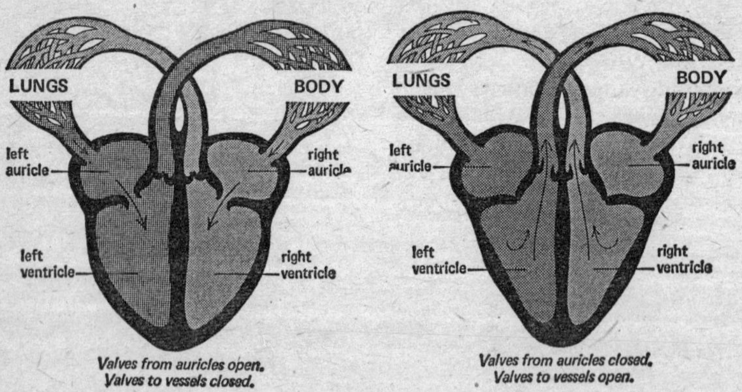

minute. Each beat has a double sound, usually described as 'lub-dup'. The 'lub' is caused by the closing of the two inlet valves and the 'dup' by the closing of the outlet valves.

The healthy heart has great reserves of power, illustrated by racing on the flat when the heart may be beating at over 200 times a minute to keep the horse travelling at 57 kmph (36 mph). Steeplechasing and point-to-point racing may appear to be more strenous than flat racing but the pace is slower and the pressure on the heart considerably less. Horses doing ordinary work seldom need to call upon their heart's reserve powers but it is comforting to know that there is a wide safety margin if a horse is suddenly required to make unusual and strenuous efforts.

Heart disease Heart diseases may occur in the muscles, the valves or the timing controls. Obstruction in the blood vessels can also cause serious trouble.

A horse owner's reaction to a suggestion that his animal's heart is not quite normal is to ask if it is safe to ride or might it possibly fall down dead.

Very few horses do fall down dead. It does happen from time to time, but so rarely that the event is widely publicized. The cause is usually a broken blood vessel or a stroke and the horse pulls up before its tragic end. Injuries to riders from horses falling down dead are the rarest form of accident.

The other question – is the horse safe to ride – requires rather more discussion. Some heart troubles are serious and continuing to ride the horse would be inadvisable for both the horse and the rider. Many of these cases may be incurable but some heart complaints, even serious ones, can be cured and, after treatment and convalescence, the horse may be safe to ride again and return to normal work.

A great many horses have slightly unusual heart sounds that have no effect whatever on the animal's health and performance. A vet examining such a horse is in duty bound to mention these peculiarities to his client who will want to know their significance. If they are not recognizable as major defects and do not become worse with exercise they may be ignored, bearing in mind the huge reserves of power that are inherent in normal horses' hearts. Absolute certainty as to the significance of these heart sounds can only be reached by repeated examinations. If the conditions noted are similar in six months' time they are certainly causing no harm. If after such an interval they have become worse the position would have to be re-assessed.

Signs of a failing heart Horses with a poor heart performance show a lack of interest in their work, with a falling off in confidence and ability that may eventually cause the animals to stumble, reel or collapse. Ordinary exercise causes them to become short of breath; uphill work distresses them and, when pulled up to rest, they continue to breathe fast with obvious pumping action from the chest wall for much longer than usual. Horses with a bad circulation show a reduction in appetite and fall away in condition. They develop swellings under the jaw, between the forelegs and around the sheath or udder, and the fetlocks enlarge with the swellings extending up the back of the legs to the knees or hocks. Filled legs are one of the earliest signs of circulatory disturbance which may be traceable to heart trouble, but is, more frequently, a simple indication of insufficient exercise in relation to the food being consumed.

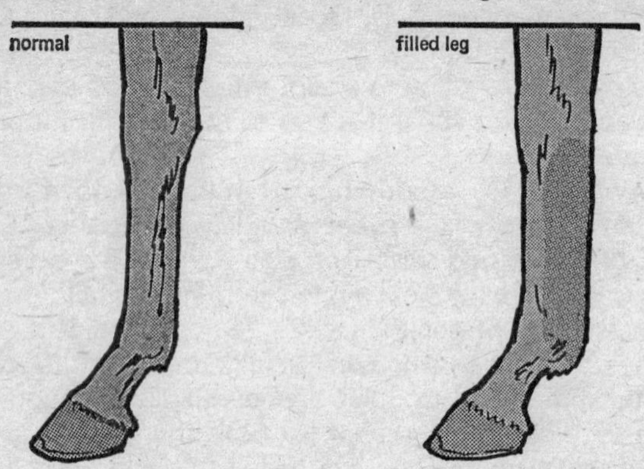

Heart muscles The heart is composed of about 4 kg (9 lb) of muscle which is capable of circulating the blood supply for 30 years or more without rest or interruption. The left side of the heart which delivers blood to all parts of the head, body and limbs has much thicker muscles than the right side which only has to supply the lungs.

Extra work produces stronger muscles. With regular work the 4 kg (9 lb) heart can be increased to 6 kg (13 lb) or more but there are limits to this development and if the horse is overworked the heart walls eventually stretch and become thin and weak.

If diseases such as leaking heart valves or an obstruction in the circulation throw more work on the heart muscles, they become stronger for a while. If the extra demand continues for a long time they stretch and weaken. If it still continues, the muscle tissues degenerate and the signs of a failing heart appear.

Infectious diseases put pressure on the heart because an increased circulation is necessary to support the body's defences against the invading bacteria or viruses. These diseases produce toxins which poison all the organs including the heart. The muscles of the overworked and poisoned heart are liable to weaken and degenerate rapidly so that death from an infectious disease is often preceded by signs of a failing heart.

Defective valves There is an inlet and an outlet valve on each side of the heart. Any of these four valves may become defective either because it leaks, which means that the heart must work harder to compensate for the leakage, or because it becomes narrowed and again the muscles have to work harder to pump the necessary amount of blood through smaller openings. Leaks may be the result of valves torn by accident or sudden exertion or damaged by infectious diseases or by worm larvae, or they may also be due to weakening and slackening of the muscle walls which prevent the valves from closing the gap. Narrowed valve openings result from scarring after disease or injury or from thrombus formation. As defective valves cannot recover or be repaired their effects are permanent. Serious defects throw heavy strain on the heart muscles and they will respond in their usual way by enlarging to meet the demand of extra work but, if the effort is too great, sooner or later they will weaken and finally degenerate to progressive heart failure. Minor defects may only require such slight adjustments from the heart muscles that the horse can continue in full work for a normal lifetime.

Heart murmurs When the heart valves are working normally it is almost impossible to detect, with the stethoscope, the faint rushing noise made by the blood as it is pumped through them. When the valves are defective the blood can be heard spurting back through an incompletely closed valve or gushing through a narrowed opening. These sounds which vary in length, pitch and volume are all classed as murmurs. Murmurs have been studied extensively and it is possible, by applying the stethoscope to various parts of the chest wall over the heart and by relating the timing of the murmurs to the 'lub-dup' of the heart beats, to determine which valve is defective and, quite often, to form an opinion as to the significance of a particular murmur. The interpretation of murmurs is complicated by the fact that in young horses some murmurs only indicate a developing heart, and other murmurs may be heard in horses that are frightened or excited signifying nothing more than that the heart is sharing in the nervous reaction.

Nevertheless, the general conclusion is that persistent murmurs are due to a fault in the blood flow. As long as the heart is absorbing the extra load thrust upon it the horse remains healthy and can do its normal work and this can often continue indefinitely. If the heart begins to fail because of valve trouble there is little that can be done to prevent further deterioration.

Murmurs can be recorded on an electro-phonographic apparatus which relates them to the heart sounds and presents their length and intensity as a tracing on a moving sheet of paper.

Jugular pulse A jugular vein runs down each side of the neck just under the skin in the jugular groove. When the intake valve on the right side of the heart is leaking a small ripple or pulse runs up each jugular vein with every heart beat. This is interesting as the only indication of a defective valve that can be observed apart from the heart sounds and it is a simple aid to accurate diagnosis.

Thrombosis Thrombosis is the obstruction of a blood vessel by a blood clot. Damage to the lining membrane of a blood vessel or to the heart membranes may be caused by disease processes, by an injury such as a fall or kick, or it may follow a surgical operation. The commonest of these injuries in horses is caused by one of the red-worms, *Strongylus vulgaris*, whose larvae spend part of their development in the walls of blood vessels. The damage to the vessel lining, whatever the cause, has to be repaired, and blood and fibre cells clot together forming a cover under which healing can take place. This protecting clot is a thrombus and its effect, partially or completely obstructing the flow of blood, is thrombosis.

Thrombosis of the coronary artery which supplies blood to the heart muscles may interfere seriously with the heart's action. When it affects the heart valves it may prevent their proper closure, while thrombosis in vessels in the abdomen and pelvis can cause colic and paralysis.

A condition known as iliac thrombosis causes complete paralysis of a horse's hind quarters so that the animal collapses and cannot get up. In many of these cases the blockage clears, or the blood finds another route to the affected muscles, and within a few hours the horse gets up and appears to be perfectly normal though similar attacks may follow.

If thrombosis is suspected the vet may suggest the intravenous injection of preparations of salts to reduce the size of the obstructions. A sensible precaution is to keep the worm burden of all horses to a minimum though not all cases of thrombosis are traceable to damage by worms. Horses known to have blood vessels injured by accident or by surgery should be given long convalescent care to avoid the results of thrombosis and the risks of embolism.

Embolism Embolism is the result of a completely blocked blood vessel. The formation of a thrombus on the wall of the heart or a blood vessel consists of a scab-like covering over a damaged area. As happens to other scabs, pieces of the thrombus break off and each piece, now an embolus, flows with the blood along the branching and narrowing blood vessels until it reaches one so narrow that it blocks it completely. This is embolism. The part of the body supplied by the vessel is completely deprived of its blood supply. In some cases blood manages to reach the part through other vessels and normal activity is restored. In others there is no alternative route for the blood and the bloodless part withers up and is replaced by scar tissue. If only a small area is affected, adjoining cells multiply to fill the gap and take over the duties. Large emboli may cause paralysis if they affect muscles or nerves. Embolism in the brain can cause a stroke resulting in sudden death or paralysis of some part of the body.

Embolism in small vessels in the heart muscles is serious. The small scars that result interfere with the timing controls of the heart beat which may become erratic and result in heart block.

Treatment and prevention of embolism are similar to those suggested for thrombosis of which embolism is a sequel.

Heart infections *Endocarditis* The membranes lining the heart and covering the valves may be attacked by bacteria or viruses spreading in the blood from infections in other parts of the body. The organisms causing endocarditis may settle on the heart membranes because these have already been damaged by worm larvae causing ulceration or thrombosis.

The signs of endocarditis are often vague. The horse loses interest in its work and falls away in condition. The heart sounds are often normal but the organ beats unusually fast after slight exertion. A history of recent disease due to an infection may help the diagnosis or a laboratory blood examination may find indications of bacterial or virus activity. Treatment consists of rest and a course of antibiotic injections. If some improvement follows there is hope that further antibiotic treatment may effect a cure. Animals that do recover from a debilitating disease of this nature need a convalescent period of at least six months before a gradual return to work.

Pericarditis Pericarditis is an inflammation of the fibrous capsule surrounding the heart, usually due to an infection spreading from some lung condition. The pericardial sac is distended by an excess of fluid produced by the inflammation making it difficult for the heart to beat under the extra compression. The horse's temperature is raised, the animal becomes distressed if put to any effort and the heart beats are muffled by rustling noises which are friction sounds from the movement of the inflamed membranes.

Treatment consists of antibiotic medication and rest until the signs of the disease have disappeared. Pericarditis does not usually occur as a separate condition. In most cases treatment will also be required for any accompanying disease.

Heart beat timing The heart beat rate is controlled by the brain and nerves which vary the speed according to demands from all parts of the body. The main heart nerve tends to run the heart fast while a secondary one keeps the speed down. This balanced arrangement seldom goes wrong, although, because the main nerve leading to the heart is bundled together part of the way with a nerve leading to the stomach, it may accidentally share a reaction to indigestion and produce a purposeless rapid heart beat. The heart also has a built-in pace-maker completely independent of the nervous system. This can take over in an emergency and keep the heart beating until control of the nerves is restored. The pace-maker occasionally jumps in unexpectedly giving extra heart beats.

Rapid heart beats The resting heart rate of 35 to 40 beats each minute is increased by nervousness and excitement as well as by physical demands. Records have shown that a race horse may have a heart rate of 40 in the stable, 130 in the starting-stalls, up to 210 during the race, back to 130 when unsaddling and down again to 40 beats a minute within half an hour after the race. The heart is not harmed by beating at these high speeds provided it is only for a short time.

Palpitations is the name given to short spells of rapid heart beats at 60 or 70 beats a minute. They occur in periods of excitement or even indigestion, this last being due to a fault in nerve transmission, as mentioned earlier. Some horses, after severe exertion, have palpitations for spells of up to 40 minutes during the next few hours. There do not appear to be any lasting effects.

The rate of the heart beat is raised in feverish illnesses such as pneumonia, laminitis and azoturia and in most acute infectious diseases. In painful conditions such as colic the heart rate may rise to about 60 per minute and in cases complicated by toxaemia up to

80. Beyond this figure a colicked horse's life is in danger.

After a bout of illness, when the heart has been required to beat persistently fast for days on end, a long convalescence is required for the heart muscles to regain their tone, strength and reserves. It should not be assumed that, because the temperature and heart rate are normal, the horse can go back to ordinary work. A simple reckoning is to allow four days' convalescence for each day's illness.

Triple heart beats When listening with a stethoscope to the heart just after a horse has completed a fast gallop, and the heart rate is likely to be over 100 a minute, the beat may be heard in a triple form as a 'dup-er-lub' instead of the usual 'lub-dup'. This is normal and, as the heart slows down to below 100, it can be heard, quite suddenly, to switch from the triple to the double beat. The extra sound is caused by the heart cavities reaching the limit of their expansion as they fill. This sound is not heard during the slower beat because it is made up of two quite separate faint sounds. These are superimposed on each other at the faster rate and then become clearly audible.

Slow heart beats A slow heart beat, sometimes down to 25 or even 20 to the minute, occurs in horses that are in a poor state of health from continuing disease or starvation and the condition is likely to be accompanied by the signs of a failing heart. Many of these cases are beyond treatment. They are not helped by attempts with medicines to make the heart beat faster. If the basic cause of the horse's illness can be dealt with, the heart rate will improve.

Dropped heart beats The heart of a resting horse, beating at 35 to 40 to the minute, may miss a beat now and again. The heart is simply idling and the occasional missed beats are not a sign of any disease. There is sometimes a faint first sound, the 'lub' without any following 'dup'. If the horse is spoken to sharply or turned round in the stable the heart beats steadily again until the effect of the stimulus passes.

Extra heart beats An extra heart beat is occasionally thrust into the steady series of beats, having the effect of a stutter in the usual rhythm. The explanation is that the heart's emergency pace-maker has been wrongly alerted by some minor upset and produces the unnecessary stimulus. The tonic effect of a change of work, food or surroundings for the horse may eliminate the extra beats. If they persist or increase the horse and its heart should be carefully examined in case they are an early sign of a condition of heart block.

Heart block In heart block there are large and irregular gaps between the beats. The condition is due to the ordinary impulses to beat failing to reach the heart because the nerves are injured or diseased, or, if they do reach the heart, failing to be properly distributed in the muscles because of scarring from embolism or other heart disease. The heart's own pace-maker complicates the picture by filling in the gaps with erratic extra beats. Horses with a heart block condition lose interest and ability, and are unsafe to ride. They may keep in good condition and appear normal except when put to work when they rapidly become exhausted. The chances of improvement in these cases are not good unless the cause can be traced to a curable condition.

Tracings from an examination of the heart with an electrocardiograph are helpful in assessing the severity of heart block cases.

Heart fibrillation In fibrillation the muscles of the heart that help to fill the main cavities with blood lose their power to contract and fall into a state of constant trembling. In consequence the main cavities only receive enough blood to pump onwards at irregular intervals. Heart beats can be heard, with the stethoscope, occurring singly or in groups quite erratically. The electro-cardiograph shows tracings of the trembling muscles and the confused heart beats.

Fibrillation occurs quite suddenly. An affected horse shows no signs of illness and appears quite normal while idle in the stable or out in a field but is reluctant to work and becomes exhausted very quickly. The cause is discovered as soon as a heart examination is made. The disease only seems to occur in big horses, especially those engaged in galloping and jumping though it is occasionally met with in the slow moving heavy breeds.

In a few cases the heart reverts to normal spontaneously. The cause of this disease is not known. Treatment in a veterinary hospital with carefully controlled doses of digitalis and quinidine can be effective in causing the heart to revert from fibrillation to the usual healthy rhythm. Recovered horses are capable of normal work, even to galloping and jumping again but the state of fibrillation usually recurs before long. It is only exceptionally that treatment is worthwhile.

Electro-cardiographs and phono-cardiographs Electrocardiographs (ECGs) are produced by apparatus that passes a small electric current through the horse's chest and traces, with an oscillating pen on a moving strip of paper, alterations in the current caused by the heart's activities. The waves on the ECG tracing can be allocated to each section of the heart beat and these are spaced on the chart against marked time-intervals. This gives a record of the rate of beats, the regular or irregular spacing between the beats, the period of time occupied by each part of each beat and the occurrence of dropped beats, extra beats, heart block and fibrillation.

Phono-cardiographs (PCGs) similarly trace, on a time-marked paper strip, all the heart sounds picked up from the chest wall by a microphone. They record the pitch, intensity, persistence and regularity of the 'lub-dup' beat as well as various subsidiary sounds and the whole range of murmurs relating them in time to the normal heart sounds.

While ECGs and PCGs are each extremely useful in helping to discover what is happening to a faulty heart, together they act as an especially powerful aid to diagnosis.

Telemetry in heart examinations In the past the stethoscope, electro-cardiographs and phono-cardiographs could only be used to take records from stationary horses. Examinations of hearts beating at speed had to be confined to a short period after a strenuous gallop or to horses whose hearts were beating fast because of some disease. With telemetry, essential pieces of cardiographic and phonographic apparatus can be strapped on to horses and the heart's electrical and sound impulses conveyed by radio to stationary receivers housed within convenient range. The horse can then be ridden, lunged or allowed to exercise freely while the ECG and PCG waves are observed on a screen or recorded on the paper strips.

Heart pace-makers Electrical pace-makers are frequently implanted in human hearts when the natural controls are proving inadequate. This technique does not appear to have been practised on horses yet but scientists studying horses' hearts have found that they can reach the heart quite simply with pace-making equipment through the jugular vein. With this apparatus they can cause the heart to produce extra beats or to beat at increased speeds at will. This has no application at present to the treatment of heart troubles but for research workers it is an advance on telemetry and enables them to make investigations previously impossible. These have already thrown light on some of the diseases that affect horses' hearts.

The stethoscope Electrical aids to heart examinations may make the stethoscope appear inadequate as the only aid used in the examination of a horse's heart. However, professional and legal authorities are agreed that, in the hands of a properly experienced veterinary surgeon the stethoscope is the most suitable instrument to help in forming an opinion that a horse's heart is free from signs of disease or has signs of disease. If the heart is free from disease further investigations are not likely to be of value. If the heart does show signs of disease and the cause is not readily ascertained then the owner may well require further investigations by more sophisticated techniques and these are readily available at veterinary schools and equine hospitals.

Bleeding When accidental bleeding occurs, the walls of the torn and injured blood vessels close up and shrink back into the surrounding tissues reducing the flow of blood which eventually clots in the narrowed vessels so that the bleeding stops. The veins are thin and their walls close over easily as the blood in them is not under pressure. The arteries have stout fibro-elastic walls and the blood is being directly pumped through them by the activity of the heart muscles. Their elasticity helps them to close but occasionally even this does not overcome the force of the blood flow and cut arteries may continue to pump out blood for an alarming length of time. It is sometimes possible to grip the end of such a pumping artery with forceps so that a ligature can be tied around it. In most cases even very severe bleeding stops spontaneously, though the horse may before then have collapsed to the ground from the severe blood loss. This reduces the blood pressure and may enable the blood to clot and prevent further bleeding.

It is a help, in cases of severe bleeding, to apply pressure to the bleeding surface by covering it with clean dressings and bandaging them in place. Bleeding in large deep wounds may be helped by plugging the wound up with clean dressings or cloths.

Tranquilizing drugs may be a help in keeping the horse quiet and so reducing its blood pressure. There are no medications that can reasonably be used to help the blood clotting mechanism which every horse is able to call upon if it is required.

Haemophilia, blood-clotting failure, is so rare a disease in horses as to be virtually non-existent.

Internal bleeding One of the causes of sudden and unexpected death in horses is internal bleeding. Some fairly large blood vessel in the chest or abdomen has ruptured. The signs are that the horse falters in its work, pulls up and after some few minutes collapses to the ground and after a few more minutes gives a little struggle and dies. The mouth and eye membranes can be seen to be paper-white.

A post-mortem examination usually reveals a burst artery that may at some time have been severely damaged by worm larvae in the blood vessel, or it may be found that some comparatively minor disease process, such as an abscess in an abdominal organ, has penetrated through into an adjoining blood vessel.

The stresses of giving birth to a foal sometimes cause the rupture of an artery in the womb and it is extremely distressing to all concerned when a mare, shortly after foaling satisfactorily, collapses on to the floor and dies within a few minutes.

There is no treatment for these cases which cannot be anticipated, though a satisfactory routine of worm control would prevent some of the fatalities.

Haematomas Bleeding sometimes occurs under the skin or into a muscle following a bruise or a fall that has injured a blood vessel. Usually the blood clotting mechanism works and the bleeding is arrested leaving a swelling under the skin or causing a muscle to bulge. Such swellings may resemble an abscess. The contents of the swellings can be checked by drawing off some of the blood from a haematoma or pus from an abscess with a hypodermic syringe and needle.

Haematomas may be minute or reach a size larger than a football. They are harmless and the blood is gradually absorbed back into the horse's system. The large ones may be a nuisance preventing the horse from doing useful work. They can be opened, after a few days, and the blood clot and serum removed through a rather large opening at the lower part of the swelling. The few days' delay is necessary to ensure that the injured blood vessel has had time to heal up. The large opening is needed to remove all the clots, and drainage from the cavity should be established. The skin has usually been stretched by the swelling and a neater healing is obtained if an elliptic section of skin is removed through which to empty the haematoma.

Anaemia Anaemia is a condition in which the blood runs thin having an abnormally low content of blood corpuscles. The horse's eye and mouth membranes are seen to be pale and the heart beats are faster than normal, the sounds being sharp and clear. Anaemia from blood loss is soon overcome by further supplies of blood corpuscles mostly from the bone marrow, but animals suffering from persistent anaemia are hampered in their growth and ability. Such cases may be due to infection of the blood by trypanosomes or piroplasms which feed on the red corpuscles or by worms and bots that live in the intestines by sucking blood or robbing the horse of its food supply. Anaemia may also be caused by infections whose toxins hamper the production of new corpuscles, or it may be the result of Warfarin poisoning. When severe haemorrhage occurs the blood volume in the vessels is maintained by absorbing fluid from other parts of the body. This restores the circulating activity of the blood but the number of blood corpuscles is seriously reduced. Normally horses have about 10 million red corpuscles in each cubic millimetre of blood. This may fall to 5 million without serious consequences but the animal's life becomes at risk when the corpuscle count falls between 2 and 3 million.

Purpura haemorrhagica In purpura haemorrhagica large, painless swellings develop on the horse's head, body and limbs usually when the animal has been suffering for a considerable time from a serious bacterial or virus disease and it was hoped that the horse would be entering a convalescent stage. Blood spots are seen on the membranes of the eyes and lips. The cause of purpura is some poisonous effect from the toxins of the primary disease. Blood transfusions may be helpful but treatment is usually confined to careful nursing. Some cases make a spontaneous recovery within a few days or after a longer period of illness but many end fatally.

Dehydration In dehydration the horse's body tissues are being deprived of sufficient fluid to function properly. The shortage of fluid may be because the horse is not drinking enough or because fluid loss is excessive from sweating or diarrhoea. If dehydration is part of a disease process, proper treatment of the disease must include fluid replacement.

A healthy animal may become dehydrated by exertion or sweating, both of which may occur during long journeys or strenuous exercise, especially in hot weather. A dehydrated horse appears dull and lethargic, with sunken eyes and sometimes trembling muscles: even when the horse is cooled off and rested for a quarter of an hour, rapid heart beats and respirations persist instead of settling in that time to the normal 35 to 45 heart beats and 10 to 14 respirations per minute. Dehydration is accompanied by a loss of skin elasticity: if a fold is picked between finger and thumb it takes quite a time to flatten out again, instead of springing back immediately.

Treatment of dehydration Dehydrated horses should be cold-hosed for a few minutes or sluiced down with a bucket or two of cold water, scraping off the water and covering them with a rug over a layer of straw while they are drying off. They should be given 4–5 litres (1 gallon) of water to drink at intervals of 15 minutes until they are satisfied. It is an advantage if 25 g (1 oz) of common salt and 100 g ($\frac{1}{4}$ lb) of glucose can be added to the water each time: these help to replace substances lost by sweating and exertion. If a horse refuses this mixture it should be allowed plain water which is the main requirement. Horses that are so exhausted that they cannot be persuaded to drink at all should be given the salt and glucose solution by stomach tube, 4–5 litres (1 gallon) at a time at intervals of a quarter of an hour. In really collapsed cases glucose saline, a 5 per cent solution of sodium bicarbonate or a proprietary electrolyte mixture may have to be given by intravenous injection. When a few litres have been given in this way the horse may recover a normal thirst and drink naturally.

Dehydrated horses require a long rest and a carefully controlled reconditioning period the length of which depends on their signs of returning fitness.

Prevention of dehydration in healthy horses Horses put to strenuous tests must be properly fit for such exercise and, if the work is prolonged for more than three hours, regular rest periods should be arranged. At least half an hour is required to benefit the animal; this allows the heart and breathing rates to return to normal and to remain there for some time, after which the horse may drink freely. Journeys by horse box must be broken for half an hour's rest every three hours so that the horse can be walked out for a while, watered and rested.

Thumps or diaphragmatic flutter Horses under stress from long journeys in hot weather or from exhausting work may develop a condition known as thumps, their breathing being accompanied by a repeated thumping sound (like a very loud heart beat) which is caused by spasmodic contractions of the diaphragm. Horses showing this condition are near collapse. Work must be stopped immediately and the horse comfortably stabled and given plenty of time to recover. Treatment consists of an intravenous injection of a calcium borogluconate solution, 200 ml (7 fl oz) to half a litre (1 pint) according to the size of the pony or horse.

Horses that develop thumps are usually dehydrated and they should also be treated for that condition.

5 The digestive tract

Food and feeding

A horse's natural food is grass. This statement has unexpected support from some dictionaries which throw the responsibility back on the horse by defining grass as the herbage eaten by horses.

The herbage that horses eat is by no means a simple substance. It consists of the true grasses which supply long thin leaves for plain nourishment and stalks for the less digestible roughage necessary to keep the intestines active. This herbage is eaten green at pasture or dried and taken as hay in the stable. The energy needed for working horses is derived from the seeds of oats or other horse-corn plants which also belong to the grass family. Horses prefer herbage, whether green or as hay, that is a mixture of true grass and a variety of other plants. These plants, which are wild flowers to the botanists but weeds to the farmers, add spice and flavour to the diet and many of them provide vitamins at those times of the year when the grasses are vitamin deficient. Grazing horses also pick up an amount of earth or soil with their food and this is a source of necessary minerals. Horses in stables miss these condiments and, if they have been off pasture for a long time, instead of eating grass when they are turned out, will often go directly to the edge of the field and eat soil from the hedge banks. Horses also enjoy browsing, that is eating twigs, shoots and bark from hedges and trees for the variety of flavours and especially for the bitter taste of the bark, to such an extent that young trees in horse pastures are soon killed by being deprived of their bark unless they are fenced off.

Horses are widely influenced in their growth by the grassland they are raised on. Young horses need to develop slowly, and rich fertilized pastures suitable for dairy cattle or fattening sheep are bad for horses, in that they encourage rapid growth and spongy bone formation. Such rich grazing may lead to the development of chronic laminitis especially in ponies. Old chalk land seems best because the soil contains suitable amounts of calcium, and the natural herbage, which is unlikely to be too nourishing, consists of a wide variety of grasses and other plants. Leys, which are cultivated fields of new grass from seeds, do not produce attractive grazing for horses, and hay from such fields, consisting of nothing but true grass, is uninteresting and lacking in flavour. Agricultural seedsmen can supply mixtures for horse pastures which contain seeds of a variety of suitable grasses and selected herbs. They have a wide choice as there are over 150 species of wild grasses in the British Isles alone.

Grassland for horses should be permanent pasture, that is land which is not ploughed up frequently and sown with other crops.

However, horses should not be kept continuously on these fields as they are untidy feeders and spoil certain areas by depositing droppings and urine. To keep permanent pastures useful for horses the field should be grazed for a short while and then mown, to knock down any weeds or rough grass that the horses have left and this should be followed by close grazing by cattle or sheep.

After a period of rest and recovery the field can again be grazed by horses and the process repeated. With a number of paddocks the horses can have a succession of fresh short grass crops through a long grazing season. Horses thrive better on short grass than they do in long, overgrown pasture. The smaller the area of land available the more attention is needed to keep the pasture in suitable condition for the horses' growth and development. This system of rotation; grazing, cutting, close feeding off by other stock and resting before putting horses back in the paddock also has the advantage of preventing the land from carrying a heavy infestation of worms likely to infect the horses. Many of the worms are eaten up by the cattle and sheep, in which they cannot survive, and many more are dried up and die in the sunshine because the grass is short. This does not reduce the advisability of treating all horses on the premises for worms at least four times a year.

Grass or hay and oats supply the horse's food requirements of proteins, carbohydrates and fats. Minerals and vitamins are essential to health and growth and, at grass, these are readily available from sunshine, herbage and soil. For stabled horses, fed only on hay and oats, minerals and vitamins need to be added as food supplements. There is great difficulty in deciding the amounts required as it is impossible to assess which items are in short supply in the food available. Even though the firms which supply these food additives often err on the side of generosity, the amounts suggested on their packages are not likely to be dangerous. Nevertheless feeding a supplement for 365 days in the year may build up accumulations of some items that could be harmful. Supplementary feeding is not important in the summer months when most horses have access to some pasture grazing and the feeding of vitamin and mineral supplements can well be stopped at that time of the year, not only as a sensible economy but to the advantage of the horses as it gives them an opportunity to balance their requirements by natural grazing. Most brands of horse nuts or pellets have vitamins and minerals added in reasonable quantities and horses fed on this type of food are not likely to require any supplementary feeding. They will, nevertheless, enjoy a run at grass just like other horses. Horses usually do well on limestone land which provides the calcium necessary for good bone development. In countries where there is little or no lime in the soil soft bones may be produced which, rarely and only in extreme cases, show as bulging facial bones in grown animals or, more frequently, as rickets in foals and yearlings. A calcium supplement should prevent this tendency. Calcium requires phosphorus but not too much of it. Both are present in bone flour but this contains too high a proportion of phosphorus. To obtain the right balance an ounce of ground limestone or chalk and an ounce of sterilized bone flour should be mixed in the feed daily. The bone flour must be sterilized as otherwise it is a possible source of anthrax and other diseases. The amount of these supplements actually fed must be adjusted according to the soil conditions in the area.

Hay Hay comes in great variety. Some hay is made from the grass on grazing land, but a lot of hay is grown as an agricultural crop on land that is never grazed. This hay, grown as a crop, is often a mixture of rye-grass and clover or lucerne, producing a very nourishing feed for working horses. Variations in hay are also brought about in the process of haymaking.

Every experienced horseman and stock-farmer must be an authority on hay because there are no reliable guides to help in assessing its quality. It is interesting that when farmers and agricultural scientists are asked to evaluate hay, their appraisals are only remarkable for their extreme variety of opinions and it has frequently been shown that if the choice is left to the horses they usually go greedily for the samples that nobody has had a good word for. The experts explain this by saying that the hay the horses select may be the tastiest but it hasn't the nutritive value of their selections. The argument can be continued by asking what nutritional benefit will the horses get from hay they won't eat.

Most hay is reasonably nutritious. The important thing is to recognize bad hay and refuse to accept it. If a bale of hay is opened and its contents are pale and dry and crumble to pieces when handled it is too dry to be palatable or nutritious. This hay has probably been cut too late in the season when it was over-ripe or else it was left lying in the field and rained upon for weeks before being gathered up.

If the opened bale throws out clouds of fine dust when struck or shaken it is mouldy, not having had long enough to dry off before being baled. The dust from such hay irritates the lungs and may lead to broken wind. The mould also irritates the kidneys and causes the horse to pass excessive quantities of watery urine.

Dark brown hay that smells like plug tobacco has not been wilted enough and has heated after baling. Most horses go crazy for it. Its feed value is lower than good hay and it may cause kidney irritation. It is so attractive to horses that a little of it mixed with poor quality hay encourages them to eat up the lot – if there is poor quality hay that must be eaten.

If the opened bale smells of new-mown hay and shows slightly green leaves and long stalks with flower heads still attached, it is good hay. If the hay is a clover or lucerne mixture some of the stalks will be black and rather wooden. This is good hard hay, suitable for strong, hard-working horses but not suitable for pony feeding or for ageing brood mares whose teeth and gums may not be quite up to the crisp bite. By contrast with the hard hay, meadow hay is soft and feels as though it could easily be compressed to make a material like felt. The permanent pasture grasses that continue to crop year after year have soft stalks and the weed mixture adds to the soft quality. Soft hay is considered to be more suitable for cattle than for hard-working horses but it is nutritious and easily digested and horses enjoy it. It should be of a good colour, sweet smelling and free of dust.

Any sudden change from one batch of hay to another may put horses off their feed. If possible the new load of hay should be delivered before the previous load is finished so that the change can be made gradually by mixing the different hays for a few days.

Horses naturally feed from floor level and prefer their hay on the floor. This wastes an awful lot of hay that is trodden into the bedding or soiled by droppings or urine. The old fashioned way was to keep hay in the loft over the stable and push it down into racks fitted on to the stable wall. This system is now discontinued because it created extremely dusty conditions leading to bronchitis and broken wind and open loft floors do not fit in with the modern ideas of proper stable ventilation. Hay is best fed in nets of tarred string. Filling the nets, in the hay barn, away from the stables, shakes out a lot of the dust and the net can be tied to a ring in the wall at a convenient level. The main objection to nets is that they provide yet another hazard for the accident prone horse which may roll and hook a shoe into the loose strings of an empty net and so become cast.

Oats Oats are necessary for energy. Grass and hay provide all that is needed for a horse to maintain itself comfortably but if the horse is to earn its keep by work, oats are the extra food of choice.

Choosing oats is almost as difficult as choosing hay. A handful of oats taken out of a sack should be light in colour and heavy in the hand and quite uncrushable, by which is meant that you should not be able to close your grip appreciably once you have grasped the fistful. Good oats have a pleasant dry smell and should not give off dust when poured from the hand back into the sack. Mouldy oats, easily recognized by dust and smell if stirred around are to be avoided as they will cause indigestion, bronchitis and kidney irritation leading to the passing of unusual quantities of pale urine. Each grain of the oats should be full and plump. This is a matter for a little comparison and experience because compared with grains of wheat or barley the oats are rather thin and covered with a lot of husk. Out of several samples of oats choose the stoutest. Rub off the husks and find the actual grains to see that they are round and stumpy.

A problem arises over choosing oats. To get full value from them as food, oats are often crushed before being fed to horses. In theory the horse should be able to grind the whole, uncrushed, grains to such small particles that the digestive organs absorb all the nourishment there is in them. In practice, horses that are hungry or whose teeth are not in perfect order, rush the masticating process and swallow whole or only partly broken grains. Crushing the oats before they are fed ensures that the grains are reasonably broken up. As crushing oats involves installing and using a crushing machine, horse owners not having a large stable of horses have the oats crushed by their fodder merchant. It is quite impossible to judge the quality of crushed oats so these should be selected before crushing even though this may involve more than one visit to the merchant. Oats are an important item of diet and ensuring their good quality is worth the extra trouble involved.

Horse nuts Compounded foods, horse nuts, are available in a number of preparations. They are made of hay, dried grass, oats or other grains, with added minerals and vitamins in a variety of mixes suitable for horses and ponies in their various types and occupations. They can be a complete diet and have a number of advantages over the grass, hay and oats – traditional feeds – in their ease of handling, convenient storage and consistency, though this may vary slightly even in a branded and named supply. A further advantage is that they can be used as a convenient adjunct to traditional feeding.

Horses which are allergic to stable dust and subject to broken wind may be safely fed on horse nuts, though their bedding should be peat or sawdust, not straw, since animals on horse nuts are inclined to eat their bedding or even stable doors as their idea of supplementary feeding for essential roughage. One Californian owner who adopted 'horse chow' as routine feeding for a large stable of horses, complained at the bill he had to pay for timber and planking to replace the fittings that his horses were eating at, apparently, no harm to themselves. Such habits can be harmful, leading to impaction of the intestine and colic. Some roughage seems to be necessary. Grazing provides the best answer but if horses must be stabled fresh cut grass should be fed to them. If hay must be fed through the winter the utmost care should be taken to ensure that it is as nearly dust free as possible.

Nourishing and invalid foods Horses that are being built up from a debilitated state due to illness, worm infestation, overwork or neglect, need a light, nourishing and attractive diet until they have recovered sufficiently to return to normal working rations.

Grass Fresh green grass is an ideal feed for sick horses, and if they can be allowed out or be led out to graze, even for only a few minutes at a time, there is a noticeable tonic effect from natural grazing in the open air. Great care should be taken if grass is cut and taken to the stable to be fed to horses. It heats and decomposes very quickly even in small quantities. Heated grass may cause indigestion and colic. Lawn mowings are particularly dangerous because, being short and compact, they heat up very quickly.

Chopped hay Chopped hay is long hay chopped up for convenience so that it can be mixed with mashes or gruels. It stops horses gulping down small tasty feeds and encourages them to chew their food properly.

Bran-mash Bran used to be a nutritious feed but modern milling produces a bran with no flour in it and it was the flour that was nutritious. Bran-mashes have a great reputation as a feed for tired horses. Their only real value is that when the bran has been well steamed and fed warm, it gives the horse a warming, slightly laxative food that goes down easily. Horses are not particularly fond of bran. Bran-mashes, like chopped hay, are used to add bulk to something more appetizing, such as barley gruel or boiled linseed.

To make a bran-mash, mix 25 g (1 oz) of salt with 2 kg (4 lb) of bran in a bucket. Pour on 2 litres (3½ pints) of boiling water and stir up thoroughly. Cover with a thick cloth pressed down firmly on to the mash and leave to self-cook for at least half an hour. Mix with other food and feed when cool enough and make it palatable by mixing in a double handful of oats. Wet bran soon goes sour, so bran-mashes should always be freshly prepared.

Gruel Barley gruel and oatmeal gruel are made by mixing 0.5 kg (1 lb) of either meal in 5 litres (1 gal) of cold water with 25 g (1 oz) of salt and stirring it on the stove until it boils. It should simmer for a quarter of an hour and then be thinned down with cold water to make a warm drink.

Linseed Linseed must not be fed raw. Even very small amounts can cause colic that can be fatal. Linseed must be boiled to a jelly before feeding. It makes an exceptionally palatable and nutritious addition to the rations. Linseed is troublesome as it sticks and burns in the pan unless stirred constantly for the three hours necessary to cook it. Many stables and stud farms use large double cookers which do away with the need to stir, to prepare linseed mashes for winter feeding.

Linseed mash Linseed mash is prepared by boiling 0.5 kg (1 lb) of linseed slowly in 5 litres (1 gal) of water for three hours. The resulting half gallon of jelly is mixed with 1 kg (2 lb) of bran and 25 g (1 oz) of salt, covered over with a cloth and allowed to stand until cool enough to stir together again and feed.

Linseed tea Boil 0.5 kg (1 lb) of linseed for 3 hours and make up to 7.5 litres (1½ gal) with cold water with 25 g (1 oz) of salt to make a warm and nourishing drink.

Linseed mash and chopped hay This makes a good winter feed for brood mares, young stock and hunters. Prepare boiled linseed and thick barley gruel, cover them with a layer of bran and salt and cover that with a layer of chopped hay. If a large quantity is required top up with further layers of boiled linseed, gruel, bran and chop and cover it over. The depth of foodstuff holds the heat for a long time during which the meal is softening up to make a warm feed when all the layers are mixed together.

Sugar beet pulp Sugar beet pulp is the residue after the sugar has been extracted from the beet. The pulp makes a good fattening food for horses but great care must be taken as it requires soaking in water for eight hours before being fed. It takes up water like a sponge, swelling in the process. If fed dry to horses it swells up in the gullet or stomach causing choking and colic and the result may be fatal. Accidents occur when someone has forgotten to put the beet pulp to soak or when, in an emergency, horses are being fed by someone unfamiliar with beet pulp. It is usually given, after soaking, mixed with chopped hay.

Milk Cow's milk is a good invalid food for horses of any age except for new born foals. Horses may be reluctant at first to drink milk neat but they may be encouraged by watering it down and adding a teaspoonful of salt to each 4½ litres (1 gal). Horses may benefit from 10 litres (2 gal) a day. Cow's milk may infect horses with tuberculosis but it is quite safe to use in countries such as Great Britain, where cattle tuberculosis has been virtually eliminated.

Eggs Hen's eggs are sometimes used to help a horse build up its strength. They may be given whipped up in milk or mixed with gruel or mash feeds. A start may be made with 2 or 3 eggs a day increasing to a dozen which makes a reasonable ration.

Digestion

As early as three weeks after conception the developing embryo, which is to become a horse, is a tube of cells less than 1.25 cm (½ in) long surrounding two smaller tubes, one to become the brain and spinal cord and the other the digestive system. When completely developed the digestive tube begins at the lips and mouth, continues down the neck and through the chest as the oesophagus or gullet and expands into the stomach. From the stomach's pyloric valve the tube continues as the small intestine and, after another junction, the ileo-caecal valve, it becomes the large intestine which blends into the rectum and ends at the anal orifice. From the stomach to the anus the digestive tube is familiarly known as the bowels. The total length is about 30 m (58 ft); the mouth 30 cm (12 in), the narrow oesophagus 1 m (3 ft), the stomach 60 cm (24 in) holding about 20 litres (4 gal) of foodstuff; the small intestine 20 metres (22 yards) long but only 5 cm (2 in) wide when not distended; the large intestine 8 metres (26 ft) long with a capacity of 100 litres (20 gal) and, finally, the rectum about 45 cm (18 in). The bowels of the average horse are dealing with 100 to 150 litres (20 to 30 gal) of a vegetable broth at any one time.

Food from a dietetic point of view consists mainly of proteins, to be built into living tissue; carbohydrates, for energy and heat; and fats, for immediate energy or for storage. The process of digestion consists of changing the food mechanically to very small particles and chemically to simpler substances so that nourishment can be absorbed as the food passes along the bowels. The chemicals come from glands in the wall of the digestive tube or from larger organs such as the salivary glands, the liver and the pancreas, all of which are developed from the original digestive tube. In the mouth the food is masticated into small particles by the molar teeth and thoroughly mixed with saliva from the salivary glands which are distributed around the mouth and throat. The salivary glands weigh 700 gm (25 oz) and produce about 2 litres (4 pints) of saliva during the quarter of an hour it takes a horse to eat 500 gm (18 oz) of hay. The saliva begins the process of digesting carbohydrates, altering the cellulose in grass, hay or oats to starch and then to sugar. The food is swallowed from the mouth to the stomach in small boluses. A bolus can be seen sliding down the oesophagus in the groove on the left side of the neck each time the horse swallows. The stomach wall produces hydrochloric acid to emulsify fats and pepsin to break down the proteins to the simpler amino-acids which are eventually built up again to form the particular proteins the horse's body requires. The food then passes through the pyloric valve to the small intestine where bile from the liver and digestive juices from the pancreas and the intestinal glands combine to act on all the types of food, protein, carbohydrates and fat. The liver and the pancreas each contribute about 10 litres (2 gal) of digestive juice during any twenty-four hours. Finally, in the large intestine, the residue is dealt with by a massive mixed population of bacteria and other small organisms which feed on the remainders and by their digestive processes break down resistant cellulose into forms of starch and sugar that can be used by the horse.

The walls of the intestines are covered by millions of finger-like processes less than 1 mm ($\frac{1}{20}$ in) in length giving the surface a velvety appearance and these absorb nourishment as the simplified foods are churned and squeezed along by rings of muscle which constrict and constantly activate the bowels in the direction of the rectum. Each tiny finger-like process is covered with cells and has a central hollow core. The fats are taken into this core in an emulsified state, reformed into fat globules and passed to the lymphatic vessels which deliver them to the blood stream. Proteins, broken down to amino-acids, and carbohydrates as various sugars, are absorbed by the cells lining the intestine and taken by the blood stream to the liver for storage. The blood stream, acting as a general carrier, takes up and delivers foodstuffs directly from the wall of the intestine or from depots in the liver to meet the requirements of cells throughout the body. The large intestine filters off excess moisture which is transmitted to the kidneys for disposal. The partially dried indigestible remains are passed periodically from the anus as droppings.

Diseases of the digestive tract

Urticaria A horse with urticaria is found to have developed quite suddenly a rash of flat-surfaced raised areas on its neck and body. The spots vary in size from less than the area of a finger-nail up to the size of a saucer. They are not irritant and the horse is not distressed by them. Rarely the swellings affect the throat and cause breathing trouble.

Urticaria is due to indigestion or follows a sudden increase in the quantity of nutritious food being given to a horse that is being prepared for extra activity, or the rash could be due to unsuitable food or a reduction in the exercise the animal is being given. Whatever the cause, the food is not being completely digested. Some components of partially digested food are toxic and when they are absorbed into the blood stream they have the effect of causing this urticarial rash.

Treatment of urticaria is to administer a laxative, reduce the ration and give reasonable exercise. In most cases the rash will disappear in a few hours. Those cases in which the breathing is obstructed may require adrenalin injections or even tracheotomy to allow air to reach the lungs. Some horses are unable to consume quantities of highly nutritious food without breaking out in urticarial eruptions. These animals are consequently unable to compete in events that require them to be highly fed for strenuous work but they remain healthy if they are fed normally and put to work at a less ambitious level.

Chronic indigestion The feeding of horses is a difficult art and many horses suffer from slight but persistent indigestion because it is generally accepted that if a horse is eating well and working well everything is as it should be. Any horse that does not appear to be in positive and excellent health is probably in need of some alteration in diet or management or is suffering from some disease. Horses look and work better if their feeding is understood and carefully controlled to avoid the long term effects of indigestion, which are a falling off in enthusiasm and ability, loss of condition, chronic laminitis and premature ageing.

Established signs of indigestion are a hidebound skin not freely moveable on the body, a coat which has lost its gloss and is dry and scurfy, and shelly horn on the feet. The mouth has a sour smell and the horse grinds its teeth, licks the walls, especially if whitewashed, and may wind-suck or crib-bite (see page 242). Wind is passed with extra frequency from the anus. The droppings are small and hard or loose and foul smelling, sometimes being streaked with yellow mucus and containing whole grains of corn. Severe indigestion may lead to colic or acute laminitis; slight indigestion to urticaria. Persistent indigestion is likely to cause chronic laminitis.

Indigestion results from faults in the food or the system of feeding, from worms, from lack of mastication due to the food being bolted or to sharp or faulty teeth. Other causes are overwork, exhaustion, exposure, and disease of the liver or intestines. The cause should be carefully sought out and cured if possible.

Recovery from indigestion is usually brought about by a run at grass, though ponies on ordinary meadow grass and horses on rich pasture may develop indigestion from simple overfeeding and it may be necessary to curtail their grazing periods. Horses turned out to grass eat quite an amount of earth probably to supply some deficiency in their diet. This need can be met for stabled horses by giving them an occasional large grassy sod in the manger, which they enjoy chewing over.

Stabled horses, showing signs of indigestion, may be started on their treatment by giving them a light dose of physic followed by 50 g (2 oz) of bicarbonate of soda given daily well mixed in the food. Your vet may find it advisable to prescribe a more active tonic mixture.

Indigestion can be avoided by careful attention to the many aspects of stable management and by relating feeding to the work being done, introducing changes gradually. Positive action should be taken if any horse is leaving its food, not working well or not looking its best.

Colic: acute indigestion Abdominal pain in horses is known as colic. A horse with colic stops feeding and indicates various degrees of pain by turning its head round to a flank, scraping with the fore feet or kicking at its belly with the hind ones. Some colicked horses stand or lie quietly between bouts of pain. In other cases, where the pain is acute, they get down, roll and get up again, or stay down, lying in various awkward positions. They may straddle their hind legs as though to pass urine, usually without success, not because, as is sometimes thought, there is an obstruction to the flow of urine, but because pressure on the bladder renews the colic pains in the abdomen. The pain may become so acute that the horse throws itself down recklessly and rolls and struggles like a freshly landed fish.

Causes of colic Anything that upsets the digestion may cause colic. Most colics are related to food and water: over-feeding; access to unsuitable foods like wheat or barley; sudden changes in diet; watering after instead of before feeding; or giving cold water in excess to a hot and exhausted horse. Other causes are worms and diseases of the abdominal organs.

The pain of colic is mostly caused by wind. The fermentation of partially digested food produces gases which distend the stomach and the intestines stretching their walls painfully and rendering them incapable of closing on the food to drive it along. As a result bowel movements and the digestive processes come to a halt. Pain also arises from toxic substances developed by worms and from the fermented food and these irritate the nerves and cause griping spasms in the muscles of the bowel walls.

Diagnosis and treatment of colic There is seldom any difficulty in detecting that a horse has colic; the signs of abdominal pain are obvious. Details of recent feeding and the work programme may give some idea of the cause and, by manual examination through the wall of the rectum, the vet can feel accumulations of food or wind that give further information. The horse is probably in pain, restless and excited. The heart beat may be raised from the normal rate of 35 to 40 to the minute to about 50 and the temperature is likely to be up to 38° or 39°C (101 or 102°F). The membranes of the eyes and mouth, usually pink, may be pale or flushed or tinged with yellow. In some cases the abdomen and flanks are distended from the pressure of wind. These are all signs of a simple colic.

In colic there is always pain and bowel stasis. Both these conditions need to be treated and in the majority of cases pain-killing drugs and laxative medicines will eventually succeed in overcoming the attack. However, there is a complication to be feared. A combination of the effects of wind, spasms of the muscles in the bowel walls and the horse throwing itself down and rolling in pain may cause the intestines to fold or twist themselves in such a way that they close the bowel as a tube in the way that a kink in a hose-pipe stops the flow of water and this folding or twisting also kinks the blood vessels so that some part of the bowel is deprived of a blood supply. Another complication with similar effects is telescoping of the bowel in which one part of the intestine overrides another, rather like a tuck in a glove finger. The length of tube affected, which may be as much as 1 m (3 ft) is now bounded by three thicknesses of bowel wall. It is completely blocked and the blood supply is obstructed.

Another complicating condition is a strangulated hernia in which some of the small intestine insinuates itself through a tear in the abdominal tissues and its blood vessels are pinched in the narrow opening. The most serious and almost inevitably fatal complication is rupture of the stomach or intestines, in which the contents of the gut are spilled out into the abdominal cavity.

When these complications occur the horse is distressed even between its bouts of pain, with anxious eyes, a drawn expression and rapid breathing. The heart rate rises to 80 or more beats to the minute and the temperature to 40 or 41 °C (104 or 105 °F). When any parts of the body are deprived of their blood supply, necrosis or death of the tissues occurs and this leads to the death of the horse unless surgical treatment is available.

Treatment of simple colic For the purpose of treatment, colic is divided into two groups: the simple cases of pain and bowel stasis which require urgent medication, and the complicated ones in which death is inevitable without surgery. Emphasis is laid on the urgency of treating the simple cases because while they continue they may at any time change suddenly to the complicated state where further medication is dangerous and surgery the only hope.

In simple colic, pain is relieved and bowel tension relaxed by using injections of atropine, acetyl-promazine and hyoscine compounds and by giving chloral hydrate by stomach tube. Wind may be evacuated from the stomach by passing a stomach tube into that organ: and from the large bowel, in extreme cases, by using a trocar and cannula (see below). Gas formation is discouraged by giving preparations of bismuth, charcoal and kaolin by the stomach tube. Bowel activity is restored with laxatives of anthraquinone, Epsom salts and common salt, and medicinal liquid paraffin may be added to the mixture if there are impacted masses of food. These masses may take several days to soften and be passed out of the bowel. This process may be helped by emptying the rectum by hand, a process known as backraking, and by using enemas of soap and warm water.

Back-raking In back-raking a gloved and lubricated hand is gently forced through the anus and the boluses of faeces within reach are pulled out a few at a time until the rectum is empty. The other hand holds the tail up and out of the way. Most horses do not resent this operation. Those that dislike it give notice of their intention to kick by trying to clap down the tail and, as the operator has hold of it, he has time to take avoiding action. Horses cannot kick while their tails are up in the air. This statement does not apply to mules.

Enemas An enema is the injection of fluid into the rectum to ease and stimulate the passing of droppings. A rubber tube is passed gently through the anus and fluid is introduced by a pump or a funnel attached to the tube. The process should not be hurried nor should force be used for fear of rupturing the bowel which will gradually expand to accommodate the fluid. 7 to 8 litres (1½ to 2¾ gal) of warm soapy water or a 2% solution of glycerine in warm water may be used.

The trocar and cannula The trocar is a pointed steel rod sheathed by a thin metal tube, the cannula. They are used to relieve wind from the bowel by penetrating together like a dagger through the horse's flank where it is most distended, into the large bowel. The trocar is withdrawn leaving the cannula as a tube for the escape of gas. The method carries some risk of causing peritonitis but may have to be resorted to as a possible means of saving life.

Nursing simple colic cases A colicked horse should be kept warm and, as far as possible, prevented from injuring itself. Rugs and a hood and stable bandages are needed. A deep bed of straw, shavings or peat, high round the walls, should be laid down in a large roomy box. The bed will need constant attention as the horse scrapes it into heaps. Two or three sacks tightly stuffed with straw are useful if the horse throws itself down or flings its head against the floor or walls. Walking the horse about has no curative effect though at times it may be the only way to maintain any control over the animal. Some colic pains pass off in a few hours, others persist for days. In most cases the violent pain can be overcome fairly quickly by suitable treatment but the need for careful nursing continues until normal digestive processes are restored. All foodstuffs should be withheld during the painful attacks as horses grabbing at food to distract their minds from pain are at serious risk of choking. Water may be offered in small amounts during the easier spells.

The treatment of complicated colic Complicated cases of colic that require surgical attention are cases of twisted gut, when the small or large intestines have folded or twisted in such a way that their blood supply is cut off; cases of telescoped bowel, strangulated hernia and rupture of the stomach or some part of the intestines. For these cases, surgery must be immediate if there is to be a reasonable chance of survival. Most of them will have been ill with colic for some time and are being poisoned by toxins from the partially digested food in the inactive bowel and are in a state of shock from their injured bowels. They are not ideal subjects for major abdominal surgery.

The twisted or folded bowels may be able to be untwisted so that the blood supply can flow again normally. This might be achieved if the case was operated on within an hour or two of the incident but the difficulties of diagnosis and the delays in deciding on and arranging for surgery are likely to have extended well beyond that period. Usually the portion of bowel involved will have been damaged beyond repair and will have to be removed, so that the healthy portions can be joined together to restore a workable tube of gut. Successful operations of this sort have involved removing as much as 10 metres (11 yards) of intestine.

The telescoped intestines reached in time could be simply drawn out to their proper length as a single tube but the usual delay means that they too almost always have to be excised and the healthy ends joined up.

In cases of strangulated hernia where a portion of small intestine has insinuated itself into an umbilical hernia and become twisted or pinched by the narrow gap in the wall of the abdomen there is a good chance of recovery as the colicky pains are soon traced to the hernia and an operation can usually be arranged before the horse's general well being is affected.

Cases of rupture of the stomach or intestines are a poor risk. Foodstuffs and digestive juices will have been spilled into the abdominal cavity and this is bound to cause some degree of peritonitis. The tear can be sewn up but the task of cleaning up the enormous areas in the abdomen is more than can be expected of any quantity of antibiotic medication or any other means that might be applied. Remarkable successes have nevertheless been achieved.

The chief problem in the surgical treatment of complicated colic cases is not the actual operation but the restoration and maintenance of the health of an animal received in a state of shock and collapse. Only too often the operation is successful but the patient dies. Surgical, anaesthetic and nursing skills and techniques are constantly improving and the percentage of successes in these, almost hopeless cases, is constantly rising.

After-care of colic cases Cases that have undergone an attack of colic are likely to be suffering from varying degrees of shock, exhaustion and dehydration. Their immediate requirements are protection from cold, rest, an invalid diet and a gradual return to normal food and exercise. The tonic effect of short spells at grass is of value if the weather is suitable. Horses in a weak state are liable to contract infections and any indications such as an increase in temperature may be countered by antibiotic injections. If the colic has lasted for several days or if the treatment has vigorously evacuated the bowel, the cultures of bacteria that help in digestion may have been seriously depleted. Administering 2 kg (4 lb) of faeces from a healthy horse in 10 litres (2 gal) of water by stomach tube replaces these and reduces the time required for the normal digestive processes to re-establish themselves. Dehydration usually corrects itself naturally but cases in which this persists may be benefited by intravenous injections of 5% sodium bicarbonate twice daily for a few days.

Prevention of colic Preventive measures to lessen the risk of colic occurring are: a regular worming programme, regular attention to the teeth and good stable management, with any necessary changes in the feeding programme being brought about gradually or preceded by two days on mash. Particular care should be devoted to horses under stress, especially those coming in exhausted and hungry, which are likely to bolt their food but are too tired to digest it.

Colic at foaling Mares often show signs of colic as a preliminary to foaling. Relief is provided by the arrival of the foal. If the colic persists without intermission and there are not clear signs that the birth is proceeding normally the colicky pains may indicate that the foal is not properly aligned and veterinary help should be obtained.

Meconium colic Foals that show colicky signs within a day or two of their birth are likely to be suffering from retained meconium. A complete recovery follows as soon as the meconium is evacuated naturally or with assistance.

Bowel stones In the 19th century, when flour was all stone-ground and quantities of bran were fed to horses, bowel stones sometimes developed in the intestines and gave rise to colic. Modern milling methods appear to have eliminated this risk. The stones developed as deposits of calcium carbonate and magnesium and ammonium phosphate around a foreign body such as a nail or a coin. Stones were found up to 30 kg (66 lb) in weight, quite round and smooth or with an irregular surface like a blackberry. Some horses suffering over a period from intermittent colic were found to be carrying one or more of these stones. It is remarkable that some of these stones could reach the size of a man's head, often without the horse showing any signs of illness before a sudden fatal colic attack.

If such stones were to occur at the present time they might be detected by a manual rectal examination or by x-ray and they could be removed by surgery.

Laxatives A laxative is any food or medicine which has the effect of softening a horse's droppings. Grass keeps the faeces moist and soft. The more nourishing and drier foods supplied to most working horses are inclined to cause the boluses of droppings to be small and hard. Firm droppings indicate a slower progress of food through the bowel. This delays the elimination of waste products and these are re-absorbed and have mildly toxic effects. This tendency is increased by sweating at work or by a high temperature from illness which both rob the bowel of some of its fluid content.

Horses' droppings may be softened by supplying adequate roughage in the form of good quality hay and by feeding fresh grass or other green foods, boiled foods, oils and bran or other mashes. 30 or 40 g (1 or $1\frac{1}{2}$ oz) of common salt in the daily ration is also a help in this direction. Medicinally preparations of anthraquinone are readily taken in the food and this is a harmless drug that combines satisfactorily with common salt. Some of the varieties of pellet feeds for horses have substances added to ensure that a slightly laxative effect is obtained which is especially useful for horses that are being shipped long distances.

Horses do not take readily to sudden changes in their diet, but such changes are inevitable when, for example, they are brought in from grass to be prepared for a season's work. They adjust to a new diet more readily if it is laxative, though many horsemen consider that this adjustment is brought about more satisfactorily if the horse is given physic, which is a purgative, before starting on a completely different feeding programme.

Physic or purgatives While laxatives hasten bowel activity and soften the horse's droppings, purgatives empty the bowel. The process of physicking or purging a horse is used to avoid digestive upsets that may occur when a horse's diet is suddenly changed. This change of diet occurs when horses are brought up from grass to go into training for preparation for a season's work or when, on account of injury or illness or other circumstances, those that are in strong work and on full rations are suddenly forced to rest. The situation may also arise when horses are being transported long distances.

Horses can adjust to a change of diet if it is introduced gradually, and they are helped in this if the diet is slightly laxative. Major adjustments in diet can be brought about in this way over several weeks. However, if circumstances demand an immediate change, physic is the proper course.

Physic consists of administering a sufficient dose of an activating medicine to cause the contents of the intestines to be diluted to a fluid and emptied out of the bowel in a state of watery diarrhoea. Physic should not be given to horses which may be suffering from any obstruction in the bowel. Horses whose droppings are small and firm should be given bran mashes and have their corn or pellet feed cut right down for a couple of days before giving the physic. This delay may be avoided if the medicine is given by stomach tube in 10 litres (2 gal) of warm water, with 250 g (8 oz) of common salt added to the mixture. The medicine used for physic is an anthraquinone preparation, and is the same as for a laxative effect, but in a larger dose. Most horses will take this drug in a feed but it is important that they should get the right dose. The drug is not poisonous but if the horse does not get the full amount there is a laxative action that may not be adequate. An overdose causes diarrhoea extending beyond the one day required. The correct dosage is assured if the medicine is given by a stomach tube and the result can be improved, being rendered smoother and quicker, by the addition of salt as suggested.

The physic is given in a reduced evening feed or at any time on day one by the stomach tube, as long as the horse has a reasonably empty stomach; that is at least three hours after a small feed. The next day is 'purging day' and the horse should be allowed hay to nibble at, free access to water and be given a small warm mash in the evening. The third is 'setting day'. Small quantities of slightly firmer droppings will be passed. The horse should have as much hay and water as it requires and be given a small mid-day feed of the new ration and a half-sized evening feed.

This programme has confined the horse to its box for two days, making the usual labour force available for other duties or holidays.

Some large stables find it advantageous to the horses' health and to the staff's morale to 'physic' over Christmas. On the fourth day the horse has a fully recovered appetite and is ready to be put on to the new feeding regime.

Physic may be helpful when it is necessary to reduce the horse's intake of food or to counter the effects of excessive or harmful food already eaten. This may apply in cases of colic, laminitis, urticaria, lymphangitis and in some cases of fever, toxaemia and poisoning.

Diarrhoea Diarrhoea is not common in horses and should always be treated seriously when it occurs. The most likely cause is a heavy worm infestation. Laboratory reports on the number of worm eggs found in the droppings, usually a most helpful guide, can be misleading on samples of diarrhoeic faeces because the enormous increase in the fluid dilutes the concentration of worm eggs. As a result a laboratory may find 'few' or 'very few' eggs per standard measure of droppings when the horse is actually carrying an excessive number of worms.

Diarrhoea may also be caused by sudden changes of food, by poisons and by bacterial infections in the bowel. Laboratory examination of the faeces may be of great help in determining the cause of the trouble. Antibiotics should be used with caution in treating diarrhoea as they may kill off the normal bacterial inhabitants of the bowel necessary to proper digestion allowing the harmful bacteria to flourish without competition. Diarrhoea, in spite of free access to water, may cause dehydration, and intravenous injections of dextrose saline or 5% sodium bicarbonate may be necessary to maintain a proper fluid content in the tissues. Kaolin, charcoal and bismuth and sulphonamide drugs are helpful in correcting this disease. A persisting diarrhoea whose only distinguishing signs are cow-like droppings and an extremely peculiar smell is attributed to an infection by trichomonads, a type of parasite. Treatment consists of a long course of medication with iodo-chloro-hydroxy-quinoline.

In convalescence a population of normal bacteria required for digestion may be restored by 2 kg (4½ lb) of faeces from a normal horse, well sieved, mixed in 10 litres (2 gal) of water and given by stomach tube. Diarrhoea occurs more frequently in foals than in older horses, and they should receive attention as described in the section on new-born foals (see page 354).

Foals are especially subject to attacks of diarrhoea while their mothers are in season. Their droppings usually return to normal in a few days but if foals become dejected and lose their appetite it is advisable to give them antibiotics, sulphonamides and kaolin. Antibiotics are suitable for treating bowel infections in young foals which do not depend on bacteria to assist their digestive processes as do older horses.

Enteritis While diarrhoea simply means loose or watery droppings, enteritis signifies an acute inflammation of some parts of the bowel, usually due to an infection and accompanied by a high temperature with diarrhoea as one of its signs. With enteritis there is likely to be blood in the motions.

A laboratory diagnosis of the cause of enteritis is urgently necessary and antibiotics may have to be used to save the animal's life in spite of the harmful effects they may have on the bacteria that help in the processes of digesting food. Tetracycline antibiotics should be avoided as they sometimes have a worsening effect on enteritis cases and no antibiotics should be given by mouth. A disease, known in America as colitis-x and apparently also occurring in the British Isles, has enteritis as its only sign. It is frequently fatal.

On post-mortem examination parts of the bowel are found to be acutely inflamed. The cause is not known though suspicion falls on salmonella bacteria associated with a virus. Colitis-x does not respond to any antibiotic or sulphonamide medicines. Some cases of enteritis arising from infection with clostridium welchii may be helped by giving sour milk by stomach tube and pulpy kidney serum intravenously. In all cases it is important to ensure that the horse does not go short of water.

Rectal prolapse – eversion of the rectum In rectal prolapse, a part of the rectum is protruded from the anus and shows as a pink or angry red fleshy swelling projecting for a few centimetres or up to 1 m (3 ft). The condition may be due to a general irritation of the bowel from unsuitable food or disease, to straining associated with colic or foaling, or following careless rectal exploration, or hot or otherwise unsuitable enemas.

The horse should be tranquillized to make replacing of the prolapse easier. In a case where the membranes do not protrude more than 25 cm (10 in) and are still pink, they should be supported by cloths soaked in warm saline, a teaspoonful of salt in ½ litre (1 pint) of water, and pressure applied gently from all sides towards the obscured anus until the whole mass is replaced. More severe cases, those out more than 30 cm (1 ft) and those in which the membranes are dark, congested and oozing, are best dealt with after the horse has been given a general anaesthetic. The prolapsed rectum, protected with warm saline cloths, should be kept above the level of the anus and shrunk by loosely bandaging over the cloths with crêpe bandage. When the warm saline has had ten to fifteen minutes to moisten and soften the membranes, some 100 to 200 g (4 to 8 oz) of domestic granulated or castor sugar, to help the shrinking effect, may be dusted over the rectum which should again be wrapped in saline and bandaged. A general pressure should then be applied towards the anus, the objective being to return that part of the rectum nearest to the anus first through the anal ring. Attempts should not be made to invert the part furthest from the anus as this would cause immediate local resistance. The operation is simplified by raising the horse's hind end so that full use can be made of gravity. When the swollen organ has all been replaced warm water should be poured or pumped gently into the rectum to ensure normal realignment and the fluid should then be drained away. Attention should be given to dealing with the cause of the prolapse and the horse kept tranquillized to reduce further straining. Feeding should be on light mashes or gruel until it is established that normal droppings are being passed without difficulty.

Salivation Saliva dropping in quantities from a horse's mouth is almost always due to some irritant in the mouth : a loose tooth crown, a broken tooth, a piece of wire, a splinter of wood or a length of bramble under the tongue. Chemicals, ulcers and stomatitis have the same effect. Washing out the mouth with dilute hydrogen peroxide may give relief if there is no foreign body that can be located and removed before professional help arrives.

Choking A horse is said to be choked when something it has swallowed becomes stuck on the way to the stomach. A ravenously hungry horse may gulp food down without mixing it with saliva so that a dry mass is swallowed that cannot slide on its way. The same thing may happen in excitement after a race or when coming round from an anaesthetic and care should be taken to prevent access to food or bedding until such an animal calms down. Obstructions can be caused by carrots, apples, thorny twigs, wire or capsules of medicine or by sugar beet pulp that has not been properly soaked.

When the object is lodged at the back of the throat the horse pokes its head forward stiffly and dribbles saliva. Sometimes this obstruction can be reached by hand or by forceps but it is usually lower down the gullet and out of reach. The horse makes repeated efforts to vomit, tucking the chin into its chest and producing violent spasms in the neck muscles. These efforts are never effective. A horse cannot reject food from the stomach and, although the gullet does make the most desperate efforts it does not seem able to return objects causing choking.

The cause of the choke may be seen and felt as a lump in the left jugular groove and massaged on its way if it is in that part of the gullet, but it is out of sight if it is passing through the chest. Its position there may be checked by inserting a stomach tube gently as far as the block and pouring down a very small amount of water or medicinal liquid paraffin to soften and lubricate the lump. Larger amounts must not be used as they are rejected and may be drawn by the windpipe into the lungs. Objects that have passed that far down the gullet are almost certain to complete their journey to the stomach though it may be a very slow process extending over hours or even days. They may be helped on by injections of an antispasmodic drug which relaxes the tension of the muscles in the wall of the gullet.

If the gullet has been previously injured so that there is a constriction in the tube at some point, choking is likely to recur frequently unless the most careful feeding programme is maintained. The same applies if the gullet has developed a diverticulum or bulge in which food can accumulate. It is not likely that either of these conditions can be treated satisfactorily.

Digestive lymphangitis Digestive lymphangitis, or Monday Morning Disease, which is the stable name this complaint goes by, comes from failing to adjust the feeding to the work being done. The latter name was particularly apt when well fed horses routinely working a five-and-a-half-day week were liable to be found with a big leg on Monday morning if they had not had their early dose of salts on Saturday and reduced rations on that day and the Sunday. The cause of these cases is simply indigestion, the toxins from overfeeding having this peculiar effect on the lymphatic drainage from one leg; hardly ever affecting more than one leg and that usually a hind one.

The leg begins to swell at the hock or knee and the swelling extends rapidly down to the hoof and up the limb to a level, all round the limb, just below the stifle joint or just below the elbow, forming a shelf beyond which it never extends, however large the limb becomes. The swelling is enormous, reaching its maximum in less than twelve hours, when the 'bone' measurement of 15 cm (6 in) may expand to 50 cm (17½ in) with the rest of the limb proportionately huge. Serum often oozes from the skin over the lower parts of the leg. Finger pressure on the inside of the thigh or forearm is very painful. The horse goes off its feed and runs a high temperature. Treatment consists of drugs to relieve pain, a purgative, antibiotics, sulphonamides, massage and gentle exercise which may need to be forced at first as the horse finds its cumbersome leg painful and mechanically difficult to move. The raised temperature and the helpful effect of anti-bacterial drugs make it clear that infection is a complicating factor, in some cases at least.

Horses under treatment should have their exercise and their feeding increased daily until they can be returned to light work in one or two weeks. Legs which have been affected usually remain slightly swollen and care must be taken to avoid further attacks, which are prone to occur in the same leg, leaving it bigger after each episode.

Prevention of lymphangitis consists of ensuring that horses which are being fed well to maintain or improve their condition while in regular work are suitably treated with laxatives and reduced rations to balance even short breaks in their working schedule.

Crib-biting and wind-sucking A horse that crib-bites grips its teeth on to the edge of the manger or crib or any other firm object, like the top of the half door, so that it can angle its throat conveniently for gulping air into its gullet. A wind-sucker is able to gulp air by raising its neck, tucking in its chin and gulping without holding on to anything with its teeth. Crib-biters are recognized by angular wear at the front edge of both upper and lower rows of incisor teeth which become marked in this way from frequently gripping on the manger rim. Wind-suckers do not bear any physical sign of their indulgence.

The practices are classed as vices, which are objectionable habits. The objection to crib-biting and wind-sucking is that the gulped air passes down into the stomach and has an effect on digestion similar to that resulting from wind in the intestines from any other source: it prevents the close application of the walls of the stomach and bowels to the food they should be working on. Crib-biters and wind-suckers become unthrifty in appearance like any other horse with indigestion.

The cause of crib-biting and wind-sucking is a mystery. The habits are attributed to the boredom of long hours in the stable and are said to be developed in imitation of other horses that already practise the vices. Once established it seems impossible to break horses of either habit. Horses out at grass very seldom make any attempt to gulp air but as soon as they are brought back to the stable they start again immediately.

A treatment for these conditions is to fasten a broad strap tightly round the throat. The strap is designed to make it uncomfortable for the horse to set its head at the angle necessary for gulping air. The strap is successful while it is being worn but it does not cure the habit. Another treatment is to remove portions of muscle from the front of the neck so that the horse is permanently unable to set its head in the necessary position. This is a major operation which is not always successful. Some owners ensure that their crib-biter has no object in the stable on which it can fix its teeth. This develops into an interesting battle of wits because the horse always finds something to bite on. Success has been claimed for electric-shock treatment by a wire from an electric-fencing battery run along the top of the stable half door. This carries a momentary current at intervals of a few seconds and deters the horse from using that particular grip for his teeth.

Dentistry

Horses seldom suffer from toothache because the sensitive tooth pulp remains deeply in the jaw beneath the massive, quite insensitive tooth. Nevertheless, horses' teeth have their share of troubles which require attention from time to time. The usual problems are sharp teeth, tooth root and tooth socket infections, tooth decay and broken teeth.

Tooth replacement Eruption of the horse's 24 temporary teeth and their subsequent replacement by up to 42 permanent ones is dealt with in some detail in the section on Telling a Horse's Age by the Teeth. The milk teeth, 12 incisors and 12 molars, are present at birth or erupt within the first year and they cause no trouble. When the time comes for their replacement their roots are absorbed leaving only the shell of a tooth that caps or crowns the erupting permanent tooth. These crowns, whether they are incisor teeth or molars, are smooth on top but their sides have sharp spikes that project downwards. When a permanent tooth protrudes far enough the crown falls off. Sometimes a loose crown is only shifted to one side and the horse bites on it driving one or more spikes into the gum. The mishap is not serious. The horse refuses to feed and dribbles saliva. An examination of the mouth reveals the offending crown which can be removed. This painful effect is prevented if loose crowns are lifted off as soon as a finger-nail can be slipped between the edge of the crown and the gum. The crown is gripped with forceps and given a slight twist. If the crown refuses to move in response to this help, it is not ready to be shed. No harm has been done and it can be lifted off a day or two later. The central incisor crowns are shed at 2½ years, the laterals at 3½ and the corners at 4½. The first and second molar crowns in each jaw are often shed together, between 2½ and 3 years and the third molar crowns a year later. Incisor crowns are sometimes caught between the remaining teeth. They are easily extracted with forceps.

Sharp teeth The molar teeth crush the food by a sideways action of the lower jaw. The surface of these teeth is not level but slopes from the tongue to the cheek on each side. The teeth wear each other away at the rate of about 3 mm (⅛ in) a year. They grow up from the roots at the same rate so their length appears constant for most of the horse's life. The grinding action of opposing teeth misses the inner edge of the lower row of molars and the outer edge of the upper row. In consequence these edges become sharp, sometimes as sharp as a razor blade. The tongue and cheeks pushing food between the molars may be cut by these sharp edges. The resulting painful wounds and ulcers can interfere with the horse's feeding to such an extent that it loses condition.

The sharp edges on the outer side of the upper row of molars and the inner edge of the lower row can be blunted and brought down to the level of the rest of the tooth table by using a file or rasp. The usual tooth rasp is 2 to 3 cm (about 1 in) wide and 5 or 6 cm (about 2 in) long mounted on a 30 cm (12 in) metal rod with a short wooden handle. This rasp is rubbed backwards and forwards along the sharp edges of the teeth until they are felt to be smoothed away. The operation is painless and most horses, having overcome the initial strangeness of the instrument in their mouths, seem to enjoy the mild vibration that it sets up. They appreciate it more if the rasp is periodically swilled in salt water.

This development of sharp edges applies to the temporary molars as well as to the permanent teeth, but whichever they are they cause little damage to young horses that are not working. As soon as a horse begins to work and receive concentrated food to masticate, as young flat race horses do before they are two years old, the effect of sharp teeth may be noticed. Rasping at intervals of three months to keep the edges smooth is better than holding major rasping sessions at long intervals during which the teeth have sharpened and caused injury and discomfort. It is an advantage to accustom young horses to the rasp as soon as they come to hand. The regular mouth inspection involved will ensure that there is no trouble from tooth crowns or other dental abnormalities. Furthermore, allowing the spiky edges to remain untrimmed leads to slight alterations in tooth alignment. This breaks the continuity of the grinding surface, allows food to be forced into gaps between the teeth and leads to serious infections of the tooth sockets and roots.

Tooth socket infection or peridontal disease As the horse becomes older the teeth fit less tightly in their sockets and the gums recede. This allows food, dirt and bacteria to penetrate into the sockets. To resist and overcome this invasion the gums inflame and new bone grows to fill up the sockets. This is peridontal disease. Most horses have some degree of this condition by the time they are six years old and it continues for the rest of their lives. The disease only causes serious trouble if it penetrates so deeply into the sockets that it causes tooth root infections. Peridontal disease is encouraged by any misplaced, broken or extracted teeth which allow food and other materials easy access to the sockets. It is impossible to prevent peridontal disease but its onset can be delayed by frequent tooth rasping.

Tooth root infection If peridontal disease reaches the sensitive tissues around a tooth root an abscess may develop. If this occurs in the upper jaw pus accumulates in the hollow sinuses of the bones of the face. The bones swell below the eye on the affected side and are painful under pressure, pus may run from one nostril and the breath has a foetid smell. The remedy is to extract the infected tooth. This allows the abscess to drain through the empty tooth socket into the mouth and the infection is overcome with the help of antibiotics and antiseptic douches.

Tooth root abscesses are less usual in the lower jaw. They can frequently be drained through an opening under the jaw so that tooth extraction is not necessary.

Tooth decay or caries Tooth decay, comparable to decay of the teeth in human beings, only occurs in horses in the upper rows of molar teeth. The 4th molar, which is the oldest tooth in a horse's mouth, is the one most often affected first, but any of the upper molars may decay in the same way. The central part of the tooth table softens and the decay spreads slowly into the tooth and extends over the table. The annual 3-mm ($\frac{1}{8}$ in) wearing away of the tooth is sometimes sufficient to remove the decaying layer and leave sound tooth exposed, so curing the disease. Usually the decay continues to spread. Rarely it may so soften the tooth that it fractures, leading to the complications of socket and root infections. If it is sought for carefully, most horses over 12 years old are found to have some degree of caries; otherwise caries is not usually discovered until after the horse's death from some other cause.

It seems that most horses do not live long enough for this disease to do them much harm and, being painless, it causes them no distress. If a case were to be treated the cavity should be drilled out, undercut and filled by the methods used in human dentistry.

Broken teeth The incisor teeth may be broken if the horse falls on its nose. Canine teeth and molars may be broken in accidents and molar teeth may fracture as a consequence of severe peridontal disease or from caries. Extraction of the teeth should be avoided if possible.

A broken incisor tooth can be trimmed level with sharp forceps. This is painless operation. The shortened tooth will not take part in the regular grinding down process and will gradually grow up level with its fellows. In the meantime, its opposing tooth in the other jaw will overgrow and this should be trimmed down eventually to restore the even line of the bite. If several teeth in one row have been broken and have had to be trimmed back it may be a reasonable cosmetic operation to clip the whole row back to one level.

Canine teeth are sometimes broken level with or below the gums. Spikes should be trimmed off and the tooth left as smooth as possible. The tooth serves no useful purpose and even when broken is unlikely to interfere with the bit. Its extraction is a major operation which is seldom required.

Broken molar teeth may have to be extracted. If they are causing no trouble they should be left alone. Sometimes a broken piece may be taken out with forceps. If a molar tooth is found to be involved in an intractable infection of one or other of the sinuses in the facial bones, extraction is probably the only satisfactory way of dealing with the problem.

Tooth extraction In very old horses which have worn most of each tooth away leaving a stump and a small root in a large tooth socket, tooth extraction merely involves applying suitable forceps and giving a twist and a pull.

Small supernumerary molars or wolf teeth appear in a great many horses in front of the first molar in the upper jaw. They are reputed to cause discomfort associated with the bit and they certainly can be troublesome if they erupt some distance away from the first molar. They usually appear tightly applied against that tooth and it would seem unlikely that they cause any harm in that position but some horse trainers insist on their extraction. Most of them come out easily enough with a twist and a pull. They have hardly any root at all.

Extracting incisor teeth is a major operation requiring a general anaesthetic. In young horses when the teeth are 8 cm (3¼ in) or more long the bone socket requires to be opened nearly all the way to the root. Attempting to remove the tooth by traction on the exposed portion is not practicable.

Molar tooth extraction is a serious operation to be carried out under general anaesthesia. Occasionally if there has been long-standing peridontal disease in the tooth socket, the tooth's attachment to the bone may be loosened. In that case the tooth may be levered by forceps out of its socket. Most teeth are too long for this levering to progress very far before the tooth impinges on the row of teeth in the opposite jaw. The portion of tooth raised up then has to be cut off with tooth shears and another 5 cm (2 in) of tooth levered up. This may allow it to be turned and fully extracted. Otherwise another piece may have to be cut off and the stump finally drawn. If the molar tooth is not already loose in its socket, forceps will not move it but are likely to break it from pressure. Such tightly fixed teeth need to be driven out. A hole is cut in the bones of the face above the tooth root and a punch is applied. The tooth can be driven

5 cm (2 in) into the mouth where it has to be cut off and the process repeated. The socket which may be harbouring an abscess can be treated by douching through the opening in the bones of the face. The operation is usually successful in such cases. The facial wound heals up within a few days. The molar tooth opposite the one that has been extracted grows unchecked and needs rasping down from time to time.

Undershot and overshot jaws The commonest tooth defect is misalignment due to the lower jaw being too short so that the upper row of incisors overlaps the lower row, causing an overshot or parrot mouth. Less commonly the lower jaw is too long so that the lower row of incisors protrudes beyond the upper row, an undershot or pig mouth. When either of these conditions is present in a minor degree the incisor teeth may meet each other but the bite is not exact. In a major degree they miss each other, sometimes by as much as 2 or 3 cm (1 in) and there is no bite.

If the teeth do not meet there will obviously be some interference with grazing, but affected animals seem to manage since most of them are unlikely to be short of food or competing for it. The condition could be serious in horses on free range in winter. The defect is important because the rows of molar teeth are also likely to overlap to the same degree and, when overshot, part of the first upper molar and the last lower molar will not be worn down; when undershot, the teeth affected will be the first lower molar and the last upper molar. These will grow spikes which need to be rasped down regularly. If this is not done the unchecked growth will develop large spikes over the years, that interfere with the bite at the front of the mouth and with mastication and swallowing at the back of the molar rows. The spikes would then require to be cut off, involving a major operation. The incisor teeth will also grow unchecked if they do not meet to wear each other down. Those that become disproportionately long can be trimmed by sharp cutting forceps without pain or stress to the horse.

There appears to be no evidence that these variations in the length of the lower jaw causing the teeth to be undershot or overshot are hereditary.

6 Poisons

Horses are seldom deliberately poisoned and, being very particular about their food and water, they seldom take poisons themselves. The commonest cause of poisoning in horses is that their attendants have used too large doses of medicines or too concentrated anti-parasitic skin dressings; next in order comes the lack of care over the use of rat poisons around buildings or weed-killers on the land; and the third cause is failure to supply reasonable food or pasture, so that the horses have no choice but to eat mouldy food (which is poisonous), poisonous plants, grass poisoned by weed-killers, or pasture having excesses or deficiencies of minerals. Closely associated with this cause is a water supply infested with moulds or algae or contaminated by industrial pollution or by salt or other minerals.

Signs of poisoning There are no clear-cut signs that differentiate a horse that is poisoned from one that is ill from some other kind of disease. Poisons affect horses in many different ways, but it will be clear to most owners when their horse is off its feed for some reason which might be poisoning. Poisoned horses are likely to show some of the signs listed:

Digestive tract
loss of appetite
salivation
diarrhoea
constipation
colic

Circulatory system
rapid heart beat
disturbed heart rhythm
pale membranes (anaemia)
red or orange membranes (inflammation)
yellow membranes (jaundice)
excessive urination

Locomotion
weakness
lameness
stumbling
staggering
collapse

Nervous system
excitement
depression
muscle tremors

Most animals that have swallowed irritant poison rid themselves of some of it by vomiting, but horses cannot vomit. Irritant poisons stimulate a horse's bowels to activity and often cause diarrhoea eventually; but the horse has many yards of bowel and the process may take several days, during which time much of the poison will have been absorbed to injure the horse's tissues. The process can be speeded by giving the horse purgatives and, if it is known what poison the horse has taken, antidotes may be available.

When a horse appears to be poisoned it is almost impossible for the vet to treat the condition unless he knows what poison may be responsible. There are laboratories that can give a confident answer in 48 hours. In the meantime the horse may have died. It is of immediate help to your vet if the containers of any medicines or chemicals which may have poisoned the horse are available for his examination. The packet itself may carry some written instructions on how to remedy such a case of poisoning.

The following descriptions of poisons are given as general information, not to encourage any 'do it yourself' ambitions; they should help owners to avoid exposing their horses to dangers of poisoning and underline the urgency of obtaining professional help.

Poison	Effect	Treatment
Weed-killers		
Borax	Diarrhoea, convulsions, prostration	2 per cent sodium bicarbonate in normal saline into vein
Dinitrocresols, dinitrophenols	Distressed breathing, jaundice, collapse	Vitamin A. 5 per cent dextrose in normal saline into vein. Chlorpromazine
Pentachlorophenol	Skin irritation, salivation	No known treatment
Phenoxyacetic acid	Loss of appetite, weakness	Saline dosing and into vein in large quantities
Phenyl urea compounds: diuron linuron monuron fenuron	Loss of appetite, weakness	Saline dosing and into vein in large quantities
Sodium chlorate	Anaemia	Methylene blue and saline into vein

Poison	Effect	Treatment
Insecticides		
Chlorinated hydrocarbons: aldrin BHC (benzyne hexachloride) chlordane DDT dieldrin heptachlor methoxychlor rothane toxaphen	Excessive salivation and urination, Nervous twitching, tremors, Convulsions, dehydration	If on skin wash off with water and detergents. If taken internally dextrose saline into vein. Laxatives. If excited give barbiturates
Derris and pyrethrum	Harmless	
Nicotine	Nervous tremors, incoordination, coma	Dose with large amounts of saline. Give laxatives

Poison	Effect	Treatment
Organophosphorous compounds: ciodrin coumaphos diazinon dichlorvos malathion parathion ronnel TEPP (tetraethyl-pyrophosphate) trichlorofon	Excessive salivation, distressed breathing, colic, diarrhoea, convulsions	Antidote : atropine sulpahte. Wash off skin with water and detergents. If taken internally give dextrose saline into vein
Petroleum products: xylene mineral oils solvents	Skin irritation	Wash off with soap and water and detergents
Sulphur and lime	Irritation and blistering	Apply soothing ointments

Poison	Source	Effect	Treatment
Acorns	Under oak trees in autumn. Poisonous in large amounts	No appetite, constipation, later diarrhoea, colic, blood in faeces, pale membranes	Purgatives, acetyl promazine
ANTU (Alpha naphthyl thiourea)	Rat poison	Weakness and coma	Phenobarbitone into vein, vitamin K, glyceryl monoacetate
Arsenic	Sheep dip, rat poison, weed killer, corn dressing, green paints, tonic medicine	Loss of appetite, bristling hair, shivering, prostration, death	Antidote : dimercapol, Epsom salts, iron oxides
Bracken	Hill grazing	Loss of appetite, swaying and stumbling, slow accumulating poison leading to eventual death	Thiamine injections. It is safe to graze on bracken for spells of 3 weeks on 3 weeks off
Common salt (sodium chloride)	Usually land near sea	Shallow breathing, weak pulse, muscle tremors, weakness	Calcium gluconate in vein. Provide fresh water
Cyanide	Rat poison, soil sterilizers, Java beans, uncooked linseed	Large doses : distressed breathing, convulsions, death. Small doses : heart weakness, fast breathing	Dose with sodium nitrite and sodium thiosulphate
Foxglove (Digitalis)	Foxglove plants green or as hay. Medicinal uses	Failing heart, distressed breathing, swollen head and throat, livid membranes	Antidote : tannic acid, acetyl promazine

Poison	Source	Effect	Treatment
Fluorosis	Rock phosphate, drinking water contaminated by industry	Bony enlargements, dry skin, cracked hooves, loss of appetite, diarrhoea	Feed aluminium sulphate. Deal with source
Lead	Rat poison, paint, batteries, lead splashes from shooting ranges, industry fall-out	Cramp, paralysis, wasting, convulsions, blindness	Antidote: calcium disodium ethylene-diamine-tetra-acetate, purgatives
Mercury (inorganic and organic)	Disinfectants, fungicides	Heart distress, muscle-spasms, excitement, diarrhoea	Antidote: dimercapol. Feed milk and eggs
Nitrates	Medicinal uses	Violent deep breathing, weak heart beat, convulsions	Antidote: 2 per cent methylene blue in saline
Phosphorous	Rat and rabbit poison	Smell of garlic, colic, convulsions, bleeding from nose, rectum, bladder	Dose with copper sulphate or potassium permanganate. Avoid oils
Ragwort	Ragwort plants (green or as hay)	Cumulative poison over months. Jaundice, loss of flesh, sluggish action	Purgative followed by light laxative diet
Selenium	Present in some soils and taken up by vegetation	Lameness, cracked hooves, loss of hair from mane and tail	Feed milk and eggs. Avoid pastures with high selenium content

Poison	Source	Effect	Treatment
Sodium fluoroacetate	Rat poison	Depression, weakness, heart failure	Antidote : glyceryl monoacetate. Phenobarbitone
Snake bite (to which horses are extremely sensitive)	Elapine snakes : cobra, mamba, coral. Viperine snakes : adder, rattle snake	Breathing paralysed, excitement followed by quiet spell then asphyxia, extensive swelling around area of bite, acute pain at intervals, depression, death	Antivenin urgently Antivenin. Apply tourniquet. Enlarge wounds and wash with pressure hose
Strychnine	Rat poison	Intermittent muscular spasms to rigidity, lengthening intervals may lead to recovery	Large doses of chloral hydrate into stomach or vein. Dextrose 5 per cent in saline into vein
Sweet clover (dicoumarol)	Sweet clover hay or silage	Bleeding into muscles and joints causing difficulty in moving	Vitamin K. Blood transfusions
Tar or pitch	Skin dressing, sheep dip, clay pigeon fragments	Depression, weakness, stupor, coma, death	Dose with sodium sulphate. Purgatives
Thallium sulphate	Rat poison	Weakness, coma	Antidote : diaphenylthiocarbazone
Warfarin and pindone	Rat poison. Medicinal uses	Stiffness and lameness due to bleeding into muscles and joints	Vitamin K. Blood transfusions
Yew	Leaves of yew trees (usually in hard winter)	Collapse and death	If suspected give purgatives

Poison	Source	Effect	Treatment
Fungi, moulds and algae living on plants or in water			
Aflatoxicosis	Moulds on ground nuts, soy beans, cereals	Loss of appetite, reduced growth	Change to clean food
Algae	Blue-green algae in ponds and lakes	Prostration, convulsions, death	Supply clean water. Move animals to shade as sunshine worsens condition
Ergot	Fungus spore pods developed on rye, grass seed heads	Trembling, incoordination, paralysis	Keep pasture short to prevent flower heads forming. Methionine in dextrose 10 per cent in saline into vein.
Lupinosis	Moulds on lupin plants in Europe, Australia, New Zealand, South Africa	Loss of appetite, Jaundice, Constipation	Grow mould-resistant (blue flowered) lupins
Mouldy corn toxins	Oats, maize	Loss of appetite, depression, staggering, excessive urination	Change to clean food

7 Infectious diseases

Infectious diseases of horses

Disease	Causal organism	Description
Infection by nose, mouth or wounds		
brucellosis	brucella bacillus	this section
anthrax	anthrax bacillus	
tetanus	a clostridium bacillus	
gas gangrene	clostridium bacilli	
haemorrhagic septicaemia	pasteurella bacteria	
vesicular stomatitis	a rhabdo-virus	
tuberculosis	mycobacterium tuberculosis	

Disease	Causal organism	Description
catarrh and coughing	herpes virus	see Respiratory diseases
influenza	myxo-viruses	
strangles	streptococcal bacteria	
chronic bronchitis	allergy and various bacteria	
glanders	pfeifferella mallei bacteria	
abscesses	staphylococci and other bacteria	see Skin conditions
botriomycosis	an actino-bacillus	
streptomycosis	streptomyces fungus	
epizootic lymphangitis	a histoplasma fungus	
ulcerative lymphangitis	a corynebacterium	
poll-evil and fistulous withers	various bacteria	
warts	papo-viruses	
foal pneumonia	a corynebacterium	See Foal diseases
new-born foal infections	various bacteria and viruses	
enteritis	clostridia and salmonella bacteria	see Diseases of the digestive tract
horse-pox	a pox virus	see Foot injuries and diseases
periodic ophthalmia	a leptospiral bacillus	see The eyes
Infection spread by insect bites		
African horse sickness	a reo-virus	this section
encephalitis	alpha viruses	
infectious anaemia	an oncorna virus	
surra	a trypanosome	
babesiosis	a piroplasm	
Infection spread by saliva		
rabies	a rhabdo-virus	this section
Infection spread during the sexual act		
dourine	a trypanosome	see Breeding (barren mares)
infectious metritis	a cocco-bacillus	
metritis	klebsiella bacteria	
coital (vesicular) exanthema	a herpes virus	
Cause of infection unknown		
serum hepatitis	–	this section
grass sickness	–	

Infectious diseases Infectious diseases are caused by minute members of the vegetable kingdom – bacteria, fungi and viruses – or by slightly larger, single-celled animals, trypanosomes and piroplasms. These tiny organisms live and multiply as parasites causing disease by feeding on the horse's tissues but, more especially, by poisoning the affected area with toxins which are by-products of their life processes. If the toxins gain access to the blood stream they are carried to all parts of the body and may poison the whole animal.

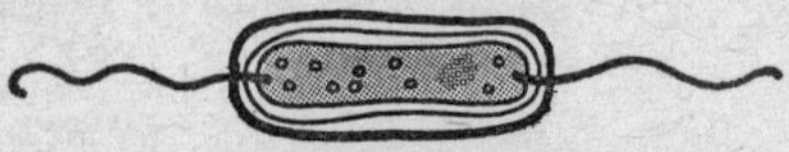

A bacterium

Bacteria Bacteria are single-celled organisms, the simplest form of vegetable life. They are mostly round or rod-like objects measuring about one thousandth of a millimetre in width. They reproduce themselves by each one dividing into two. As this can happen in as little as twenty minutes, one of these microbes could, in theory, increase to a thousand million in less than twelve hours. Fortunately their multiplication is limited by food supply.

Bacteria live on animal or vegetable matter that may be living or dead. They are widely distributed in soil and have great powers of survival in dust in which they may be carried to any situation. Some bacteria can thrive almost universally, others require very specialized nourishment. Most of them are harmless: some cause disease by accident, happening to fall into a wound where they find nourishing food; a few kinds must have living animal tissues to feed on and these may be dangerous to horses' lives because, as a by-product of their life processes, the bacteria create poisonous substances – toxins. The toxins are carried by the horse's blood stream all around the body and poison the animal's organs so that they cannot function properly. In some cases the horse may overcome these poisonous effects, in others the results are fatal.

Bacteria are present in large numbers both outside and inside the the horse's body: burrowed into the hair and skin, taken into the nose and lungs with the air the horse breathes, or swallowed with food and water. They do little damage on the skin unless they get into the hair follicles or the sweat glands where they may cause spots or pimples, but they can be dangerous if they reach fleshy tissues through cuts or wounds. The horse keeps its nose and lungs clear of bacteria by coughing them up or sneezing them away in mucous discharge, and the bacteria in the intestines are passed out with the droppings. Bacteria are especially attracted by the discharges from any injured tissues, flourishing in and around such conditions as a broken tooth, a gullet scratched from eating brambles, in intestinal ulcers caused by worms or in lungs damaged by migrating worm larvae.

Some types of bacteria are widespread, seizing any opportunity to gain access to a horse's tissues; others may crop up unexpectedly from time to time and cause an epidemic of disease, spreading from horse to horse in moist droplets in the breath or from shared food or water containers or by being carried on grooming kit.

Bacteria – identification Bacteria can be detected by selective staining, which shows them up on microscope slides prepared from animal tissues which they have penetrated and they can be identified by their size and shape. Bacteria may be cultivated on specially prepared nutritive jelly on which they form colonies like mould on jam. They can also be grown in broth. The varying appearances of the colonies on the jelly and chemical changes that they cause in the broth are also used as means of further identification.

Resistance to bacteria – anti-toxins When a horse is infected by bacteria and its blood stream is invaded by toxins, it counters the infection by attacking the bacteria with white blood corpuscles which engulf and digest the organisms, and it deals with the toxins by producing anti-toxins which are minute particles that unite with the toxins and render them harmless. The battle is on. If the white corpuscles and the anti-toxins can overwhelm the invaders, the horse will recover from the infection. If the invading bacteria can multiply faster than the horse can mop them up, then the horse may die of blood poisoning or of toxaemia.

Vaccination Vaccination is a means of stimulating the production of anti-toxins. The healthy horse is injected with bacteria that have been killed or treated to render them harmless. Toxins from these bacteria are sufficient to cause the horse's tissues to produce a supply of anti-toxins. If the horse is exposed to infection at a later date it already has anti-toxins mobilized which may give it such an advantage in overwhelming the invading organisms that they never establish themselves sufficiently to cause any sign of disease.

Treatment of bacterial infections Many bacteria in a horse's body can be suppressed or destroyed by sulphonamide or antibiotic drugs. These are of great value in the control of bacterial diseases but their use can upset a horse's digestion quite seriously if they destroy those bacteria which are helpfully processing the less digestible foodstuffs in the intestine.

Anti-serum is also helpful. This is serum from horses which have recovered from the disease or been vaccinated against it so that their blood is already stocked with a supply of antibodies. This anti-serum, injected into a sick horse, immediately neutralizes the disease toxins and reduces the effect of the disease for a period during which the horse can mobilize its own antibody defences.

Abscesses Abscesses are accumulations of white blood corpuscles assembled to attack and engulf bacteria which are infecting some part of the body. Some bacteria, staphylococci and streptococci, are especially likely to attract this attention. The white corpuscles gather in such large numbers that they form a swelling containing a thick creamy liquid which is pus. It is an advantage if the abscess can extend to the surface of the body and rupture and this can sometimes be encouraged by fomenting with hot cloths or by surgery. The pus discharges and carries with it most of the infecting bacteria. The remaining organisms are often swept out through the opening by the body fluids and the infection is overcome. Abscesses that burst inwards can cause severe illness, causing peritonitis if they discharge into the abdomen or septicaemia if they penetrate into a blood vessel.

Septicaemia and toxaemia In septicaemia bacteria actually enter and multiply in the blood stream, reaching it through cuts or wounds or being absorbed with food particles in the bowel. Since the blood circulates to all parts of the body septicaemia is usually a rapidly fatal disease because the bacteria produce their damaging and poisoning effects directly on the full range of tissues. Anthrax and haemorrhagic septicaemia are diseases that act in this way.

By contrast, tetanus and gas gangrene remain close to the site of infection and it is only their toxins that are carried around in the blood stream. If the bacteria can be dealt with, preventing further production of toxins, there is a much better chance of the animal's survival.

Viruses Viruses are particles of living matter that are parasitic on animals and plants. They are to be found in many body fluids and tissues but they are only able to multiply inside living cells. While bacteria measure around one thousandth of a millimetre, viruses measure one ten thousandth, or they may be as small as a hundred thousandth of a millimetre. They can only be examined by using an electron microscope which can produce screened images of the virus magnified a quarter of a million times.

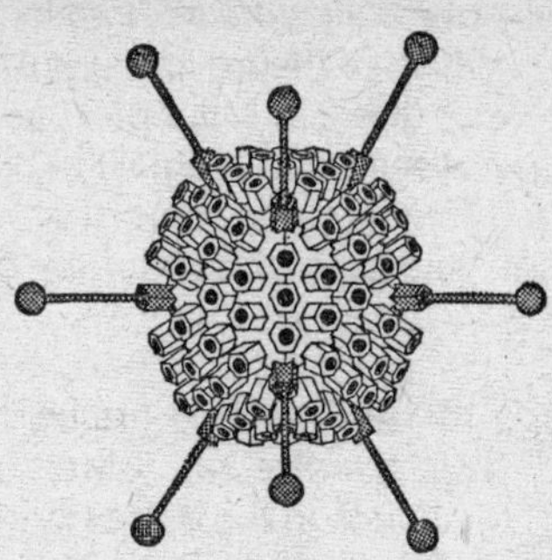

A virus

Virus diseases Over fifty varieties of virus have been recovered from horse tissues. Most of them are harmless to the horse but some, like bacteria, produce toxins that poison their host and give rise to signs of disease.

Horses deal with virus infections as they do with bacterial ones. The white blood corpuscles engulf and consume the viruses and the horse's tissues produce antitoxins to neutralise the toxins. If these activities are successful the horse recovers. Otherwise the toxins poison the horse's organs so that they cannot function properly and the horse does not survive. Vaccination of horses against influenza is widely used and has proved effective in preventing the spread of the disease in recent outbreaks.

Treatment of virus diseases Careful management and good nursing form the most important help that can be given to horses affected with a virus disease.

Viruses flourish and multiply inside the cells that make up the horse's tissues and organs, and antibiotic and sulphonamide drugs cannot be of direct help because if they penetrate in sufficient quantity into the cells to affect the viruses, they would kill the cells and, consequently, the horse. Virus diseases lower a horse's resistance to infection by bacterial diseases, so it is sometimes helpful to give a horse suffering from a virus illness injections of antibiotics, not to cure the virus disease, but to prevent secondary infection by bacteria.

Mycoplasma Mycoplasma are small organisms occupying a place in size and characteristics between the bacteria and the viruses, being about five thousandths of a millimetre in diameter.

A mycoplasm is the cause of pleuro-pneumonia in cattle, a highly infectious and often fatal disease. Mycoplasma are also associated with a number of other diseases in animals and birds but, although mycoplasma are found thriving in various organs in horses, they do not seem to be responsible for any conditions of disease in equine animals.

Brucellosis Horses with this infection are liable to go lame for no obvious cause and develop swollen joints or tendon sheaths. Persistent swelling of the bursa on the poll or swollen withers may be due to brucella infection. A laboratory test for antibodies in the blood is necessary for a firm diagnosis.

The bacterial infection by brucella abortus originates from cattle. It causes cows to abort and it is present in milk from infected animals. Human beings can become affected with brucellosis from drinking such milk and develop a disease known as undulant fever. Horses catch brucellosis from drinking milk or being in the field where a cow has aborted and coming into contact with the dead calf or its membranes. Brucellosis does not spread naturally from horse to horse, though discharges from wounds could be infectious and dressings should be disposed of carefully.

Antibiotic medication is helpful and treatment by vaccination to encourage antibody formation is sometimes successful. The course of brucella infection is always uncertain and there is a risk of a recurrence even in cases that appear to have made a complete recovery. Swollen joints or bursae suspected of being infected by brucellosis should not be opened. If they burst spontaneously they are more inclined to remain discharging persistently than to heal up.

Prevention by vaccination has been extensively used in cattle but has not been adopted for horses. A vigorous campaign of testing and slaughtering infected cattle is in its final stages in the United Kingdom and this will shortly remove most of the risk to horses.

Anthrax (*Bacillus anthracis*) Anthrax is a bacterial disease which occurs sporadically and is almost always fatal. Horses do not seem to be as susceptible to anthrax as cattle and sheep. The signs in horses are a high fever and either a violent colic or swelling around the throat so extensive that it causes suffocation. In both types of the disease the victims are unlikely to live for more than twelve hours from the first indications of illness. Cases occurring in Great Britain must be notified through the police to the Ministry of Agriculture, whose officials will supervise the proper and safe disposal of the bodies. Other countries have similar rules.

Anthrax bacteria are world-wide in their occurrence, being especially prevalent in the tropics where the disease frequently occurs in cattle and sheep with fatal results. The bodies are seldom burnt or buried but are disposed of by jackals and vultures. The bacteria left on the ground form themselves into spores which survive for many years, being remarkably resistant to destruction. The disease is contracted by animals eating anything containing these spores. The shipping of fertilizers and foodstuffs containing blood and bone meal, and hides and wool, some of which may be from animals killed by anthrax, is one way in which the infection may reach temperate lands. Cases also occur from animals that have died locally, whose bodies have not been disposed of correctly. Some pieces of land are known to be infective and give rise to fresh cases if precautions are forgotten. There is no satisfactory method of rendering these places safe.

If a case of anthrax does occur it is almost certain to be fatal but in-contact animals or others at risk may be saved if they are treated with anthrax serum, penicillin and sulphathiazole as soon as, or preferably before, a rise in temperature is observed. An anti-anthrax vaccine is also available but its protection takes several days to develop.

Tetanus The signs of tetanus in horses are an increasing stiffness of movement that progresses until the limbs are rigid, the head poked forward and the tail raised. If a hand is placed under the horse's jaw and the head forced up, the third eyelid extends from the inner corner of the eye to cover half the eyeball. Horses that progress within twenty-four hours from the first signs of stiffness to such rigidity that they cannot be persuaded to move at all are not likely to recover. Those in which the onset is slower have a good hope of recovery. With such help as can be given the chances of survival are about fifty per cent.

Tetanus cases are best moved to a dark box or stable where they are not likely to be disturbed. The muscles are in a state of spasmodic contraction but they relax a little in peaceful surroundings. Quietness is essential, because each time somebody shouts or a door bangs the muscles are set off into a new series of spasms. The jaws are likely to be clamped shut, which gives the disease the name lockjaw, so sloppy mashes and drinking water should be placed at a level where the horse can put its muzzle in the bucket or a shallow vessel and sup up some nourishment and liquid through the side of its lips. Sedative and muscular relaxant drugs and tetanus anti-serum at intervals will aid in recovery and anti-biotics are also needed. Horses that get down on the floor should be left for a few hours before being disturbed if they are lying comfortably in the usual resting position or fully stretched out. After three hours they should be encouraged to get up or, if that is beyond their ability, they should be turned on to the other side by attaching ropes to the pasterns and pulling them over. It is more likely that horses that get down will lie on their side with the legs stiffly projected like a wooden toy. Such cases are serious but they would have a better chance on their feet and may have to be raised with professional help in slings after they have been given sedatives to reduce their awkward struggling while being lifted. The longer a tetanus case can be kept alive the better the chance of recovery. This is a slow process but any sign of improvement may be considered hopeful. Recovering cases very gradually relax their contracted muscles. Horses that are unable to take any food or water should be given thin nourishing gruel by stomach tube. When a case of this sort is able to drink for itself recovery is almost assured, though it may be a couple of months before normal activity is restored. Horses that recover do so completely.

The cause of tetanus is a bacillus, *Clostridium tetani*, which lives in soil and thrives in horse manure. The disease occurs when the organism gets into the horse's body tissues through a wound. Clostridium tetani thrives best away from air, so the wounds most likely to be favourable to its development are deep punctured ones, such as might be caused by barbed wire or a nail, where the dirt containing the germs is tucked away from any access to fresh air. Wounds around the feet are a likely way of admitting the disease as the feet are naturally in close contact with soil and horse droppings. Sometimes no wound is found. In these cases the tetanus germs may have entered the horse's system from the bowel, where they are present in large numbers, harmless until some worm damage or ulcer in the wall of the intestine allows them access to the horse's tissues. If a wound is discovered it should be washed with antiseptic solutions. The vet may open it further to ensure cleanliness and drainage.

Every horse should be vaccinated annually with a vaccine, tetanus toxoid, which creates anti-bodies ready to deal with any tetanus infection. Toxoid takes some days to stimulate any reaction and so, if an unvaccinated horse suffers any wound, however small, it should be given an immediate injection of tetanus serum which already contains the necessary antibodies. The effect lasts two or three weeks. However as horses are constantly cutting or injuring themselves they would need frequent injections of tetanus serum. It is safer to use an annual tetanus toxoid injection to cover all eventualities.

Gas gangrene Gas gangrene is the result of wound infection. It is caused by bacteria of the clostridium group (*Clostridium chauvei, Clostridium oedamatiens, Clostridium septique,* and *Clostridium welchii*), all of which live in soil and thrive and multiply in animal tissues. The name gas gangrene comes from the ability of these bacteria to produce gas causing the affected area to swell enormously. The gas penetrates under the skin so that the part creaks and crackles if pressed. The bacteria remain in the affected muscle, not usually spreading through the body, but their toxins are taken up by the blood stream and poison the horse's system. The disease is also called black-quarter and quarter-ill, because the affected area of muscle is infiltrated and stained with black clots of blood. One of the hind quarters is the usual site of infection, though it may appear on any part of the body.

The disease is insidious in onset and develops so rapidly that a horse may just be found dead with a very swollen limb. Cases detected early should be treated with antibiotics. Sheep and cattle are very susceptible to gas gangrene and are frequently vaccinated routinely against this infection. The disease is not common in horses but vaccination should be carried out if gas gangrene appears to be prevalent in a particular area.

Prevention is by absolute cleanliness of surgical methods and the careful treatment of accidental wounds, especially if they are deep or pocketed. The clostridium bacteria multiply best without oxygen. In deep wounds they are tucked away from the air. In pocket wounds, those without drainage, the oxygen is used up by other bacteria. If drainage is established these bacteria are washed away with the discharges and the conditions are not so favouable for gas gangrene to develop. Antibiotic injections to prevent infection developing are frequently used when horses are operated on surgically or are suffering from wounds.

Haemorrhagic septicaemia Haemorrhagic septicaemia is a bacterial disease caused by *Pasteurella multicida*, an organism present in richly cultivated soil in various parts of Europe, Africa, Asia and America. Infection is usually from food or from drinking contaminated water. Once the bacteria have gained access to the horse's tissues through the bowel wall or by wounds they multiply rapidly in the blood stream and are carried to all parts of the body, poisoning the tissues with their toxins.

Signs of the disease are a very high temperature, up to 42°C (108°F), very rapid heart rate and breathing rate, complete loss of appetite, and collapse. Swellings may occur under the jaw and along the belly. Death follows in three or four days after the first onset.

Treatment is by antibiotics, but the rapid onset of the disease and its almost immediate spread to all parts rate the chances of success as slender. Vaccination against this disease is practised but, up to the present, there are grave risks that vaccination may actually produce the disease in a high proportion of cases.

Improved hygiene, especially by ensuring that the horses are supplied with clean water to drink, seems to give most hope for reducing the incidence of this disease.

Vesicular stomatitis Vesicular stomatitis is a virus disease occurring only in the Americas. It produces inflammation and watery blisters in the mouth and on the tongue of horses and donkeys causing them to go off their feed and drip saliva from their mouths. The disease is not a serious one though it is very infectious, spreading by the bites of flies or through food or drink contaminated by saliva. Treatment is not usually necessary. A swab soaked in dilute hydrogen peroxide may be used to wipe discharges and foodstuff from the ulcers in the mouth. Recovery is usually complete in less than a week.

Vesicular stomatitis is of interest because of its similarity to foot and mouth disease. Horses do not suffer from foot and mouth disease, but both vesicular stomatitis and foot and mouth disease affect cattle and pigs and both cause blisters in the mouth and around the feet. It is urgently necessary to know which disease it is, as an outbreak of foot and mouth disease requires the speedy application of control by vaccination or by slaughter and quarantine, while vesicular stomatitis is not serious. Laboratories can now give an accurate diagnosis. Before laboratory help became generally available if cattle or pigs developed mouth blisters some of the discharge from the blisters was rubbed on a horse's tongue. If the horse went off its food and developed blisters in a day or two the diagnosis was vesicular stomatitis but if the horse, not susceptible to foot and mouth disease, continued to eat and remained healthy, the diagnosis was foot and mouth disease. Laboratory tests are more dependable.

Human beings can be infected from horses or other animals with vesicular stomatitis. There are no mouth blisters, only the symptoms of a mild attack of influenza that pass off in a day or two.

Tuberculosis Tuberculosis is a bacterial disease which particularly affects the abdominal organs, appearing as abscesses in the lymphatic glands and notably in the spleen. The source of infection is likely to be cow's milk given as a supplementary food to foals and yearlings. Signs of the disease, which may not appear for several years, are a gradual loss of energy and condition, with slight rises of temperature from time to time. The skin loses its bloom and becomes hidebound. The neck bones are liable to be involved in a tubercular arthritis and horses affected in this way turn stiffly and show signs of pain if the head is forced round towards the saddle. A definite diagnosis is difficult to establish as the skin test for this disease, most accurate in cattle, is difficult to interpret in horses. Sometimes the abscesses on the spleen can be felt by making a rectal exploration. Although streptomycin and other drugs are successful in treating tuberculosis in humans, the disease is always too far advanced in horses before it is diagnosed for any current treatment to arrest it and destruction is the only sensible course. In some cases a tubercular abscess opens into the blood stream so that the bacteria are carried to the lungs giving rise to innumerable small abscesses. These cases are rapidly fatal.

Tuberculosis is, fortunately, becoming rare because national campaigns to eliminate the disease from cattle have achieved an extremely high rate of success. Tuberculosis in horses is now only a problem in those countries which do not regularly tuberculin test their cattle.

African horse sickness African horse sickness is caused by a reovirus and is spread by night-flying biting insects. The disease is constantly present in central and southern Africa and periodically spreads to North Africa and Middle Eastern countries. In 1966 cases occurred in Spain but did not reach any other part of Europe. Horses and mules are very susceptible to the disease while donkeys are rarely affected.

Signs of horse sickness appear about a week after infection. In most cases the disease is rapidly fatal. It appears in two forms, one drowning the lungs with fluids, the other causing swelling of the fore quarters. In the lung condition breathing becomes rapid with coughing and a frothy discharge from the nostrils. The temperature rises to 40.5 to 41.5°C (105 to 106°F) and the animal collapses and dies, often within twelve hours of the onset of the illness. The swollen form is less acute: the temperature rises to 40°C (104°F), the mouth and eye membranes become inflamed and swellings appear on either side of the forehead. These swellings spread over the face and down the neck to the forelegs. Breathing becomes rapid and death may occur within a few days of onset. In both types of the disease the horses continue to feed until they collapse.

In the past, in affected countries, locally bred horses were not so severely affected as imported horses and some local horses survived infection by horse sickness. This rendered them immune to further attacks. They were known as salted horses and were highly valued. Nowadays vaccination provides an excellent protection and this is routinely applied in affected areas.

Encephalitis There are several arborviruses that cause encephalitis, an inflammation of the brain, in horses. The signs of the disease are unusual excitement, irregular movements and a high temperature which continues until death, except in those few animals which throw off the disease, although their recovery is seldom complete. The later stages of encephalitis are characterized by loss of sight, partial or complete paralysis and a lapse into unconsciousness. Large doses of anti-serum are the only remedy but prior vaccination in areas where these diseases are liable to occur has been found to give good protection.

Some arborviruses live in a harmless state in birds from which they are spread, by biting insects, to horses. The disease occurs in the Central American countries from infection by the Eastern, Western and Venezuelan encephalitis viruses; in Australia from Murray River virus; in the Near East from the West Nile virus, which is spread by ticks; and in Japan from a Japanese virus which is spread from humans to horses by insect bites. This disease is a mild complaint for people but a fatal disease in horses.

Changes in environmental conditions favourable to the viruses cause epidemics from time to time. In Japan, 4,000 horses died of encephalitis in 1949. Over half the equine population there is now regularly vaccinated and this has brought the annual average death rate down to two or three horses. In 1970, 6,000 horses died in Mexico – but that outbreak was also rapidly brought under control by vaccination. Serum and vaccine would be readily available to deal with any epidemic of this disease that might occur, through the veterinary section of the Food and Agriculture Organization of the United Nations, which constantly monitors infectious diseases of animals throughout the world.

Infectious anaemia (swamp fever) Infectious anaemia, which only occurs in horses, is caused by a virus of the oncorna group. It is spread by biting insects. The disease may appear in any part of the world where there are marshy and wooded areas supporting a large insect population. Horses imported into the British Isles have been found to be infected with swamp fever but there is no record of any transmission from them to other horses.

Infectious anaemia cases lose their alertness, tire very easily, so that they stagger at the least exertion, and are found to have a high temperature that may reach 41.5°C (106°F). The membranes of the mouth and eyes become yellow or bronzed and are marked with numerous blood spots. The heart beats very fast and quite irregularly, the legs fill below the knees and hocks and swellings appear on the belly. Some affected horses rapidly become worse and their death occurs within one or two weeks of the first signs of illness. Other cases recover from this first attack but relapse at intervals and at this stage the horses show extreme pallor from anaemia, and further deaths occur. Those that survive may appear to recover completely but they become carriers and infection can be spread from them to other horses by biting insects especially in the summer and autumn. The disease is also easily spread by hypodermic needles. A disposable syringe and needle should be used each time a horse is given any injection.

There is no treatment for infectious anaemia. Diagnosis of the disease can be confirmed by a laboratory test on a sample of blood. The disease is so persistent in carriers and so readily spread that affected horses must be destroyed. Vaccination has not been found to produce a satisfactory resistance. Control can only be by draining marshy land to reduce the insect population and by fly-proofing the stables.

Trypanosomiasis Trypanosomes are single-celled animals that live in the blood stream causing anaemia and wasting. Various types of trypanosomes are distributed in the world's tropical regions

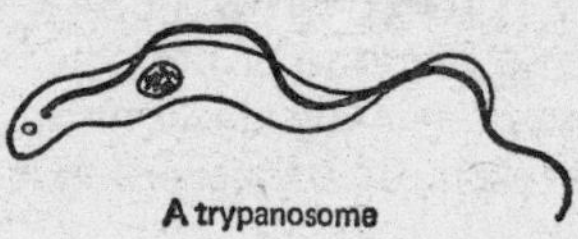

A trypanosome

causing sleeping sickness in man and a number of diseases in animals. Wild animals are often infected without showing signs of disease but severe and often fatal anaemia is caused when the trypanosomes are spread by biting flies to man or to domestic animals. Trypanosomes cause surra, mal de Caderas and dourine in horses. This last disease is exceptional in that the infection is spread, not by biting flies, but from horse to horse during the sexual act.

Trypanosomiasis (surra) Surra is a tropical disease, not unlike malaria, that is caused by a blood parasite, *Trypanosoma evansi*. It is found in the blood of cattle, pigs and buffalo in which it seldom causes disease, but when spread by biting flies to camels, horses, mules or dogs it causes serious anaemia, wasting and frequently the animal's death. Diagnosis is by laboratory examination of blood in which the trypanosomes may be identified.

Treatment is by injections of specific trypanocides. In many parts of the tropics susceptible animals cannot be used because of this disease or they can only be worked seasonally. Camels, which carry out a lot of heavy transport work in the northern Indian plains for eight months of the year have to be moved up into the hills 960 km (600 miles) away for the four months of the rainy season when insects are active. Horses require to be stabled behind fly-proof screens during the same period.

Piroplasmosis Piroplasms are minute single-celled animals occurring in red corpuscles of the blood, particularly in those corpuscles retained in the spleen. Two species are found in horses' blood: *Babesia equi*, which multiplies in the corpuscles by dividing into four pear-shaped parasites, and *Babesia caballi*, which divides into two before transferring to other blood corpuscles.

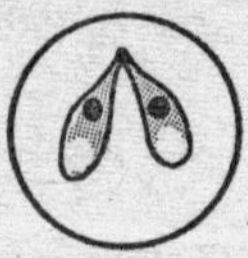

Babesia in a blood corpuscle

Babesiosis (biliary fever) The piroplasmosis of horses, babesiosis, is spread from animal to animal by the bites of ticks. Infection is widespread in many parts of the world, up to fifty per cent of the horse population being found to be affected in parts of India, but the great majority of native animals show no signs of disease. Horses imported from areas free of babesiosis may, when they become infected, suffer acutely from anaemia, diarrhoea, body and leg swellings, a low temperature, collapse, and death. In its milder form the chief indications are anaemia, fever, and a deterioration in condition. Babesia parasites are occasionally found in the blood of horses in the British Isles.

Diagnosis of babesiosis is by seeing the parasites in the blood cells under microscopic examination or by a simple laboratory serum test. Control is by hand dressing horses to keep them free of ticks or by the avoidance of tick infested pastures. In clinical cases rest is essential and treatment is by injections based on quinine derivatives.

Rabies Rabies is a virus disease liable to affect human beings and all warm-blooded animals including horses. Foxes and other wild creatures are the most common carriers of the disease, which is spread in their saliva – usually by means of a bite. Since the time of Pasteur it has been known that any animal showing signs of rabies is certain to die: but it is also known that the signs may not appear for as long as two years after exposure to the disease. Vaccination against rabies is available and the development of the disease is so slow that, if a person has been bitten or has come into contact with an animal suspected of carrying rabies, there is plenty of time for a course of vaccine to be given, almost always with success.

The horse is as susceptible to rabies as any other animal. The first sign of the disease is a marked change of temperament. This may be followed by colic or lameness, progressing in one or two days to total recumbency. The prudent owner who lives in a rabies infected area will not investigate strange illness too closely. He will remove all other livestock and, without taking risks, try to confine the horse in an escape proof area and place further responsibility on his vet. As rabies develops the horse becomes agitated and paddles with all four feet. Some cases, not recumbent, become uncontrollable, kicking and biting anything within reach and damaging themselves recklessly. Mercifully, death then follows within a few hours, less than a week after the first indication of illness.

The cause of death should be checked by a laboratory examination of the animal's brain and if rabies is confirmed care must be taken to ensure that any human beings who may possibly have been infected by the horse are vaccinated, while other animals at risk will be dealt with by the veterinary authorities of the country concerned.

It is interesting that Britain, at present free from rabies, insists that imported small animals should spend six months in quarantine, while horses, equally susceptible to rabies, are allowed in from countries where rabies exists without any precautions against introducing this disease. It is not that the horse industry, being a multi-million dollar international one, is using undue influence; but simply that while small animals are frequently responsible for fresh outbreaks of rabies, horses are so constantly under control and observation that there has never been an outbreak of this disease attributable to spread by horses even in countries where rabies is rampant.

Serum hepatitis – cause unknown Horses with serum hepatitis, a liver inflammation, go off their food and appear dejected. The membranes of the eyes and mouth become tinged yellow with jaundice and a number of minute blood spots may be seen on them. Within a day or two the animal becomes distressed, breaks out into sweating and moves with difficulty. The pulse is usually fast, over eighty to the minute, and the temperature below normal. Most cases end with collapse and death due to severe damage to cells in the liver.

Serum hepatitis can be caused by the injection of medicines containing horse serum if the serum was from a horse with this disease. Pharmaceutical houses take infinite care to avoid this risk but it remains a possibility. The disease can also be spread from an infected horse to others by biting flies or by hypodermic needles which is one of the reasons why veterinary surgeons use disposable syringes and needles.

Serum hepatitis is thought to be due to a virus but, as yet, the cause has not been isolated or identified.

Not all cases of hepatitis, resulting in inflammation of the liver and jaundice, are necessarily due to this serum infection. Similar illnesses may be caused by parasites in the liver or by the horse eating quantities of the plant, ragwort.

Grass sickness – cause unknown Grass sickness is a disease of horses which is nearly always fatal. It is met with in spring and summer among horses turned out to grass, as is suggested by the name. The disease is thought to kill about 200 horses each year, mostly in eastern and central Scotland, but its occurrence is widespread in Great Britain. Grass sickness also occurs in Scandinavian countries and there have been a few cases reported from Normandy.

Signs of grass sickness are extreme depression, very inflamed membranes around the mouth and eyes, difficulty in swallowing and a complete cessation of bowel activity. Some food and water is swallowed but cannot reach the intestines. A tube passed down the gullet may recover several gallons of fluid held under pressure in the stomach. Breathing is accompanied by a loud snoring sound and the breath becomes foul smelling. Saliva accumulates and dribbles from the mouth, and green slime runs from the nostrils.

The abdomen is drawn up and the horse becomes herring gutted. No droppings are passed. Manual exploration of the rectum reveals hard packed masses of foodstuff in the large bowel. The membranes in the rectum are dried up and so sticky that the plastic sleeve the operator is wearing while making a rectal examination is liable to be retained when he withdraws his hand. Horses affected with grass sickness rarely show any signs of pain.

Acute cases of this disease may die a few hours after the first signs of illness. Others may survive for a few days or, if they have not been destroyed on humane grounds, sometimes for weeks before they die from starvation and exhaustion. A few horses are known to have survived the disease but only as useless shadows of their former selves.

There is no treatment for grass sickness. Investigations suggest that horses are less likely to become affected if they are brought in from pasture daily and fed in the stable for a few hours. The significant point seems to be that their grazing and concentrate feeding should be supplemented by several pounds of hay each day. This may deter them from grazing close to the ground and eating dead stalks and earth which are a possible source of this disease.

8 Respiratory diseases

Sinusitis Sinusitis is due to abscesses developing in the hollow bones of the face which extend from below the eyes to above the front molar tooth. They become infected from diseases of the nose or throat, from accidental injury or from a diseased tooth root. The condition is recognized by the discharge of creamy pus usually from only one nostril. The bones below the eye on the affected side may be swollen and tender.

Treatment by antibiotics and sulphonamides is not usually effective unless the abscesses can be drained by making openings in the bones of the face from which the pus can escape. Two holes are usually made so that the abscesses can be flushed out with antiseptic solution syringed into an upper opening and draining out by a lower one. The openings in the facial bones heal up rapidly when the treatment is completed. A thick ointment smeared on the face prevents the discharges scalding the skin and stripping off the hair. In some cases satisfactory drainage may only be established by removing a molar tooth. If the sinusitis is caused by a diseased tooth this operation is essential. It is described in the section dealing with dentistry.

Nose bleeding Nose bleeding occurs occasionally in horses during or after fast galloping. It may even happen to a horse resting in the stable. There are three known causes: bronchitis, a blood vessel tumour in the nose, and ulceration in the guttural pouch (see below).

In the early stages of broken-wind, which is a form of chronic bronchitis, the horse may not show the contraction of the abdominal muscles towards the end of each breath that calls attention to the disease so that it may not be known that the lungs are diseased. In this state a number of the air vesicles in the lungs are blocked with discharges and are put out of use. If the horse is then galloped putting unusual demands on the lungs, some of these shut-down vesicles are torn open with a loss of blood which is later coughed up and appears as blood-stained mucus trickling from the nostrils. If such horses are put to the extreme effort of racing a considerable amount of blood may be blown in froth from the nostrils during the race. They require treatment as broken-winded cases.

At the back of the nostrils are the turbinate bones which consist of thin plates of bone covered with a membrane well supplied with masses of blood vessels. This arrangement exposes a large area to act as a radiator and warm the air on its way to the lungs. An overgrowth or tumour of the blood vessels in this part can occur and bleeding may result from some shock which can vary from a sudden sneeze to a fall while racing. Bleeding is likely to be copious and prolonged. There is no treatment for this condition and there are considerable risks of severe haemorrhage at any time.

A cavity, the guttural pouch, extends from each side inside the throat to below the ear. A fungus infection is liable to occur in these pouches causing ulceration which may extend so deeply that a large and thinly covered blood vessel is ruptured. This mishap may occur without being triggered off by an accident or extreme effort. In some cases the horse bleeds to death immediately. In those which have survived it is possible to ligature the artery that is at risk. This has the effect of closing down that blood vessel and its functions are able to be taken over by other arteries. The fungus infection must also be treated.

First aid for horses that are bleeding from the nose is to confine the patient in a quiet area. Applying cold water swabs or injecting blood clotting agents are not likely to be helpful. Plugging the nostrils will cause the blood to flow into the lungs and drown the animal. The only course is to keep the horse absolutely quiet and wait for the bleeding to stop of its own accord. All is not over if it collapses on to the ground from loss of blood. The blood clots more readily as the quantity is depleted and, with the horse recumbent, there is a beneficial lowering of the blood pressure. No attempts should be made to persuade the horse to get up until it does so in its own good time.

Horses which suffer periodically from some minor nose bleeding appear to be helped by an injection, during the day preceding some special effort, of a 1 in 1,000 solution of adrenalin or by the injection of the diuretic, frusemide.

Soft palate disease – choking-up – 'tongue swallowing' When galloping fast some horses suddenly check in their stride, at the same time making a gurgling noise in the throat. In a few moments they recover and are able to continue their activity but in competitive events they have fallen well behind.

This trouble is not due to 'tongue swallowing' as was thought at one time but has been traced to the edge of the soft palate which is a membrane concerned with directing air from the nostrils into the larynx. If this membrane is slack it vibrates, causing the gurgling noise, and obstructs the air flow. As the lungs become short of air the horse gasps and slows up.

The lack of tension in the soft palate can be overcome in several ways. Some horses recover spontaneously from the condition as their fitness improves. Many persistent cases have been successfully treated by the surgical removal of a piece of the edge of the soft palate or by injecting substances into it that cause scarring. Both these treatments increase the soft palate's tension. An operation to shorten muscles on the front of the neck alters the positioning of the larynx in relation to the soft palate and this has been found to overcome the obstruction to the air flow in a number of cases.

Roaring and whistling (laryngeal paralysis) This disease is known as 'sawing' in French, an apt name as the noise made by affected horses closely resembles the intermittent rasping of a hand-saw. Horses affected by roaring or whistling make this rasping noise during the intake of each breath. The noise is caused by the left vocal cord which is paralysed and flaps loosely in the larynx instead of being drawn to the side to allow the air a clear passage on its way to the lungs. The distinction between roaring and whistling is only a matter of degree, whistling sometimes altering to the louder roar. The noise is heard most clearly when the horse is cantering or galloping and is most obvious if the animal is worked with the chin pulled in to the neck on a tight rein.

Roaring or whistling is most common in light horses over 15 hands high that have worked for 2 or 3 or even more years. The nerve controlling the left vocal cord takes a long and rather unexpected route from the spinal cord to the larynx, actually passing around the base of the heart, while the nerve on the right hand side which is not involved in this disease runs by a much shorter and direct route. It is thought probable that the left nerve in these bigger horses becomes stretched or damaged during their growth and activity and gives rise to the paralysis. Roaring and whistling are listed as hereditary diseases by the British Ministry of Agriculture.

Horses do not recover from this paralysis. Whistlers may continue to make a slight noise or they may slowly or rapidly change to roaring. The disease does not interfere with ordinary activities but it restricts air intake and causes affected horses to be short of breath when they are asked to exert themselves. The noise is also objectionable because it publicly announces the disability.

Hobdaying The most frequent treatment of roaring and whistling is by an operation, ventriculectomy, devised by Williams of New York and modified by Hobday of London. In this operation the offending vocal cord is bound permanently to the side of the larynx leaving the passage uninterrupted for the flow of air. Hobdaying is satisfactory in many cases but the claims of success, based on performance, seldom exceed 50% greatly improved, 25% improved and 25% no change, with somewhat similar figures for a reduction in the noise produced.

Tubing (*tracheotomy*) Another operation for dealing with whistlers or roarers is to insert a tube into the wind-pipe or trachea, a short distance below the larynx. The tube allows air directly into the trachea through an opening about 3 cm ($1\frac{1}{4}$ in) in diameter, so that there is no shortage of air available for the lungs in spite of the obstruction in the larynx above. The tube has a stopper which is kept in place, except when the horse is being worked, to prevent dust, foodstuffs or water getting to the lungs.

This method is extremely successful and completely overcomes the impediment. Unfortunately there are objectionable features. The tube irritates the skin and the windpipe and there are often discharges that require frequent attention to the operation site: in spite of mechanical ingenuity the horse may lose or get rid of the tube and, if worn for long periods, it may cause inflammation and growths on the rings of cartilage that form the trachea. For these reasons the tube is removed when the horse's seasonal activities are over and the hole in the neck closes up by scarring so that, for the next season, another operation has to be carried out lower down the neck. As a short term aid to performance tubing is excellent but in the long term the disadvantages are serious.

Strangles Strangles is an infectious bacterial disease, caused by *Streptococcus equi*, which only affects equines. The first signs are a creamy discharge from the nose and a raised temperature soon followed by swelling of the glands around the throat and under the jaw. The horse goes off its food, partly because of the illness and also because swallowing, especially dry food, is painful. In a week or ten days the abscesses burst and discharge quantities of yellow pus. The animal then rapidly recovers its appetite and the temperature returns to normal.

Treatment consists of rest from work, feeding with easily swallowed food such as grass and sloppy mashes, and fomenting the throat with cloths wrung out in hot water to hasten the ripening of the abscesses.

It is advisable to let the disease take its normal course. Antibiotics interfere with the ripening of the abscesses so that they are unable to discharge and may enlarge to cause greater pressure on the throat and a dangerous prolongation of the disease. In an outbreak of strangles antibiotics may be useful to prevent the disease spreading to in-contact horses if given to them before they show signs of the disease.

In some cases, strangles abscesses occur not only in the throat but in the lungs or abdominal organs and such cases are extremely difficult to detect and require the most expert treatment if they are to survive.

Strangles used to be a disease almost entirely confined to young horses because the older ones had been infected in their youth and were immune. Any young horse going through a dealer's yard caught strangles as a matter of course. Strangles became less common in Britain in the 1930s and 1940s and about 1950 it disappeared altogether. It has now returned and since few horses have immunity to the disease from an earlier attack, it affects old and young indiscriminately.

Vaccines against strangles used to be obtainable but there was some doubt as to their value. The outbreaks of this disease are not frequent enough at present to warrant vaccine production and use.

Coughing Horses cough occasionally when a morsel of food catches in the throat, and at exercise they may give a cough to clear their air passages and follow it up with a good snort through their nostrils. This is healthy coughing.

Horses that develop an intermittent or a persistent cough require attention. Coughing is nearly always caused by unusual quantities of mucus being brought up from the lungs because they are inflamed. If the cough is considered to be due to a slight cold, which is a virus infection, the horse should at least be rested until the cough and the accompanying runny nose have cleared up. If the horse is off its feed and its temperature is above 38°C (101°F) the cough is likely to be an indication of influenza, virus cough, or pneumonia. If the horse is eating reasonably and the temperature is normal but coughing persists it may be due to broken-wind or a lung worm infection. Giving cough medicines or cough electuary will not cure any of these diseases. The coughing should be investigated and suitable treatment arranged. Coughing horses should never be sent out to work, as exercise is likely to throw further strain on the already diseased lungs and may have damaging consequences on the heart.

Influenza Influenza is a disease of horses caused by a virus infection. Epidemics of equine influenza periodically sweep through the horse populations of countries or continents. In the intervals small outbreaks occur from time to time until, after a few years, conditions occur which are favourable to produce another epidemic. When it occurs in a stable it may spread to every horse within forty-eight hours.

Affected horses first develop a temperature up to 40°C (104°F), then they go off their feed, develop a runny nose and a moist cough. The eyes may also discharge tears down the face. The lungs are inflamed and the rate of breathing is increased, which is especially noticeable if the horses are exercised.

Treatment of influenza cases is by rest and careful management. Horses on rations suitable for hard work should have their feeds reduced and should be put on to a laxative diet, kept warm and allowed plenty of fresh air. In a few days the appetite returns, the temperature falls to normal, the cough and nasal discharge decline and in 10 to 14 days from the first sign of disease the horse appears to have recovered. It must be remembered that the lungs have been damaged. Putting such horses back to strong work may cause such strains on the lungs and heart that permanent injury is done and in some cases they may die of heart failure. At least a month of quiet exercise is required followed by another month of increasing work before any strenuous tasks are undertaken.

All cases of influenza do not react by recovering in two weeks. Virus infections always lower a horse's resistance to bacterial disease. While a horse is suffering from the influenza virus, a bacterial infection may occur. The chief indication of this is that the temperature, instead of falling nearer to normal each day, begins to rise again. The horse will show continuing signs of illness and the cough and rapid breathing may both increase. Such cases require even more careful attention and nursing. They are likely to respond satisfactorily to treatment by antibiotics.

Veterinary advice in a stable may be that any horse affected with influenza should be given antibiotic treatment to avoid the risk of secondary infection by bacteria. The particular circumstances will decide if this is required and which of the many antibiotics is most suitable.

Vaccination against equine influenza is extremely satisfactory. A dose of vaccine is given, followed by a second dose in two months' time and an annual booster is required. Stables that have adopted this method have either escaped infection altogether in an outbreak or have had a case or two in a very mild form of the disease. Horses that race internationally are only allowed to travel from country to country if they have documents showing them to be properly vaccinated against equine influenza.

Virus coughing (rhino-pneunmonitis) There are several viruses, in addition to the influenza virus, that cause coughing in horses. The most widespread virus causes a disease known as rhino-pneunmonitis. The signs of this infection are not as striking as those of influenza. In rhino-pneunmonitis cases there is a moist cough and some running at the nose. The appetite and temperature are not noticeably affected. The lungs are slightly inflamed and, consequently, the horse does not work as well as usual. If affected horses are rested they lose the cough and nasal discharge in a week or ten days but their lungs take longer to recover and may suffer serious damage if the horses are put back to work too soon.

Rhino-pneunmonitis is difficult to detect. Sometimes the only reason to suspect its presence is that the horse loses some ability and this diagnosis can be confirmed by laboratory findings of antibodies to this disease in blood from the horse.

Vaccination is of little value as its effects only last for a few weeks. The horse's own natural resistance to the disease is equally transient and an animal which has recovered from rhino-pneunmonitis may catch it again in 2 or 3 months' time. In a large stable the infection may be constantly passing from horse to horse.

Rhino-pneunmonitis has occasionally, but only occasionally, been found to be responsible for mares at stud developing a partial paralysis and aborting their foals.

The most satisfactory way of avoiding infections by the rhino-pneunmonitis virus is adequate ventilation and plenty of fresh air. The virus flourishes where horses are kept together in large numbers especially if the stables are poorly ventilated. Small numbers of horses kept largely in the open air are not likely to be affected by this particularly difficult disease.

Pneumonia Pneumonia is the name given to inflammation of the lungs. It is caused by infectious organisms, streptococci, viruses and fungi or by fluids, such as medicines, accidentally passing down the windpipe and inflaming the lungs. Pneumonia may affect only part of the lungs spreading from bronchitis, broken-wind, nasal catarrh, glanders, or lung-worm – or the whole of the lung tissues may be inflamed in cases of acute infection.

The signs of pneumonia are coughing, an increased rate of breathing, and a high temperature. The inflamed lung tissues produce discharges which make the breathing sounds louder as the air forces its way through them and coughing is caused as they are brought up and discharged from the trachea. Later the inflammation may produce so much congestion of blood in the small vessels and discharges in the lung tissue that air cannot penetrate and no breathing sounds at all can be heard from that part of the lung.

Horses with any degree of pneumonia must be rested. Even gentle exercise is liable to spread infection in the lungs. Easily digested green food, soft hay and warm mashes should be fed. Water and ample fresh air should be available and rugs may be needed for warmth. Pneumonia cases always need veterinary attention. Medication with antibiotics is usually helpful but it will have little effect if the disease is due to a virus infection. If the pneumonia is a complication of some other condition, that will also need to be treated.

The horse's own powers of resistance to disease can be helped by good management and careful nursing which consists of encouraging the animals to eat and keeping the stable clean, warm and comfortable. Cases that are accompanied by a harsh cough may be relieved by steam inhalation. A steam kettle may be boiled for half an hour four or five times a day near the horse's head or a kettle of boiling water may be poured over a bucket of hay placed under the horse's head. Surrounding the head and the bucket with a light sheet gives a higher concentration of steam. A teaspoonful of turpentine, oil of eucalyptus or Friar's Balsam may be added if advised but these may cause the horse to be less cooperative. The really beneficial effect is from the steam. Oxygen is sometimes a life-saver in dealing with pneumonia in foals and it can be equally helpful in dealing with the disease in older animals. It needs to be led to a funnel held loosely over the animal's nostrils in spells of 15 minutes on and 15 minutes off for several hours to be of significant value.

Convalescence after pneumonia must be a long process to allow the lungs and the heart to recover from the serious strains they have suffered.

Hypostatic pneumonia is an accumulation of blood in the lower part of the lungs in recumbent horses. The blood cannot be driven on because the horse is not able to help the circulation by its usual frequent changes of position.

A horse lying on one side because of injury or illness or because it is cast is likely to develop hypostatic pneumonia in the lower lung after only a few hours. That lung gradually drowns in the steadily mounting mass of blood. Recumbent horses should be turned on to the other side at hourly intervals to prevent hypostatic pneumonia developing. Whenever possible they should be encouraged to stand up and it may be necessary to support some cases in slings.

Broken-wind Broken-wind is a form of bronchitis caused by dust irritating the minute air pockets deep in the lungs. The small air tubes in the lungs become blocked with discharges. The condition has now been given the descriptive name chronic obstructive pulmonary disease (COPD). This process continues until the lung becomes so inefficient that the horse can only obtain sufficient oxygen to keep itself alive by forced breathing, that is, helping the lungs to contract by bringing its abdominal and flank muscles into play each time it breathes out. This gives a double expiration : the normal chest contraction followed by muscle contraction in the flank.

Other signs of broken-wind are a deep cough, well described as a 'churchyard cough', and thick creamy discharge brought up from the lungs and coughed out of the mouth or down the nostrils. If the top half of the stable door is open these discharges are often splashed on to the ground outside.

The above is a description of an advanced case of broken-wind. In the early stages there is an occasional but persisting deep cough and a falling off in performance. The double breathing action may be seen after exertion and the stethoscope may detect crackling sounds at the edges of the lungs.

Not all dust produces this disease. It must have mould or fungus spores in it to cause the particular irritation in the lungs. These spores come from hay or straw. Damp and badly harvested hay or straw are the most prolific source of these spores but they are present in large numbers even in good quality supplies. This means that, unless special precautions are taken, any stable dust contains quantities of these spores.

Only certain horses are sensitive to these spores. It is not known why some horses are sensitive and some insensitive, but the fact remains that some horses exposed to stable dust become broken-winded while others remain healthy under the same conditions.

Horses will recover from the early stages of broken-wind if they can be removed from the dusty atmosphere. Turned out in a field a slightly broken-winded horse will cease to cough and will, in many cases, pass the most careful examination as perfectly healthy as regards its wind but, within a few days of being stabled again, it will cough as before and the disease will steadily become worse.

There is no treatment for established cases of broken-wind. Many of them become quite incapable of doing any useful work. Some settle down to a chronic condition and may be used for light duties or as brood mares. These animals should be stabled as little as possible not only to avoid the dust which always has the capacity to worsen the condition but because, being deprived of a great deal of lung capacity, they manage better in the open air.

Horses that are sensitive to the fungus spores in dust may still be stabled if they are fed on horse nuts and bedded on sawdust or shavings, thereby avoiding coming into contact with hay or straw in which the spores develop.

Many horse stables are badly designed with hay lofts above or fodder stores alongside the horse boxes so that the air is inevitably dusty, while lack of ventilation allows no opportunity for the horses to breathe anything approaching fresh air. Such stables encourage virus coughing and other respiratory diseases as well as broken-wind, and they are detrimental to any horse's health.

Glanders and farcy Glanders is a disease affecting the nose, throat, and lungs, causing ulcers and abscesses with blood-stained discharges. Farcy is another form of the same disease affecting glands all over the body which rupture and appear as ulcers on the skin. These diseases affect the horse family primarily and they can spread from horses to human beings and to cats. The cause is a bacillus known as *Pfeifferella mallei*.

Glanders has been a scourge ever since man associated himself with horses and has been responsible for untold numbers of deaths in horses and their attendants. The cause was traced to *Pfeifferella mallei* in the 19th century, and early in the 20th century a skin test was discovered whereby infected animals, even though showing no signs of the disease, could be detected. An extract from cultures of *Pfeifferella mallei* is injected into the skin near the horse's eye and if the animal has the disease the eyelids swell and the eye discharges. By widespread use of this test and destruction of all infected animals the disease has been eliminated from every country that has an effective veterinary service. This test is still frequently used when horses are being moved from one country to another to guarantee that there is no possibility of re-introducing the disease into the importing country.

9 Parasites

Worms All horses have worms. This statement is literally true. The worms range from minute threads (only visible with the aid of a microscope), that live in the blood stream, in the skin, or in the connective tissues, to worms as thick as a lead pencil and twice as long. Nearly all of them spend part of their lives in the horse's intestines, where they lay immense numbers of eggs. Regular worm dosing helps to keep their numbers in check but no treatment can ever eliminate all the worms. Some healthy horses are able to put up with the damage that their worms are causing but there is always a risk that conditions may favour the worms, so that by sheer numbers they will rob the horse of so much nourishment that it sickens. Untreated horses are also a menace to other horses because their droppings contain vast numbers of worm eggs which hatch into larvae that spread on to the pasture grass and even into food in the stable.

Horses, cattle and sheep each have their own variety of worms and they are not interchangeable. A great variety of worms infest horses.

Red worms (*Strongyles*) About 30 varieties of strongyle worms live in the intestines. They are stout worms from 1 to 5 cm ($\frac{1}{3}$ to 2 in) long. They are popularly known as red worms because many of them suck blood and are red in colour when well fed. Although most of the strongyles are comparatively harmless, one of this group, *Strongylus vulgaris*, is the most damaging worm of all. This species needs to spend a part of its life in the blood vessels causing such obstructions in the path of the circulating blood that colic, paralysis, heart disease, or sudden death may be the result. The arteries of foals and yearlings are especially liable to suffer this damage and the consequences, if not fatal, remain for the rest of the animal's life. So general is this damage that a post-mortem examination on a horse, at any age and dead from any cause, can be expected to show signs of obstruction to the flow of blood caused by these worms. The wonder is that so many horses perform so well for so long handicapped by this interference with their circulation.

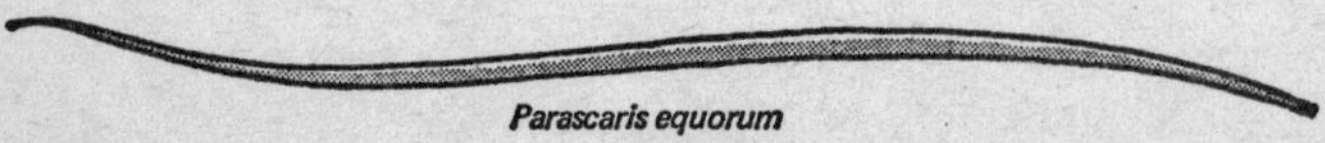

Parascaris equorum

White worms (*Parascaris equorum*) White worms may be up to 30 cm (1 ft) long and as thick as a lead pencil. They are particularly dangerous to foals and yearlings from their size and numbers which may completely block the bowel. Their young forms spend a period of time in the lungs and they may not only damage these organs by their activities but may carry infections to them from the intestines. In this way they may be responsible for a type of pneumonia in foals at 4 to 6 months old which is usually fatal. The eggs of the white worm are laid in the horse's intestines in millions and are passed out in the droppings. These eggs are particularly tough and may lie on the pasture or in stable dust for many months. Consequently horses that are never out at grass can acquire a heavy infestation of these worms by picking up the eggs in hay or straw from the floor of the stable.

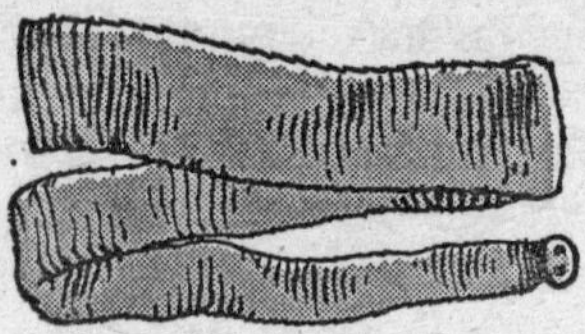

Anaplocephala magna

Tapeworms (*Anaplocephala magna*) Tapeworms seldom cause trouble in horses though, in large numbers, they may give rise to indigestion or signs of poor health. Each tapeworm consists of a small head followed by a number of broad flat segments joined together. They grow to a length of 5 to 8 cm (2 to 3 in), and are occasionally seen in the droppings.

Pin worms (*Oxyuris*) Pin worms have a white body up to 5 cm (2 in) long. These worms live in the large bowel and are chiefly objectionable because they lay their eggs around the horse's anus in a paste that causes the horse so much irritation that it may rub all the hair from the back of the tail. These worms affect stabled horses as well as those at grass.

Lung worms (*Dictyocaulus*) Lung worms live most of their lives in the bronchial tubes of the horse's lungs, causing irritation and frequent coughing. The eggs are laid in the bronchial tubes, are coughed up in the mucus and swallowed to pass out with the horse's droppings. Lung worms are common in donkeys in which they cause much less coughing and illness than in horses, but lung worm infection is probably the reason why donkeys are much more severely affected by lung disease when epidemics of influenza occur. Donkeys should be regularly treated for lung worm infestation for their own sakes and because they are a source of this trouble spreading to horses.

Filarial worms Filarial worms are minute, thread-like worms, some only visible under a microscope. They are found in various parts of the horse's body, in connective tissues, in tendons, inside the eyes and in the skin. Filarial worms living in the skin sometimes give rise to crops of small bleeding points described as bloody sweat. Filaria in the eye can be dealt with by surgically puncturing the eye, when the worm is flushed out with the eye fluids which are soon replaced.

Worm eggs.

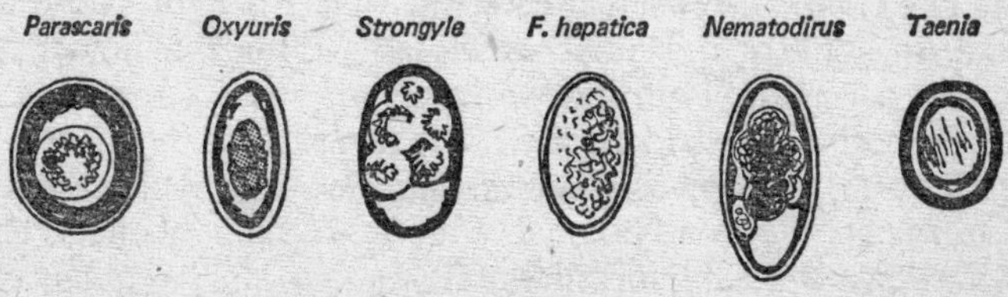

Worm numbers Worms are sometimes seen in the droppings. The 30 cm (1 ft) parascaris is spectacular. Occasionally a fresh dropping is seen to be covered with a number of small red worms, or a tapeworm may appear. These are definite signs of the presence of worms but they are no indication of numbers. Worms thrive in the intestine where they normally persist, laying vast quantities of eggs which pass out with the horse's droppings. The most useful guide to the extent of a horse's worm infestation is a laboratory examination of a sample of droppings. The laboratory reports on the number of eggs found per gram of faeces for each of the main groups of worms. Less that 100 eggs per gram indicates that the horse is fairly free of worms. Regular worm treatment should establish and maintain this low figure. Horses with around 1,000 eggs per gram are requiring treatment. Counts beyond a few thousand eggs indicate a severe infestation and the worming routine and general management of the horse should be overhauled. Laboratory reports need to be considered carefully in conjunction with the horse's general state of health. In cases involving diarrhoea their findings can be deceptively low.

Signs of worms The effect of worms in horses, if they are present in large numbers, is that the coat loses its shine and the skin becomes harsh and dry and does not pick up in a soft fold from the underlying tissues; there may well be anaemia, shown by the pallor of the membranes of the mouth and eyes; and the droppings are likely to be looser than usual. Wormy horses develop a fickle appetite, lose condition, and may become pot-bellied. A number of young horses die because this condition is not dealt with early enough. Some of these signs may be due to other causes, but if several of them are present worms are probably contributing their share to the horse's poor appearance. It is a serious matter to allow a horse to reach such a condition because a large worm burden causes damage not only to the bowel, but to the liver, lungs and blood vessels during the migration of immature worms and may cause acute or chronic illnesses associated with coughing or colic. This is especially the case in foals and young horses which may well be handicapped for life.

Worm treatment Worm treatment must be a part of every horse's routine. In spite of the great variety of worms that infest horses treatment is simple, with modern preparations squeezed as paste into the mouth or given in the food. The two really dangerous worms, the red worm, *Strongylus vulgaris*, and the white worm, *Parascaris equorum*, can now both be dealt with by a single medicine chosen from a variety of satisfactory preparations. One small problem arises: that worms become resistant to any medicine that is used repeatedly, so the choice of mixture must be varied to maintain good results from worm dosing. Most worm medicines are based on fenbendazole, mebendazole, thiabendazole, dichlorvos, or haloxon. Parasitologists believe that all horses should be dosed every 4 to 6 weeks. This is harmless to the horses but is expensive and some of it may be unnecessary. The minimum requirement for all horses should be:

March – a bendazole preparation
June – haloxon
August – a bendazole preparation
October – dichlorvos

Mares should also be dosed with a bendazole preparation a month before foaling. Foals should have a bendazole dose at 4 months and from then on they should be given one or other of the preparations mentioned at intervals of 6 weeks until they fall into line with the general dosing of all the horses in March. Two or three extra doses during the summer while they are yearlings are also advisable.

The advantage of regular treatment of all the horses on the premises is that the horses are kept reasonably free of worms and the stables and pastures are not heavily contaminated because the droppings only contain small numbers of worm eggs. Re-infestation is constantly occurring but at a much lower level than would be the case if any of the horses were to be left untreated for a long period.

Worm control Pastures are the most prolific source of worm infection. The young worms hatched from eggs in the faeces can live in damp shady places for weeks waiting to be eaten. Their numbers on the ground build up to enormous figures in spring and summer weather. Horses that are regularly wormed will not spread so many worm eggs, but one untreated horse can rapidly create conditions for massive infection of all the other horses grazing or stabled with it. Danger lies in forgetting to treat the family donkey or the trainer's hack or allowing a visiting horse that may not have been wormed regularly to share in the grazing.

The numbers of young worms in a field are greatly reduced by lapse of time, dry weather and frosts. If a field can be divided into four paddocks and the horses grazed for a week in each paddock in rotation, each area is eaten down short and then has three weeks' rest. Droppings, averaging 12 droppings per horse, should be picked up daily. This is very effective and helps to keep the whole pasture grazed evenly. Whether this is done or not, as soon as each paddock is vacated it should be mown and harrowed. This cuts down the weeds and tufts left by the horses and spreads the droppings so that the young worms have less cover against light and sunshine and so are reduced in numbers. If it can be arranged that the small paddocks are kept free of horses for longer than three weeks this will further reduce the worm numbers, but the fast growing herbage needs to be used up in some way particularly as horses keep their condition better if their grazing is from short grass. This need can be met by using cattle to eat the grass down as required and this also removes a large proportion of the larval worms, none of which affect cattle.

Well trimmed fields lose practically all their worm population through the winter, provided horses are not grazed in them during that time. The real dangers arise in the spring and summer when favourable conditions to the worms can soon turn a worm-free pasture into a heavily infected area even when a strict programme of regular worm treatment of all the horses is combined with good pasture management.

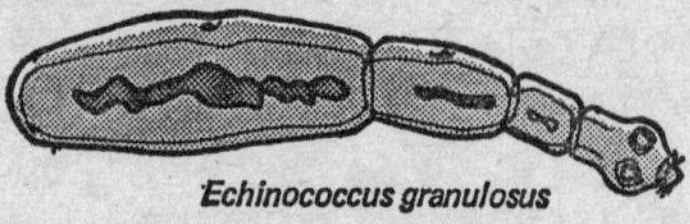

Echinococcus granulosus

Bladderworm disease In this disease cysts or bladders develop in the substance of the horse's liver, from a hazelnut to a coconut in size, and varying greatly in numbers. The cysts are the result of the horse swallowing eggs from a particular type of tapeworm (*Echinococcus granulosus*) that occurs in dogs' intestines. The worm eggs are passed in the dog's faeces which dry up and scatter as dust, some of which may reach land that horses are grazing over. Taken in as dust on the food the eggs hatch in the horse's stomach, penetrate to the liver and develop there as cysts. The cysts contain a form of the tapeworm which can infect dogs but they remain as intact cysts in the horse until its death. If they are numerous they may cause jaundice, general unhealthiness and even the death of the horse; but in many cases the horse remains apparently unaffected and dies eventually from some other cause. If the affected liver is then fed to dogs in an uncooked state, tapeworms develop in the dog.

There is no treatment for this bladderworm disease in the horse. Its continued existence depends on dogs gaining access to raw liver from horses. Prevention of the disease demands the regular dosing of dogs to eliminate tapeworms and especial care that all horse flesh, especially liver, fed to dogs is thoroughly cooked to kill off this infection.

Warbles Warble flies (*Hypodermia bovis*) are cattle parasites which can lay their eggs on horses by mistake. The fly resembles a small bee, having a yellow, black and orange body, brown wings and an ominous buzz. This is the gad-fly that sets cattle galloping on hot days in the summer and its presence is also irritating to horses though it does not stampede them. The eggs are laid on single hairs, sometimes as many as a dozen on one hair. The larvae hatch in a few days and, after boring through the skin, they migrate, one species to the oesophagus and another to the spinal canal, where they grow through the winter. In the spring the grubs migrate again and come

A warble fly, larva and egg

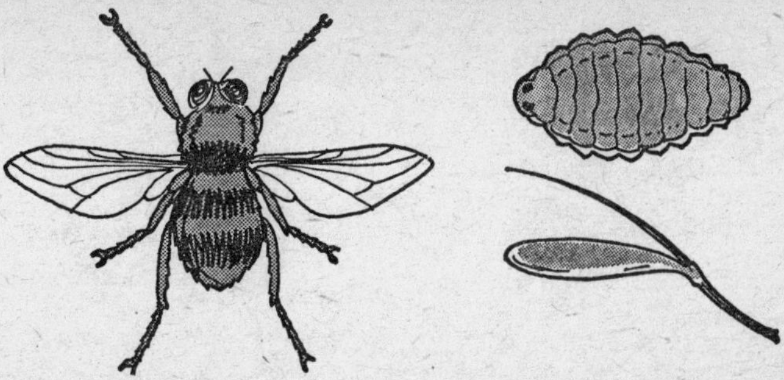

to rest under the skin of the back where each one forms a swelling with a central breathing hole. In April, May or early June the swellings discharge the full-grown grubs which fall to the ground and pupate under cover to emerge as mature warble flies in three weeks. Horses seldom develop more than one or two warble swellings. It is doubtful if the grubs that have developed in horses ever reach maturity, their normal host being cattle.

Warbles have a nuisance value in horses in that the ripening swellings usually occur under the saddle causing a discharging sore that is painful and may become an abscess. As soon as a swelling is noticed it should be poulticed to encourage it to discharge the maggot. Squeezing the grub out of a ripe swelling may help but too much pressure could spread infection under the skin and lead to the formation of an ugly sore that heals slowly.

Cattle, which may develop two or three dozen warble swellings, are treated in late autumn or early spring with a systemic insecticide which is absorbed through the skin. This is not recommended for horses because horse warbles are not a common condition and because there are risks of poisoning. Warbles are most likely to occur in horses which have run at grass with cattle during the previous summer. Any campaign to eliminate warbles from cattle should have incidental benefits for the horse population.

Bots The horse bot flies (*Gasterophilus species*) are a little larger than the common housefly, thick-set and hairy with a black and reddish brown body. Bot flies appear during the summer and lay their eggs on the hair of a horse's limbs. In about three weeks the eggs are ready to hatch and probably cause some irritation because the horse licks its legs and swallows the tiny grubs. These attach themselves to the stomach wall, sometimes in large numbers, and

A bot fly, larva and egg

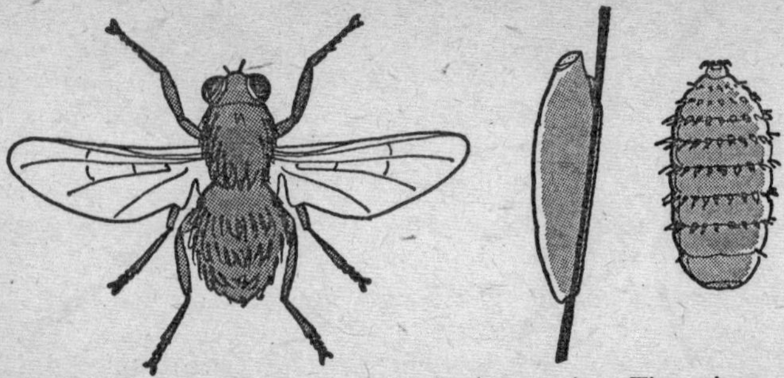

there they feed until fully grown in the late spring. They then release their hold and are passed out in the droppings as stubby pink or brown segmented grubs about 1.5 cm ($\frac{5}{8}$ in) long. After pupating in the ground for three weeks they emerge as mature flies. Bots in large numbers deprive the horse of a considerable amount of nourishment and interfere with its digestion. They cause stomach ulcers and these may rupture the stomach wall giving rise to peritonitis, severe colic and death.

Horses are not worried by bot flies, but are less exposed to their attentions if there is a shed to shelter in during the heat of the summer days. Infection with bots can be reduced if the creamy yellow eggs are scraped off the legs daily with a bot knife which has a serrated edge designed to strip them from their attachment, or they may be wiped off with a warm sponge. Brushing does not remove them: it actually stimulates them to develop to a stage suitable to be swallowed by the horse or its companion. Bots, the grubs which are feeding in the horse's stomach, can be got rid of in the autumn by using a worm treatment containing dichlorvos, which is suggested as part of the routine worm treatment for all horses and ponies.

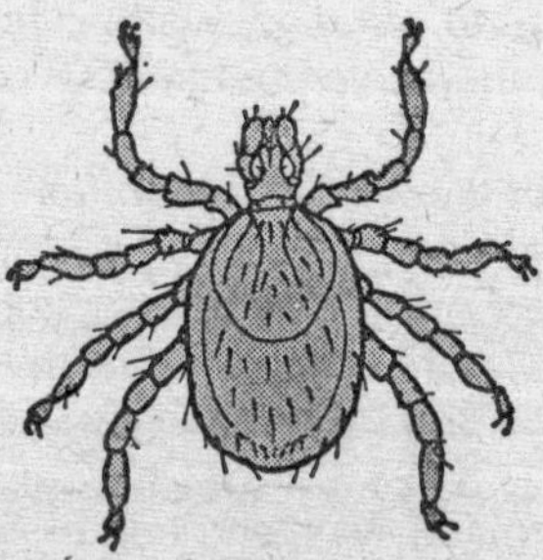

A tick, *Ixodes*

Ticks The common tick, *Ixodes ricinus*, is almost world-wide in its occurrence, being found especially on rough pasture. It attacks any of the domestic animals. It may be found on a horse's skin, usually around the head, as it attaches itself while the animal is grazing. This tick is oval and grey and is known as the 'castor-bean' tick from its resemblance to a small bean. Ticks live by sucking blood and may grow to nearly 1.25 cm ($\frac{1}{2}$ in) in length before dropping off to lay their eggs. In the tropics other varieties of tick occur on horses and are responsible for spreading equine biliary fever, a blood disease that causes anaemia and jaundice. A few cases of biliary fever have been reported in Britain.

Individual ticks may be dealt with by wetting them with turpentine or paraffin oil or snipping them off close to the horse's skin with scissors. They should not be pulled off as this may leave an ulcer.

Ticks in numbers may be destroyed by spraying or washing the affected parts of the horse with gamma benzene hexachloride. Tick attacks can be avoided by keeping horses off rough grazing likely to be tick infected.

The hair may grow white at the site of a tick bite and in some tropical countries many of the native ponies' coats are flecked with white from this cause.

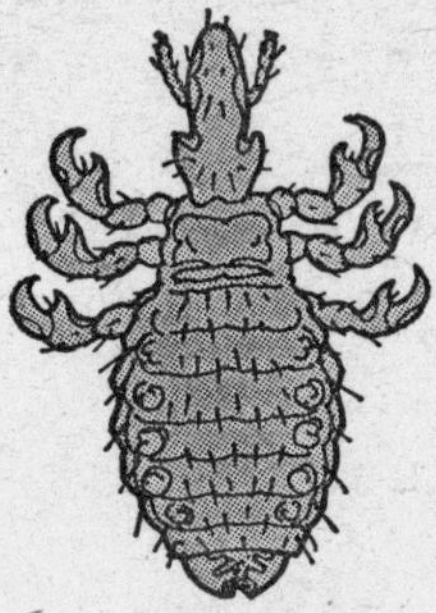

A louse, *Haematopinus*

Lice Lice are small wingless insects about 2.5 mm ($\frac{1}{10}$ in) long and pale brown in colour. Three kinds of lice affect horses: *Trichodectes equi* and *Trichodectes pilosus* being biting lice, and *Haematopinus asini* a sucking louse. The sucking lice gather in the mane and tail and the biting lice occur more usually on the legs. On neglected horses any of them may spread over the head and body. Lice cause itchiness and rubbing, and if the affected parts are examined the lice can be detected moving among the scurf and their eggs or nits seen attached to individual hairs. Lice are likely to occur in the rough coats of horses turned out for the winter; though they may not be noticed until the spring, when the warmer weather leads to a rapid increase in their numbers, and the horses begin to rub and bite at their itchy skin.

Lice can be destroyed by dressing the horses with a wash or spray of gamma benzene hexachloride, repeated several times at intervals of ten days, to ensure the destruction of any that hatch from the nits. Grooming and clipping are also helpful in restoring a good coat. Biting lice are harmful in large numbers since they derive their nourishment at the horse's expense. Severe lice infestations can cause such loss of hair from the mane and tail that they may take months to appear respectable again.

There is an old wives' tale that lice cross over daily from one side of the horse to the other, to follow the sun for warmth, so it is only necessary to apply a louse dressing along the spine and this will catch them all. Scientific observations do not confirm this economical suggestion.

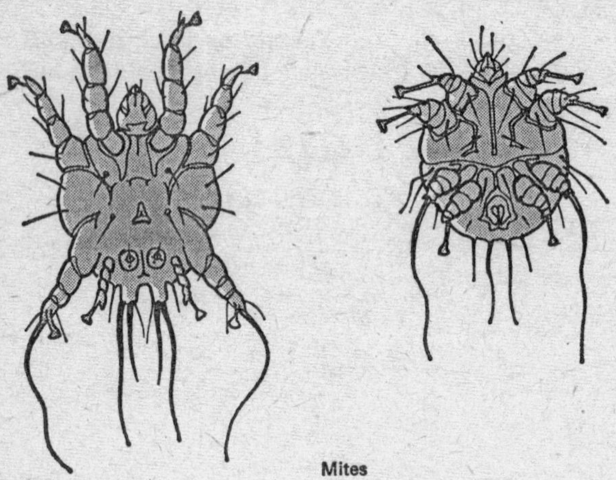

Mites
Chorioptes and *Sarcoptes*

Mange Mange in horses is caused by mites which live on the surface or burrow into the skin. They are about 0.5 mm ($\frac{1}{50}$ in) long, white in colour, and almost round, with biting parts and four pairs of legs. They lay eggs in the horse's skin. These hatch in a few days and the larvae develop so rapidly that they are laying eggs in their turn in less than a fortnight. Mange mites cause intense itching and the skin becomes bare, thickened and scabby. Three kinds of mite affect horses: sarcoptic mites occur over the head, neck and body, being especially troublesome in the spring; psoroptic mites affect the mane and tail, and one type of *Psoroptes* is found in the ears; chorioptic mites occur on the legs of horses with feather or long hair about the fetlocks and pasterns. These mites cause incessant rubbing, stamping and biting.

Mange can only be diagnosed with certainty by a laboratory identification of the mites taken from skin scrapings. In Great Britain cases of sarcoptic or psoroptic mange must be reported to the Ministry of Agriculture through a vet or the police. Chorioptic mange is not notifiable.

Mange is best treated with a spray or wash prepared with gamma benzene hexachloride, applied several times at intervals of a fortnight. Grooming kit and harness should be disinfected or fumigated. Bedding should be burned and stables thoroughly cleaned out and disinfected. Mange is only likely to occur in horses that are dirty and neglected, though it can readily spread by contact or by grooming tools to horses in good condition.

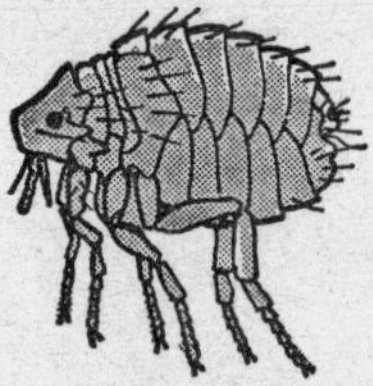

A flea, *E. gallinaceae*

Fleas Fleas (*Echidnophaga gallinaceae*) are not commonly found on horses in temperate climates but they may spread to them during plagues of fleas. In tropical countries, stick-tight fleas and jigger fleas can cause severe damage by setting up ulcers in the skin. Treatment is by dusting or shampooing the horses with derris powder and it is equally important to clean the stables thoroughly with particular attention to the floor where the young fleas can develop in accumulated filth.

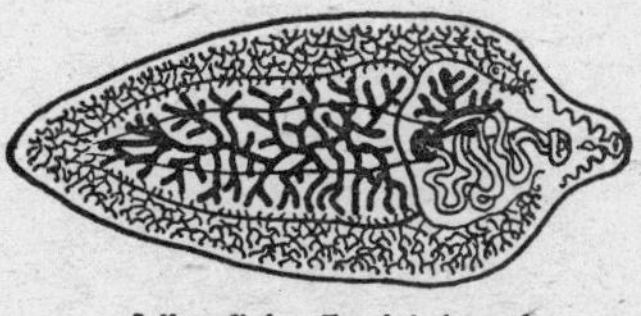

A liver fluke, *Fasciola hepatica*

Liver fluke Liver flukes (*Fasciola hepatica*) live in the bile ducts in the liver. They are flat, leaf-shaped parasites about 2.5 cm (1 in) long and 1.25 cm ($\frac{1}{2}$ in) wide. Their chief hosts are cattle and sheep, but they also occur in horses which have been grazed with those animals on low-lying or marshy land. Wet land is necessary for the spread of these flukes as they spend a part of their life in a mud-snail. The signs of the disease in horses are loss of appetite, listlessness, watery droppings, anaemia, and muscle wasting – though, unless the infestation is heavy, many infected horses show no deviation from normal health. The disease can be confirmed by finding eggs of the parasite in the faeces. Treatment with oxyclozanide by stomach tube is effective. Horses should be removed from infected pastures.

10 Skin conditions

Wounds Wounds heal by forming a blood clot which is penetrated by tissue fluids and cells to form a scab. The skin cells at the edge of the wound multiply and spread under the scab until they meet and so complete a new skin-cover.

A fresh wound should be covered with a clean cloth or cotton wool and firm pressure applied to stop the flow of blood. When the bleeding has stopped, the wound can be inspected and soil, grass, splinters of wood, or any other foreign body, picked out or washed out of it with a weak antiseptic solution or with clean water to every 4.5 litres (1 gal) of which a tablespoonful of salt has been added. Pressure hosing with cold water for 10 to 15 minutes is very effective. Apparently clean wounds should be treated similarly. Horses live in such close contact with dirty conditions that it is never safe to assume that any wound is clean. After bathing the wound, it should be dusted over with antiseptic powder and covered to protect it from dust, dirt, and infection.

When there is any infection in a wound, fluids from the horse's tissues seep into it to wash out the disease organisms. If these discharges can drain away easily they soon clean the wound and it heals up. When the drainage is not satisfactory, fluids accumulate, healing is delayed and there are discharges of pus. Surgery is needed to ensure that the pus drains away by gravity. If drainage is satisfactory pus is not to be seen. Tubes are sometimes used in deeper wounds to assist in draining them.

Surgery may also be applied to tidying up the wound so that long hair or tags of torn skin do not interfere with healing. Stitching may be necessary but there are several reasons for avoiding this if possible in horses: their damaged skin is very liable to swell up so that a neat repair on the day injury occurred is likely to be a gaping hole with torn out stitches the following day; tetanus infection develops more readily in a closed wound than in an open one; and drainage is all important and must not be impeded.

The wound should be covered with an absorbent dressing held in place by bandaging. If the wound is in a part that cannot be bandaged, plentiful and frequent dressings with a soluble antiseptic powder will give considerable protection against infection; Antibiotic injections are advisable to protect the horse from infections that might spread from the wound.

Any wound in a horse may give rise to tetanus which is often a fatal disease. An injection of tetanus serum is, consequently, a necessary part of wound treatment unless the horse has already been vaccinated with tetanus toxoid which, with an annual booster, gives constant protection against this disease.

Wound sinuses If there is something in a wound that cannot be washed out by the body fluids, such as a chip of bone, an air-gun pellet, or a piece of gravel, the wound may heal up except for a channel running from the object to the surface of the skin. The channel is known as a sinus and its outer opening continues to discharge a thin fluid. The only treatment for sinuses is by surgery to extract the object causing the trouble.

Ulcers A shallow wound only affecting the surface layers of some body tissue is usually called an ulcer. The word ulcer carries a morbid association because, while most superficial wounds affecting the skin, or the eye, or the mouth heal up rapidly, those that do not heal but spread to adjoining areas are called ulcers or even 'rodent ulcers' – hinting at a gnawing extension of the injury.

Ulcers need careful inspection of their edges to discover why the wound is widening instead of healing normally and reducing in size. The cause may be persistence of the original cause of the wound – rubbing harness, grit under an eyelid or a pinching bit; or the horse may find the wound irritating and worsen it by rubbing or licking. The healing tissues may be unable to function because of some infection in the wound or because the medication applied is too strong. Some cancer growths take the form of ulcers. Ulcers in the mouth cause eating problems and may lead to food being refused or rejected or accumulating between the teeth and the cheeks, causing a foetid smell.

The treatment of ulcers depends on finding the cause and removing it or preventing its recurrence. Sometimes surgery may be necessary to remove the edges of an ulcer so that healthy tissue can take over and proceed to heal the wound. Ulcers on the eye usually leave a permanent white scar when they have healed. Unless these are large they do not usually interfere with the horse's eyesight.

Thorns Hunters and other horses working in rough woodland are frequently pricked by thorns from shrubby trees. These, especially from blackthorn, can be extremely painful, causing acute lameness. If projecting, they should be pulled out with tweezers. They are often impossible to extract but can be encouraged to work their way out if the area is well poulticed. A small injection of local anaesthetic over the area will relieve the acute pain for some hours.

Foreign bodies Foreign bodies are objects which cause trouble by involving themselves with the horse's tissues causing wounds, ulcers or irritation. Examples are grit under an eyelid, brambles, wire or broken teeth in the gums or tongue, stones under the shoe, nails or sharp flints penetrating the frog or the sole of the foot, gravel working up in the white line between the sole and the wall of the foot (see page 191), and a variety of objects penetrating the skin and into the muscles such as sharp pieces of fencing, stable forks, and bullets or pellets from guns.

Attention is called to the presence of foreign bodies by tears from the eyes, saliva running from the mouth, blood from wounds, and lameness from foot or limb injuries. In most cases, removal of the object relieves the animal. Some objects are difficult to shift and local or general anaesthetics may be required.

Foreign bodies that have penetrated into deep tissues often announce their presence by causing a discharging wound or sinus requiring surgical treatment.

Abscesses Abscesses are not confined to the skin. They may occur in any part of the body, being accumulations of pus made up of white blood corpuscles gathered to overwhelm an attack by infectious bacteria. The natural tendency of abscesses is to erupt through the skin as a means of discharging and ridding the body of the infection. In consequence most abscesses eventually bulge under the skin and they may be encouraged to discharge by using hot fomentations to soften the skin or by cutting through the skin surgically.

Small abscesses may occur in the skin due to infections occurring in its grease and sweat glands or in the hair follicles. These are discussed under spots and pimples (see opposite).

In most cases in which abscesses occur, the horse may be helped to throw off the infection by the use of antibiotics, though established cases of strangles are an important exception to this generality.

Poll-evil (A variety of bacteria including *Fusiformis necrophorus* and *Brucella abortus*) Poll-evil is the rather dramatic name given to an abscess affecting the bursa or synovial capsule that lies between the skin and the poll at the highest point of the skull. This prominence is sometimes bruised by the horse striking its head when passing through a low doorway, and the resulting swelling is liable to be infected by various bacteria turning it into an abscess. The infection is more serious if the horse has brucellosis. The name 'poll-evil' reflects the difficulty in treating the abscess, which is liable to involve the exceptionally large ligament attaching to that part of the skull. A wound persistently discharging pus is likely to develop and, in spite of its elevated position, drainage from the abscess is difficult to arrange; quite complicated surgery is sometimes required. Antibiotic treatment is helpful if used in the early stages, but chronic abscesses which have had time to develop thick fibrous walls cannot always be reached by these drugs so that cases of poll-evil remain a problem, and a challenge to veterinary skill.

Fistulous withers (A variety of bacteria including *Fusiformis necrophorus and Brucella abortus*) There is a bursa capping each of the upright bony processes that form the withers. These may be bruised by falls or by the saddle or simply by a tight rug and, as occurs in poll-evil, they may be infected by bacteria and turn into abscesses which are more serious if complicated by brucellosis. The drainage problem is difficult as the abscesses tend to spread down under the shoulder blades. This gives the name to the condition, a fistula being a deep-seated abscess discharging through a narrow passage Downward drainage, so important in the treatment of abscesses, is difficult to arrange. There is a story of one stubborn and persistent case of fistulous withers that defied treatment until the abscess extended down so far that it developed a swelling between the forelegs. The abscess was opened there, downward drainage was established and recovery was uneventful ! Antibiotic treatment may be helpful but as described under poll-evil, treatment of these infected bursae is likely to be difficult and is not always successful.

Spots and pimples The horse has a very sensitive skin that flushes up readily into a swelling in response to injury, infection, or poison. Skin swellings from being struck by a whip, bitten by insects, stung by nettles or scratched by brambles usually disappear in a few hours. Applying a mild antiseptic lotion or ointment may help to prevent an infection developing if the skin has been broken.

If an infection does develop the spot may discharge a few drops of pus before forming a scab and healing up. If a large pimple appears it may be helped to discharge its pus by bathing with hot water 2 or 3 times a day or by applying a poultice. Even such small infections as these give rise to a risk of tetanus, though this would not be a likely development if the horse was already vaccinated with tetanus toxoid. Isolated spots do not usually affect the animal's general health but a rash of spots or pimples might cause a high temperature for which antibiotic treatment would be required.

Faulty feeding sometimes causes a rash of raised areas on a horse's neck and body. This is urticaria, described in the chapter on Digestion. Pimples on a horse's back caused by the emerging grubs of the warble fly are described in the chapter on Parasites. Rashes and spots in the heels are described in the chapter on the Feet.

Acne Minute hard pimples may occur in the skin on a horse's neck, shoulders and quarters, singly or in groups or lines. They are due to bacterial infection of the hair follicles. If picked off they leave a tiny ulcer. These pimples are not irritating but they spoil the look and feel of the coat and skin. They are a bacterial infection due to *Staphylococcus aureus* and other bacteria and are spread by vigorous grooming. They are extremely difficult to treat. A course of antibiotic injections is usually necessary. Grooming tools should be thoroughly disinfected and grooming conducted with softer brushes or restricted to rubbing over the affected areas with a cloth until the pimples have dispersed.

Sweet itch Sweet itch appears as a moist eczema affecting the mid-line of the mane and the root of the tail. Affected horses and ponies show signs of desperate irritation and frequently rub the areas affected so that raw ulcers are formed. The condition may spread to a continuous line from the poll to the tail.

The cause of this condition are small biting flies, usually *Culicoides* midges, which swarm for an hour or two before and after sunset from May to September. The varieties of midge concerned bite particularly along the animals' upper mid-line. Most horses and ponies are insensitive to these bites but some are allergic to the midges' saliva and suffer each summer.

Applications of benzyl beuzoate cream are helpful. The most satisfactory control appears to be by bringing susceptible animals into the stable at four o'clock each afternoon and turning them out again in the morning through the summer months.

Actino-bacillosis Actino-bacillosis, like actinomycosis, causes fibrous swellings in and around accidental or operation wounds that have become infected with one of the pus-producing bacteria, *Staphylococcus aureus*. The growth increases steadily in size, becoming lumpy with frequent small cavities which discharge a gritty pus. These growths may occur on any part of the body, the common sites being the scrotum, following castration, and the shoulders of draught horses where the skin has been damaged by the collar. Actino-bacillosis responds well to sulphonamides and antibiotics or to sodium iodide solutions given intravenously.

Ulcerative lymphangitis (Canadian pox – contagious acne) Ulcerative lymphangitis is an infectious skin disease of horses due to the bacillus *Corynebacterium pseudotubercolosis*, though *Staphylococci*, *Streptococci* or other pus-producing bacteria may be involved. The condition appears as small swellings occurring in lines extending up the limb from a heel infection. The swellings turn to abscesses which burst to discharge a greenish pus and are inclined to join with each other to form large dry scabs. The disease is sometimes known as Canadian pox. The round dry patches may cause it to be mistaken for ringworm, and the swollen cords under the skin may suggest epizootic lymphangitis. Any doubts can be dispelled by a laboratory examination of pus from the sores.

Ulcerative lymphangitis is not irritating. Affected horses go off their food and may run a temperature of up to 40°C (104°F). They should be rested until the temperature returns to normal. The disease is unsightly, spreads rapidly from horse to horse, and interferes with their work because of their sickness and because the ulcers and scabs prevent saddles, girths and harness from being comfortably applied.

The disease may be introduced into a stable by contact with other horses. It is spread by grooming and this should be suspended while the condition persists. Treatment is by applying antibiotic dressings and injecting antibiotic medicines.

Spread of the disease must be countered by disinfecting grooming tools and saddlery, burning discarded bedding and dressings and washing the stables with disinfectant. Ulcerative lymphangitis can spread to human beings so attendants should wash carefully after treating affected horses. With reasonable care a stable should be able to clear this infection in a matter of a few weeks.

Epizootic lymphangitis Epizootic lymphangitis, caused by a fungus *Histoplasma farciminosus*, is a tropical disease which is occasionally introduced into temperate climates by imported animals. Infection occurs through abrasions on the limbs and spreads rapidly in a stable through the common use of grooming tools.

Signs of epizootic lymphangitis develop slowly. It may be two or three months after infection before cord-like thickenings appear along the course of a lymphatic vessel with a series of nodules at intervals of a few inches. The nodules discharge pus and form ulcers which bleed easily and heal slowly over a number of weeks. The lymphatic glands become enlarged and the whole leg swells – though not suddenly as in digestive lymphangitis, and not to anything like the same extent. Affected horses show no distress and remain in good condition for months or years, but later they deteriorate, become emaciated and die.

Diagnosis depends on finding the fungus in pus from the ulcers by a laboratory examination. The disease is so highly infectious, so tedious in appearing and so resistant to treatment that in most countries the only method of control is compulsory slaughter of all known cases.

Galls and sores Galls are sores produced by chafing. The chafing may be from the saddle, the girths or other harness, from rugs, hobbling ropes, or even from a rider's boots.

Chafing denudes the skin of hair and inflames the area which becomes hot, swollen and tender. If the chafing continues the skin becomes red and raw, then scabs over and heals up. If further chafing occurs the skin may be penetrated forming ulcers that require treating as open wounds and these take a considerable time to heal.

The most important part of the treatment of galls is to remove the cause so that repetition of the injury does not make the condition worse. Calamine lotion helps to cool an inflamed skin, while an aureomycin spray is useful as an antiseptic dressing. Moist skin surfaces may be dressed with an antiseptic powder or with a cream of sulphonilamide and medicinal liquid paraffin and then covered with a gauze and cotton wool pad.

Galls that have caused only superficial injury will heal without scarring. Those that have penetrated more deeply may form adhesions and scars that persist in the skin and deprive it of some of its flexibility. The hair growing on and around these healed areas often turns white, creating additional marks that may be used for identification and are described as saddle-marks, girth-marks, rope-marks and so on.

Galls occur commonly on the withers, especially prominent withers, being caused by bruising from the pommel of an ill-fitting saddle or, much more commonly, from rugs which, however carefully applied, are liable to shift and tighten. With military and western saddles that are used over a blanket, galls can be caused by failing to ease the blanket over the withers before girthing up. Other causes of galls are bruising of the back from the saddle cantle due to bad saddle fitting; pinching of the skin which has not been smoothed out after tightening the girths; and the rider sitting too heavily too far back. Galls may also result from hobbling horses with ropes or shackles that injure the cannons or pasterns, or from bandage tapes that have been tied too tight or that have tightened by becoming wet, and have cut into the skin of the legs or round the tail. Harness horses may develop galls from an ill-fitting collar or from chafing caused by any part of the harness not correctly placed. Pack-saddle blankets on ponies, donkeys and mules used for transport in mountain country often cover large, raw gall wounds. Being out of sight, they are out of mind. Galls may develop, even when harness and clothing are correctly fitted, simply from excessive use and they are a constant menace in endurance competitions. The friction of a rider's boots may gall a horse's ribs, though this can be prevented by properly designed saddle flaps. The horse's skin gradually becomes accustomed to reasonable pressures. Young horses gall easily and special care should be taken that their training is conducted in short spells of work and that they are inspected for tender areas of skin which are the first sign of galling.

Dirt is an important contribution to the formation of galls, since the accumulation of scurf, shed hairs and sweat in the coat, or dust and grease on the harness, increase the amount of friction that inflames the skin.

Pressure on the skin should be relieved gradually. The compressed skin is deprived of blood. When pressure is removed the blood rushes back suddenly and for a while the skin is in a state of inflammation and easily injured. This condition can be avoided if the saddle, after a spell of work, is loosened and lifted but left in place for half an hour or so to allow the circulation to be restored steadily. If further work is intended the saddle can then be girthed tight again without the risk of galling or, if work is finished, the saddle can be removed knowing that circulation has been gently restored. Horses that have had their legs tightly bandaged for support should have these bandages removed as soon as is convenient, but the bandages should immediately be replaced, more loosely, and over cotton wool to prevent the restoration of the blood supply too suddenly.

Galls are nearly always an indication of faults in management. They happen in the best of stables where work and training are in progress but they are detected early and given every opportunity of healing quickly so that no permanent damage is done. Their prevention is a constant responsibility for all who have horses in their care.

Sit-fast Sit-fast is the name given to a saddle gall that appears on the mid-line of the spine and persists. It is curious that it usually occurs in horses in such good condition that the mid-line is in a hollow between the long muscles of the back; it is difficult to imagine how a gall should occur in such a position. However, such galls do appear and remain static, probably due to the mid-line being poorly supplied with blood as it is at the end of blood supply from either side. These sit-fast scabs do little harm, but they are unsightly, a nuisance when grooming and a worry in case they become infected and erupt as an abscess. Sometimes the circulation can be activated by applying a blistering ointment so that the abscesses heal up and shed off the scab, but they usually have to be removed surgically, leaving a raw wound which needs very careful attention during healing as, being in a hollow, there is no gravity drainage to clear away any discharges.

Sebaceous cysts The sebaceous glands in the skin produce a grease that puts a gloss on a well-groomed horse and helps to form a waterproof covering in the thick coat of a horse at grass in the winter. One or more of these glands may occasionally become blocked. Its cells continue to produce the grease which cannot escape and forms a swelling in the skin. This may grow to the size of a hen's egg. Sebaceous cysts are usually harmless but unsightly, though they may sometimes interfere with harness. On the nose they may obstruct the proper intake of air.

Small cysts may be punctured so that they discharge the accumulated grease. Larger ones may have to be removed completely by surgery.

Leucoderma White patches sometimes develop on hairless parts of the body where the skin is usually dark. The parts affected may be the angles of the eyes, the lips, nostrils, anus, vulva and the sheath or the udder. The patches are irregular and quite small, usually no larger than the area of a finger nail and they alter in size and shape over long periods. They are due to the activity or lack of activity of cells in the skin which produce melanin, the dark pigment of skin and hair. Leucoderma is not a condition of disease. It is quite harmless and has no effect on the horse. Leucoderma on the lips may follow the use of rubber bits but, in general, the cause is quite unknown.

Warts Horses produce a variety of warts. Foals and yearlings and sometimes older horses may develop a crop of pale flat warts round the nostrils or lips. These are caused by a papovirus infection. There are numerous traditional remedies for these, all quite successful because, treated or not, warts disappear in a few weeks. They occasionally cause trouble by being pinched by the bit.

In older horses larger warts, often reaching the size of a walnut, may grow by the lips, ears, sheath or udder, or round the anus. In grey horses as they age and the hair becomes white, shiny black warts appear in these locations. These are melanomas, their growth being connected in some way with the disappearance of pigment from the hair of the coat. All these warts are harmless unless the harness impinges on them so that they bleed. They should be left alone if possible. Taking them away, even by the most careful surgery, usually stirs up the tissues to produce a larger crop in the same place. The melanomas may become unsightly on grey horses but they often continue to work well for up to twenty-five years without being hampered by their warts. In some cases melanomas also develop in the abdominal organs and these may cause severe loss of condition leading to debility and death.

Warts on the skin that do interfere with a horse's work may sometimes be removed satisfactorily by cryosurgery – that is operating under intense cold which does not cause reactions in nearby tissue.

Ringworm Ringworm is an infectious skin disease caused by various types of fungus that grow inside individual hairs causing them to break off, leaving bare patches of skin. In the horse ringworm is caused by *Microsporon* fungus almost anywhere on the body, or by *Trichophyton* fungus which usually occurs at the girth or on the neck. The first sign of infection is a matted tuft of hair which falls out after a few days, by which time adjoining matted tufts are forming. The patch extends outwards leaving a bare central area in which, after a while, new hair growth appears. The affected patches do not usually extend beyond 4 or 5 cm (1¾ to 2 in) in diameter, but they may be so plentiful that they join upto form large scabby denuded areas. Ringworm does not usually itch and affected horses are not inclined to rub or bite at the affected skin; but it can be very troublesome, leading to painful sores if the diseased skin is chafed by girths, saddles or rugs.

Ringworm is very infectious, being spread on the animal or from horse to horse by grooming and other contacts. The disease is liable to have infected a number of horses in a stable before the patches on the first horse have developed sufficiently for the condition to be recognized. Spread can be controlled to some extent by having a separate set of grooming kit for each horse, by using saddle cloths and by putting plastic covers over the girths. Ringworm can be suspected with some certainty by the typical appearance of the disease. A laboratory examination of skin scrapings will confirm the cause of the disease by finding spores of the fungus in and around the broken hairs.

Treatment of ringworm is by giving griseofulvin orally and it can be obtained as a pre-mixed food additive. This is not recommended for pregnant mares. Dichlorophon spray or gentian violet solution may be applied to the affected parts at three-day intervals. Gentian violet has the advantage of brightly colouring the lesions and making it easy to detect newly forming and uncoloured eruptions. Sodium iodide given intravenously is also an effective treatment.

It is difficult to determine when an animal is free of ringworm infection as the fungus can be found on the skin of horses which do not develop the disease. Horses cannot really be declared clear until hair is growing again up to the edges of all the denuded areas, and this may take two or three months from the beginning of an attack.

Horses that have had ringworm develop a resistance to the infection and are not likely to be infected by the same fungus for quite a number of years. Unfortunately there are four varieties of *Microsporon* and four varieties of *Trichophyton* fungus that may occur on horses and the resistance is likely to apply only to the particular variety by which the horse has been affected. Attempts to produce resistance by some form of vaccination before the horse's active term of years has begun have, so far, not been successful.

The spread of the disease often occurs at gatherings of horses when grooming kit, saddlery and clothing are used on various horses. A strict adherence to the rules of stable management will reduce this risk considerably.

Horse ringworm can affect human beings. In them it is an unsightly but not a dangerous disease. Reasonable care and cleanliness should guard against such infection.

Sporotrichosis Sporotrichosis causes a series of hard nodules to develop around the fetlock area. One after another they ripen, scab over a collection of pus and recede leaving a small scar. Antiseptic dressings and antibiotics do not affect the process which may continue indefinitely. The cause is a brachycladium fungus. Treatment with sodium iodide injections given intravenously is usually successful or griseofulvin may be given by the mouth.

Rain scald Horses exposed to heavy rain for long periods without shelter, especially in tropical conditions, may develop a condition in which the skin over the back and quarters becomes spongy and the hair peels off in large patches leaving bare, raw areas. Various bacteria and fungi may thrive in the matted hair and the sodden skin. Bringing the horses into shelter is frequently all that is necessary for the skin to dry off and the hair to begin to grow again. Cases that show persistent discharges require antibiotic dressings or injections to deal with bacterial infections and dosing with potassium iodide or intravenous injections of sodium iodide to counter the fungi. Neglected cases fall off rapidly in condition and may not recover if treatment is delayed.

Bursati (summer sores – swamp cancer) Bursati causes the development of large ulcers on the skin of horses in the tropics.

The edges of any small wounds that may occur become fibrous and thickened and the wounds, instead of healing, develop into ulcers, sometimes as much as 25 cm (10 in) across, surrounded by a ridge of hard tissue in which gritty red or brown particles are formed. These are known as kunkers. The kunkers vary from less than a pin-head to the size of a pea, and appear to act as a stimulant to the skin to produce more fibrous tissue. The common sites for bursati are on the face, especially around the eyes and lips; on the front of the chest; and on the sheath or udder. Most bursati sores heal up in cooler weather but the large ulcers only scab over thinly and are liable to break out again and spread even further, on the return of hot weather.

Bursati is caused, in some areas, by a minute *Habronema* worm that spends its early life in the maggots of flies and its adult life in the horse, causing the ulcers described as well as thickened and fibrous growths in the stomach and intestines. In other districts bursati results from infection by a fungus, *Hyphomyces destruens*. Laboratory assistance is needed to determine the cause because heavy doses of thiabendazole are required for the cases due to the presence of worms, while the fungus cases need to be treated with potassium iodide or griseofulvin by mouth or by intravenous injections of sodium iodide. In both types of disease the ulcers heal more readily if the fibrous edges can be cut away surgically.

The occurrence of bursati cases can be reduced by good stable hygiene, early attention to even the smallest wounds, fly-screening the stables and the disposal of manure, in which flies develop, away from the stables.

Photosensitization (blue nose) Photosensitization is an inflammation of the skin which occurs when sensitized skin is exposed to strong light. The skin can be sensitized by grazing or feeding in the stable on a number of plants such as St John's wort and other hypericum species, lucerne, alfalfa, some types of clover and lupins and dried up plants of buckwheat. Some pasture plants only have this effect when they are infected by a fungus disease.

The condition is only seen when the horses that have eaten the sensitizing food are exposed to strong sunlight. Any areas of pink skin which are covered with white hair become flushed and tender. They soon thicken and swell and develop a purplish hue. This has given rise to the name 'blue nose' for the disease, because most horses with white marks have white on the face and muzzle. The affected parts itch to such an extent that the horses rub their noses on the ground, and other areas against fences and trees, tearing the skin. In some cases the surface of the skin peels off but the hair follicles remain and the coat is restored as before. White heels may become cracked and require careful attention. Horses with large areas of white hair may suffer from shock, with a staggering gait, rapid pulse and a temperature raised to 40.5° or 41.5°C (105° or 106°F).

Affected horses should be stabled, giving them immediate benefit from shade and removing them from access to the herbage that is sensitizing their skin. Laxatives should be given to hasten the elimination of the poisons already eaten. Cases showing shock should be treated with injections of antihistamine.

Prevention of photosensitization depends on discovering which plants are responsible. They may sometimes be eaten by dark-haired stock whose skin is not affected by the bright sunlight, but this should be done with caution because the sensitizing plants in some cases also have a damaging effect on the animal's livers regardless of the colour of their coat.

Non-sweating (dry coat) In tropical areas that are both hot and humid, horses are liable to develop a condition in which they lose the capacity to sweat. In the early stages of the disease an affected horse sweats excessively at work and is easily exhausted. As the disease develops the capacity to sweat is steadily reduced over several months until the horse does not sweat at all. The coat becomes harsh and dry and distressed breathing, a rapid heart rate and a high temperature develop with exercise. The horse falls off in performance and condition and becomes useless. The disease is considered to be a failure of horses accustomed to a temperate climate to adapt to extreme tropical conditions.

Horses removed from the heat and humidity gradually return to normal if their hearts have not been permanently damaged. Most horses brought into tropical conditions for high quality performance such as racing and polo are liable to some degree of non-sweating and dry coat. This can be alleviated by keeping them in air-conditioned stables, feeding a good ration of fresh green food daily as well as their more concentrated feed for energy and ensuring an adequate intake of salt, 50 or 75 g (2 or 3 oz) a day, which may have to be given by stomach tube or by intravenous injection. Pressure hosing with cold water for 15 minutes several times a day is helpful. Even with these aids such horses can only be expected to maintain the robust health necessary for competitive work and an impressive appearance if they are able to spend at least six months of the year, not necessarily in one long holiday, in a more suitable climate, found in most tropical countries up in the hills.

Hidebound Hidebound skin looks and feels dry and tightly attached to the body, and it does not ripple under the fingers. It usually goes with poor condition. Starvation, bad teeth, indigestion, worms, or extreme old age may be responsible.

11 Eyes and ears

Cross-section of eye

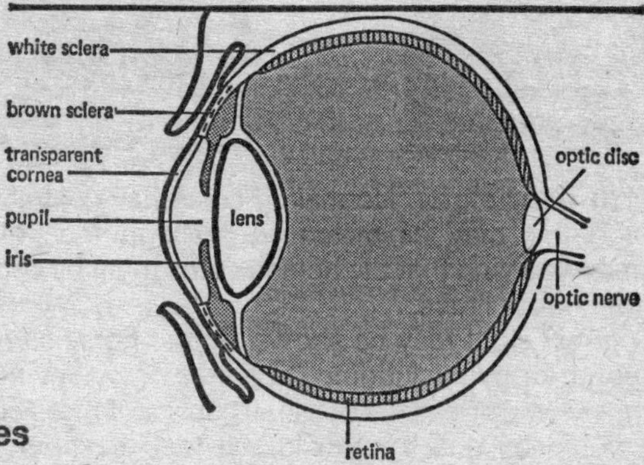

The eyes

A horse's eyeballs are about 6 cm ($2\frac{1}{3}$ in) in diameter, fractionally smaller than a tennis ball. They consist of a thick fibrous skin, the sclera, distended by some 50 ml (2 fl oz) of fluid. At the front of each eye the sclera is transparent, forming the cornea through which light enters the eye. The remainder of the sclera is white except for a diffuse band of brown around the cornea. One is seeing beyond this band when horses show the white of their eyes, opening their eyelids more widely than usual – indicating distress, fear or temper. In wall-eyed horses the iris is pale and in these cases, as well as in a few other horses, the corneal band is not brown but grey or white, giving an impression of constant surprise. Muscles are attached around the eyeballs to turn them in their bony sockets and, at the back, the optic nerves run in a thick bundle towards the brain.

Inside the eye, behind the cornea, a transparent crystalline lens is suspended to focus an image of the objects in view on to the retina, which is a layer of nerve tissue inside the back wall of the eyeball. From the retina the images are transferred by the optic nerves to the brain. The amount of light entering the eye is controlled by the iris, which encircles the front of the lens and is able to expand or contract leaving a variable open centre, the pupil. In a human eye the pupil is circular; in the horse it is an elongated strip rounded at each end. In poor light the iris draws back forming a large, almost round, pupil; in bright light it advances, reducing the aperture of the pupil to little more than a slit.

Eye in poor light
pupil enlarged

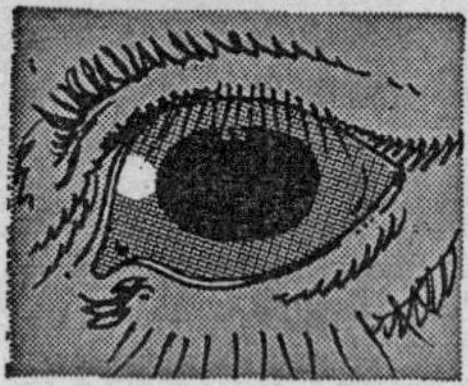

Eye in good light
pupil contracted

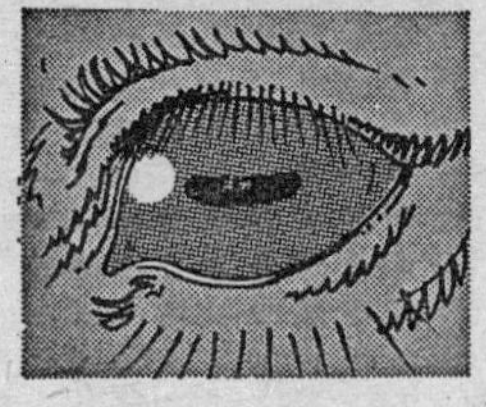

Horses with poor sight Normally horses have extremely good eyesight, and this may be tested by walking the animal over obstacles and observing that the horse avoids them by coordinating the action of all four limbs.

Lack of perfect sight may be shown by the horse stumbling on uneven ground, or by misjudging its jumps or by shying, though poor eyesight is only one of the possible causes of these conditions. Stumbling could be due to pain in the feet or shoulders; misjudging jumps to inexperience or unfitness or pain in the back, and shying to over-excitability or nervousness. A careful eye examination with the ophthalmoscope can usually reveal if there is any cause traceable to the condition of the eyes.

Cataracts The lens of a horse's eye is normally transparent. A cataract is a white deposit in the lens which interferes with sight. Affected horses may show nervousness – shying, losing confidence, and becoming less efficient at work. On the other hand, the presence of a cataract may not even be suspected until it is discovered during an eye examination. The outward appearance of the eye remains normal but the cataract can sometimes be seen by looking into the eye in a good light. With the use of an ophthalmoscope it shows up clearly as a black area in the lens. The development of cataracts is erratic. Some appear suddenly and do not enlarge; others may commence as a small spot and gradually progress until the lens is completely opaque: even then cataracts do not cause complete blindness, as some light makes its way round the lens; but the sight is limited to differentiating between light and shade.

Foals are occasionally born with cataracts. These are soft, and the white deposits can be drawn out of the lens leaving it comparatively clear, enabling the animals, in some cases, to be put to normal use.

Cataracts may develop following accidents or severe disease. The cataracts of older horses are hard and can only be removed by taking out the whole lens which leaves the horse with unreliable sight and little better off than before. It has not been found practicable to fit horses with spectacles or contact lenses to correct their sight after such an operation.

Any cataract seriously depreciates the value of a horse. Even if it does not appear to be interfering with the animal's performance there is always the possibility that the cataract will extend and lead to a degree of blindness. As the cause of cataracts is not known there are no steps that can be taken that might prevent their occurrence.

Dislocated lens A dislocated lens in the eye is not a common condition but does occasionally occur as the result of an accident or due to periodic ophthalmia. The displacement of the lens may be seen with an ophthalmoscope which shows it like a setting sun, instead of the full circle being visible. This may cause distorted vision and extreme nervousness. Some horses adjust to the peculiar vision in one eye after a time; others may work less nervously if the affected eye is blinkered or covered with a shade. The lens can be removed leaving the horse with poor sight in that eye, and this may be preferable to the sometimes frightening effect on the horse of the misplaced lens.

Eyelid injuries and entropion Eyelids are liable to injury by being caught and torn by nails or other projections. If the edges of the eyelids are involved they need very careful repair; otherwise they may heal up leaving a gap in the row of eyelashes or become turned inwards, so that the lashes rub on and irritate the surface of the eye: a condition of entropion. If entropion occurs it can usually be corrected by putting several sutures into the eyelid at right angles to the long axis of the lid. When these are drawn tight and tied they turn the edge of the eyelid out slightly and remove the lashes from contact with the eye surface. The sutures are removed a week later. Very often this temporary stitching effects a cure. In persistent cases more definite surgery may be needed.

Clouded cornea If the surface of the eye is scratched by grit or thorns or damaged by bacteria or viruses the injuries are healed by the process of inflammation. Inflammation of the cornea, the transparent front of the eye, unlike inflammation in most parts of the body, is white, not red. This is because the blood vessels on the cornea are too small for red blood corpuscles to enter, leaving that part of the eye nourished by transparent fluid that does not interfere with sight. When damage occurs and inflammatory repair is needed, the white blood corpuscles, being much more active than the red ones, squeeze through the very narrow vessels and create a white film over the area. When the injury is repaired the white corpuscles retire, leaving the cornea transparent again except for a small central scar.

Scars on the eye Wounds, injuries and ulcers on the front of the eye often leave permanent white scars when they have healed up. They interfere with the horse's vision and their effect is judged by the animal's behaviour at work. Many of these scars are of no importance and they do not increase in size. They should not be confused with cataracts in the lens which are likely to enlarge and progressively interfere with sight. Superficial scars on the cornea that are interfering with a horse's efficiency at work can be exised and replaced by a piece of transparent cornea taken from another horse's eye – a corneal graft.

Punctured eyeball Wounds of the eyeball may allow fluid to leak from inside the eye, causing it to shrink or collapse. If the internal structures are undamaged the fluid is replaced as soon as the wound heals, and the eye returns to its normal tension. Small punctures often heal without assistance. Larger wounds are likely to require stitching.

Tear duct obstruction Horses constantly produce a thin clear liquid from their tear glands to wash and lubricate the surface of the eye. This fluid is normally drained away by a tube that runs from the inner corner of the eye through a bony passage in the skull and discharges from a little round hole just inside the nostril. If this duct is blocked by thick discharges from the eye or by injury to the skull, the tears overflow the lower eyelid and run down the face. Treatment must be applied to clear up the infection or irritant that is causing the obstruction in the duct. As soon as this has been overcome, the tears will drain away again through the tube. Blockage of the duct by damage to the bones of the skull may result in a permanent discharge from one eye. This requires the regular application of a greasy dressing to protect the skin of the face from the burning effects of a constant flow of tears. In some cases the tear duct may be helped to re-establish its flow if it is gently syringed out with a mild antiseptic dressing through the lower opening in the nostril.

Periodic ophthalmia (moon blindness) In this disease there is an inflammation of nearly all the tissues inside the eyeball.

The first indication of ophthalmia is that one eye closes up and a few tears flow on to the face. This resembles any slight damage to the eye; but with periodic ophthalmia an inspection with the help of an ophthalmoscope shows that the fluid in the front of the eye is cloudy, so that the lens and the back of the eye cannot be seen. The other eye may be affected to some degree or not at all. The inflammation subsides in a week or ten days, though the ophthalmoscope may show that the cells that caused the clouding in the fluid in front of the lens have settled as a white deposit low down in the eye and the pupil may be a little mis-shapen. The upper eyelid, instead of forming a smooth curve, develops a central peak giving the eye a slightly triangular appearance.

The disease is likely to recur after an interval of a few weeks, though not as regularly as the stable name of moon blindness might imply. The attacks may recur again and again, each one leaving the eye in a worse state. The eyeball sinks a little, the lens becomes cloudy, the pupil deformed and the cornea opaque rendering the eye quite useless. Both eyes are usually involved during these later attacks and the horse becomes blind.

The cause of this disease is unknown. Atropine and physostigmine ointments are used on the eye to activate the iris and prevent adhesions. Cortisone ointment and injections may also be helpful.

Antibiotic injections are usually given in case some infection may be involved. Some workers have suggested that cases of the disease may be due to leptospirosis, a disease that is carried by rats.

Eye growths (tumours) Growths occasionally develop on the surface of the eyeball or on the eyelids. They call attention to themselves by causing the eye to discharge an excessive quantity of tears. Growths on the eye should be removed surgically at an early stage and subjected to a laboratory examination, as one variety tends to spread rapidly to adjoining tissues and glands. Radio-active implants have been used successfully to prevent recurrences.

Eye worms Filarial worms occasionally find their way into the fluid in front of the lens in the eyeball and can be observed with the aid of an ophthalmoscope. It is thought that they do no harm while they are alive but produce an irritant when they are dead, clouding the eye fluid. The anterior chamber can be opened surgically at the side of the cornea so that the fluid floods out under pressure bringing the parasite with it. The eye rapidly regains its proper tension and the inflammatory changes usually respond to cortisone treatment.

Blind horses If a completely blind horse is to be kept alive, usually as a brood mare, the animal can manage with very little extra care, finding her way about a limited and safely fenced area by smell, touch and memory, making great use of her ears to observe what is going on. Like other mares she will always be anxious over her foal and literally keeping in touch with it is important. It is a help to the mare if the foal carries a small bell around its neck.

Removal of the eye An eye that is damaged beyond repair can be removed surgically and the eye socket covered with skin from the face by a simple plastic operation. The horse is relieved of the constant irritation liable to be associated with an injured eye and the facial appearance is not unpleasant. One-eyed horses can join in a wide range of activities without detriment though they are, sensibly, not allowed on the polo ground.

Artificial eyes are obtainable for cases in which it has been possible to remove the eyeball without damaging the eyelids.

Ear conditions

A horse's ears are constantly in use, being able to turn to catch sounds coming from any direction. In the grooming process the outside of the ears should be brushed over and the inside wiped clear of dust. Horses' ears are seldom a cause of trouble.

Excess wax If a horse pulls to one side, shakes its head frequently or shows a tendency to lean the whole body to one side in the stable, all rather puzzling conditions, it may be worth while wiping out the ears daily for a few days with a wad of cotton wool soaked in equal parts of ether and olive oil, which softens the wax and allows excessive quantities that may be blocking the ear to be wiped out quite easily.

Teratoma A teratoma is a rare and peculiar growth about the size of a walnut that is found occasionally at the base of a young horse's ear. It is not usually noticed until a discharge is seen to be oozing from it. On investigation it is found to be a cyst containing hair and, sometimes, a small tooth. It is considered to be a fault traceable to the horse's development while an embryo. The teratoma is usually quite simple to remove by surgery with little likelihood of any harmful effects.

Warts The ears are one of the sites where warts are likely to occur – see Skin conditions page 299.

12 Breeding

The expectation of success

In the breeding of horses a start should be made with healthy young stock. Barren mares and infertile stallions present interesting problems to the experts, but are not likely to produce any foals. The best results are obtained with the least trouble from ponies running under wild conditions and these are nearly equalled at thoroughbred stud farms where trained staff and veterinary advisers combine to apply devoted attention and scientific aids. 90% of the mares conceiving and 75% producing live foals would be considered an excellent achievement. The difference in numbers between conception and live birth is due to early resorption of the embryo, abortion (which is usually caused by twins), and mishaps at foaling. Diseases of new-born foals are likely to reduce the final figure of production to 70%. Horses bred under less natural conditions than wild ponies or with less expert attention than at the National Stud may expect to achieve a production rate of 50%: that is, one young horse from each mare in two years. A lower figure than this probably indicates serious trouble, a stallion of sub-normal fertility, mares with chronic womb infection, or major faults in management.

Mating

Mares carry their foals for eleven months, so having a foal can conveniently be an annual event. Mares will only accept mating when they are in-season, or oestrus, which occurs for a few days at a time at intervals of three weeks from some time in March until September. Normally from October to March mares do not come into season and cannot be mated. During their days in-season mares are friendly towards the stallion's approach and will stand to be mated. At other times the stallion and the mare are indifferent to each other.

Mares in season (oestrus) The mare's coming into oestrus is controlled by chemical messengers or hormones carried in the blood stream. Stimulated by the increasing hours of daylight in the spring, the mare's pituitary gland at the base of the brain produces a hormone that rouses her ovaries to activity. There are large numbers of egg cells in the ovaries and, in response to the hormone, one of them is surrounded by a fluid follicle which enlarges until it appears like a water blister 3 cm ($1\frac{1}{3}$ in) in diameter, protruding from the wall of the ovary which itself measures about 10 by 5 cm

(4 by 2 in). While this follicle is developing the ovary sends out a hormone which rouses the mare's sexual interest, increasing its intensity over several days. The mare is coming into oestrus. The signs are a change of temperament, often to an increased excitability, but sometimes to an unusual docility; she stands from time to time with the hind legs extended and the tail raised as if to pass urine and frequently opens and closes the lips of the vulva, which is referred to as 'winking'. She is likely to squeal and kick and eject small jets of urine if touched on the flanks or behind the saddle. These signs become intense in the presence of the stallion. Oestrus lasts from 4 to 8 days, averaging five days. In the very early stages, if approached by the stallion, even though she is showing clear signs of oestrus, the mare may squeal and kick at him viciously. Later she will accept his advances, turn her quarters to him and allow mating.

During oestrus the wall of the egg follicle on the ovary becomes tense and thin and then ovulates by bursting and discharging the egg into the funnel-shaped opening of the fallopian tube. For a successful mating the egg must be met by the stallion's semen at the ovarian end of the fallopian tube and conception takes place by one of the sperm cells from the semen penetrating into the egg cell. The fertilized egg then passes down the tube to implant itself in the wall of the uterus or womb.

Oestrus terminates about forty-eight hours after the discharge of the egg cell from the ovary, and from that time the mare has no attraction for the stallion. If the mare has not been mated during that oestrus period, or if she has been mated but has not conceived, oestrus returns in about fifteen days. If she has conceived, oestrus does not occur again until after the foal is born. For conception to occur it is important that fresh semen from the stallion should be waiting in the fallopian tube. The only guide to the time the egg enters the fallopian tube is that oestrus terminates two days later. It follows that the best time for service by the stallion is two days before the end of oestrus. Since oestrus varies in length from 4 to 8 days, a satisfactory mating is ensured if the mare is served by the stallion every other day until oestrus ends and she will no longer accept him. This plan is practical and is widely adopted.

The time for mating Under natural conditions with horses running wild, the stallion controls a small harem of up to five or six mares and serving them frequently meets the requirement of fresh semen adequately, since the conception rate among groups of free-ranging horses and ponies is remarkably high.

Before the arrival of motorized horse-boxes for transport, horse breeding was largely conducted by travelling stallions which were walked around a large district during the spring and early summer, calling by arrangement at intervals of a week or more at farms or other convenient assembly points such as blacksmith's forges to serve a few mares judged to be in-season. This was a chancy arrangement that led to a very low fertility rate, only acceptable to the mares' owners because foal raising was not their prime consideration. Mares failing to conceive continued in their working capacity, as did many of those carrying foals until they became too large to fit between the shafts.

Nowadays mares are sent long distances to be mated and are required to stay at the stud farm for several weeks to ensure that they are served at the right time and to establish that they are pregnant. Allowing a mare to foal at home and then go to the stud farm means that both the mare and her foal must travel. It is usually more satisfactory to send the mare to the stud about a month before her foal is due. At that time she is not likely to be upset by the journey and she has time to settle before foaling. In addition there will be experts around if any problems arise at foaling and from then on the staff will have the mare's oestrus periods under observation and mating can be arranged at the most favourable time taking the stallion's interests into account as well as the mare's. It is usually considered that a horse can deal with up to 20 mares in his first year at stud and with 40 or a few more in subsequent years. Because some mares only show that they are in-season in the presence of a stallion, another stallion – known as the teaser – is sometimes used to check if the mares are in oestrus, saving the valuable animal for the more important duty of actually serving the mares.

Colts are able to beget foals at 2 years but they are seldom used for stud purposes until they are 4 years old. Fillies can be bred from as yearlings, foaling at two years, but this is unusual and is detrimental to their development and to the production of strong foals. Well cared for fillies can be mated as two year olds to produce foals at three but, because they are required for other purposes, many are not bred from until later in life. The delay does not seem to have a significant effect on their productivity unless they have been badly managed and overworked or, worst of all, allowed to get fat, which seriously interferes with the activity of the ovaries. As an example of late breeding a hunter mare, long retired to grass, broke out at the age of twenty-three to join a passing group of gypsy horses and produced her first foal with no trouble the following year.

The system of trying to mate mares at the right time by allowing the stallion to serve them at repeated intervals is not considered to be accurate enough on studs dealing with thoroughbred and other horses of very high value, and it involves using the stallion more than is necessary. In these circumstances a veterinary surgeon examines the mare by passing his sleeved arm into the rectum to detect the presence and condition of a follicle on the ovary. He can tell, almost to the hour, when the follicle will ripen and ovulate so that the mare can be served at the most favourable time for conception. This is now routine practice on some stud farms. The mare need not be mated frequently and the stallion's vigour is conserved.

It is an urgent matter that thoroughbred horses should be born early in the year. They are aged from 1st January; thus, in a race for 2-year-olds in June, a January-born foal would be actually 2 years and 5 months old, a great advantage in competition with a foal born in May which would only be 2 years and 1 month. Thoroughbred studs are allowed to start their mating programme on 15th February, and they put on the pressure to bring their mares into oestrus early, housing and feeding them indulgently through the winter and arranging artificial lighting in imitation of the onset of spring. Their efforts are remarkably successful and the mares come in season a month or more before the usual appearance of oestrus in late March. The first one or two periods of oestrus are sometimes prolonged and manual examination of the ovaries shows that although egg follicles are developing, none of them is ripening. In these conditions veterinary checks on the ovaries are particularly useful to indicate if mating would be worth while or quite fruitless.

The foal heat Mares that have given birth to a foal usually come into season about a week later. This is known as the foal heat. It would seem sensible to miss this oestrus period to allow the mare time to recover from the stress of foaling, but experience has shown that a number of mares suckling their foals do not come in season again for months. Mating was therefore often arranged at the foal heat because there might not be another chance. Recent investigations have made it clear that mares mated at the foal heat are more likely to lose their foals from embryonic death, that is early death in the womb, than those mated at a later date, so service at the time of the foal heat is not advised. Mares not coming into season because they are suckling a foal or for other reasons can now be treated to restore the regular occurrence of oestrus.

Artificial insemination Artificial insemination consists of obtaining a quantity of semen from a stallion and injecting portions of it into a number of mares. The stallion is persuaded to ejaculate into an artificial vagina. The semen collected in this way is diluted with preservatives and is made up into suitable doses. These remain viable, using present techniques, for long periods, some workers reporting successful conceptions after storing the semen for several years.

The main advantage of artificial insemination is that a great many mares can breed foals from one horse that has desirable characteristics, thereby rapidly improving the quality of a breed. Another advantage is that mares may be inseminated with semen transported to any part of the world without moving them from their home ground, avoiding any risks of injury to the mare and her suckling foal. Artificial insemination prevents the spread of venereal diseaes; and breeding can still continue if movement controls are applied because of epidemic disease. A less important point is that mares unable to be mated naturally because of injury or disease can still, in suitable cases, bear a foal: and, finally, the semen of outstanding horses can be put in store for use when they become incapable of service and for years after their death.

Racing authorities have not adopted artificial insemination because they fear that the temptation to breed from a few fashionable horses would cause a reduction in the number of the blood lines now available. The various blood lines allow a wide selection of characteristics and their disappearance would lead to inbreeding which would be more likely to exaggerate the faults than the perfections in a comparatively small population of horses. Thoroughbred breeders also doubt if the origin of the semen and therefore the pedigree of the foal could be guaranteed, but this fear can be overcome by the modern methods of blood-grouping horses which are so accurate that parentage can be determined with certainty.

An extensive and practical investigation at the Hanoverian National Stud Farm concluded that artificial insemination could be used successfully to overcome great distances and disease problems but that the current demand for horses did not justify setting up and maintaining the technical staff and specialized apparatus required.

Dating and synchronizing oestrus A problem with the large scale use of artificial insemination is that, with a number of mares ovulating at different times, a great deal of work is required to observe them and work out the proper time for insemination in each case. This difficulty can now be overcome by using bio-chemical preparations, so that in the breeding season any group of mares can be brought into oestrus on a given day:

On day 0 all the mares are given a dose of fluprostenol
On day 6 they are all given a dose of chorionic gonadotrophin
On day 14 they are all given fluprostenol again
On day 20 they should all be in oestrus. Whether they are or not they should all be given a dose of chorionic gonadotrophin and they should all be inseminated. Those that are not in oestrus will almost certainly be in 'silent heat' – that is, ovulating without external signs; and they should be inseminated like the others, with an equally high expectation of success.

Mares not coming into season WARNING! The most usual cause of a mare's failure to come into oestrus during the breeding season is that she is pregnant. Any treatment applied to such a mare to bring her in-season in the belief that her ovaries are inactive is likely to cause abortion.

Nothing will induce mares to come into season if their ovaries are in the state of winter inactivity, but quite a number of mares do not come into season for long periods during spring and summer. Consequently their mating is delayed until later than was intended or it may possibly be missed for the whole season. The mare is the only domestic animal in which this oestrus failure is common, and it is not confined to mares that are suckling a foal. The cause is known to be due to the persistence in the ovary of a substance, the corpus luteum, its function being to inactivate the ovary between oestrus periods and during pregnancy. Why it persists is not known, but it seems likely to be associated with some fault in the established methods of horse management, as it seldom occurs in horses running under wild conditions.

The remedy for this condition was, to quote an old veterinary guide, 'to confine the mare and let her be served by a vigorous colt' – that is, she should be put in the stocks and raped, not in the hope of conception but to restore the normal rhythm. At a later date 'arming' was substituted for the 'vigorous colt'. The stud groom would plunge his arm as far as he could reach into the vagina. The claim that these crude methods of stirring tissues into activity were frequently successful is not difficult to believe, because it has since been found that the stimulus of gently injecting 250 ml (9 fl oz) of warm salt water solution through a small tube into the uterus usually brings a mare into season in 4 or 5 days, and mating at this time is likely to be successful. This last method is in frequent use, having the advantages of simplicity and, if carefully carried out, negligible stress or risk to the mare.

The most recent approach is by bio-chemical control. A hypodermic injection of fluprostenol brings the mare into season in 2 to 5 days. Six days after the fluprostenol the mare should be mated and, on the same day, given an injection of chorionic gonadotrophin. This causes the ripening egg follicle on the ovary to ovulate and discharge its egg cell at the right time for conception to occur. The great advantage of this approach is that none of the mare's organs are interfered with by handling or by instruments. Neither saline infusions nor fluprostenol can be effective when the ovaries are in their state of winter quiescence.

Barren mares

Barren mares are those which have been expected to breed but have reached the end of the mating season without conceiving a foal.

Reproductive organs

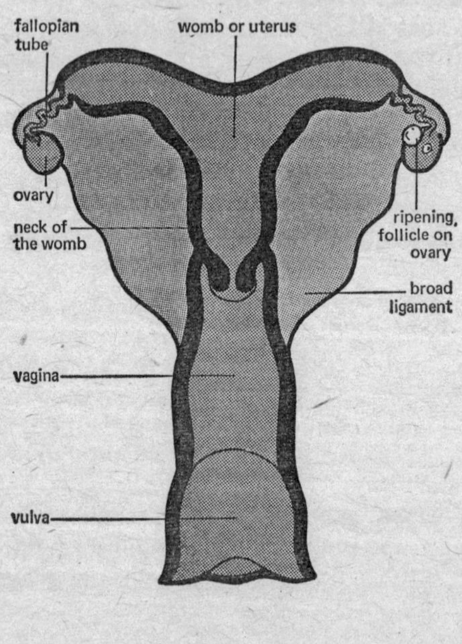

The mare's normal processes in preparation for conception are that the ovaries, small and inactive through the winter, produce a follicle in the spring which ripens and discharges an egg cell into the uterus. For a few days before this event and for two days after it the mare is in-season and permits the horse to mate with her. His semen meets the egg cell in the fallopian tube and the egg cell is fertilised.

For a mare to fail to conceive, this series of events must have failed in some respect. The two most usual reasons are, firstly, that the mare does not come in-season and so cannot be mated ;and, secondly, that she has some infection in the womb that prevents it from accepting and nourishing the embryo. These and a number of less usual reasons for a mare to be barren are discussed in the following pages.

The influence of age and condition A mare may not come into season through the spring and summer because she is too young or too old, too thin or too fat.

Well fed yearlings come into season during the summer when they are eighteen months old, and will readily conceive a foal. Mating at this age should not be permitted as over fifty per cent of any foals conceived are aborted or die at birth, and any live foal is likely to be a weakling and its mother's normal growth and development retarded. If an accidental mating at this age has taken place the pregnancy should be terminated by an injection of prostaglandin within four days of that event or, later, by dilating the passage from the vagina to the uterus. Horses running free are seldom well nourished enough for the fillies to come into season before they are two years old.

As regards old age, mares that have bred a large number of foals still come into season regularly but they have usually suffered tears or other injuries to the womb or contracted infections that prevent them conceiving. Failure to come in-season may occur in mares that have never had a foal, because their ovaries are either infiltrated with fat or are scarred up by the production of innumerable follicles. There is no treatment for these cases.

Being too fat or too thin has direct effects on the ovaries. Fat infiltrates the ovarian tissue and interrupts its activities. Animals that are thin from starvation or disease do not produce the chemical messengers, hormones, that initiate the breeding cycle. Their tissues are too fully occupied with survival to permit procreation.

Thin mares can more readily be restored to health and breeding condition than fat ones. Nourishing food, worm treatment and good management will usually cure poor condition. Fat animals need very carefully restricted diets and a graded exercise regime. The excess fat may have permanently injured the ovaries but there is quite good hope for young fat mares to be brought into production when they have fined down.

Persistent corpus luteum Two days after the mare's follicle has ruptured and discharged its egg to the uterus, the mare goes out of season and will not allow mating. This sudden change of attitude towards the horse is due to the development of yellow tissue on the ovary in the cavity left by the burst follicle. This yellow tissue, the corpus luteum, produces a hormone which keeps the mare out of season for about sixteen days, after which the tissue dissolves, and, if not pregnant the mare comes in-season again. Sometimes the corpus luteum does not dissolve and the mare remains under its control and does not come into season.

If it is clear that the mare is not pregnant, and this will be certain if she has not been mated, the corpus luteum can be persuaded to dissolve by injecting 250 ml (9 fl oz) of warm salt water (normal saline) into the uterus by gravity through a tube or by injecting a dose of prostaglandin into the mare's muscles. The mare then comes in-season in four or five days and may be mated with reasonable hope of success.

Clover feeding Clover has a substance in it that acts on a mare's ovaries rather like the corpus luteum and prevents her from coming in-season. This condition can be treated by moving the mare on to a pasture that has less clover or is free of it. The ovaries may need to be reactivated by injecting prostaglandin into the mare's muscles to stimulate the development of a follicle followed four days later by an injection of chorionic gonadotrophin which helps the follicle to rupture and discharge its egg.

Suckling a foal Mares suckling a foal that have not been mated at the foal heat sometimes do not come into season again. They should be injected with prostaglandin followed in four days by an injection of chorionic gonadotrophin and taken to the stallion on that fourth day. These mares are usually shy of showing themselves in-season but with the help of these injections which will almost certainly make the timing right, it is likely that they will accept mating by the horse.

Failure of the mated mare to conceive

Womb infection Bacteria and viruses usually enter the vagina and uterus through the vulva, carried in at mating or during the complications of foaling or gaining entry through faulty closure of the vulva. These bacteria and viruses, and others that may reach the uterus carried by the blood stream, multiply there if they find conditions suitable and cause such inflammation that the embryo cannot settle and grow.

'If they find conditions suitable' is a significant point. It is generally agreed that a healthy uterus overcomes infections. This is often the case but the uterus may succumb to infection because of old age when the natural defences weaken or because the infection is an overwhelming one, as with infectious metritis. Infection may be difficult to overcome when some of the placenta is left behind after foaling, or when the vulva fails to act as a valve so that faeces and other filth are constantly sucked into the vagina.

Pyometra and other womb infections This condition of pus in the womb is noticed by discharges from the vulva that run down and dry on the legs. Because of old age or some debilitating disease, the uterus is unable to throw off an infection. Washing out the womb with quantities of warm salt water, a tablespoonful to 1 litre (2 pints), daily for a week may be of help, followed by infusion into the womb of a suitable antibiotic and injections of antibiotic drugs into the muscles. In persistent cases a stilboestrol implant in the neck muscles will have the effect of shrinking the uterus and this will reduce the area available to the infectious bacteria and render them more accessible to antibiotic medication. After a few weeks the stilboestrol may cause objectionably masculine behaviour, such as mounting and biting other mares, and the implant should be removed.

Contagious equine metritis This metritis is a disease of the uterus and vagina which causes quantities of thick discharge to flow from the vulva. It is a highly contagious disease that is spread by infected stallions during mating. The cause is a coccobacillus now known as *Haemophilus equigenitalis*. The disease first appeared in Ireland in 1976 and in Newmarket in 1977. It appears to respond to suitable antibiotic treatment but there has not yet been time to discover how persistent this infection may be.

Other bacteria cause inflammation of the uterus with negligible discharges from the vulva. One which seriously interferes with some mares' breeding ability is *Klebsiella pneumoniae*. Infections associated with pieces of placenta left behind after foaling may cause womb inflammation and severe illness until the offending membrane has been removed. These various infections usually respond satisfactorily to douching the uterus with saline and using antibiotic treatment.

Wind suckers – fluters The vulva in a young mare in good condition lies vertically just below the anus. As the mare grows older her belly is inclined to drop and this has the effect of drawing the anus forward under the tail, dragging the upper end of the vulva with it. Before long the vulva is sloping at an angle of forty-five degrees downward and the mare's droppings slide over it as they fall from the anus to the ground. To avoid the vagina becoming infected by flith and bacteria from the faeces, the vulva must act as a very efficient valve with lips closely opposed.

Mares that have had several foals and have suffered from the stretching and sometimes tearing of the vulva that occurs at foaling are likely to have sloping vulvas with lips distorted by scars which prevent them closing satisfactorily. In ageing mares and sometimes in younger ones the vulva loses its muscular tone and the lips are loose instead of being firmly closed. When these animals trot their bellies flop down at each step and they suck in air through the vulva which makes a whistling sound at each step: from this they are known as 'fluters' or 'wind suckers'. They are not to be confused with horses which have the habit of swallowing air into their gullet, a vice also known as wind sucking.

Fluters do not suck in air alone. The air takes in with it dust and faeces and the vagina and womb become chronically infected so that the womb is unsuitable for conception.

Caslick's operation Fluters are dealt with by an operation devised by an American veterinary surgeon named Caslick. Caslick's operation consists of shortening the vulva by cutting a thin strip of skin from the upper junction of the lips and down each side for two thirds of their length and then stitching the lips together. These heal across, reducing the vulval opening to its lower third. The result is usually satisfactory. The vagina and uterus, being freed of the constant entry of faeces, clear themselves of infection and mating is able to be conducted, with some careful assistance, through the reduced vulval opening. The vulva has to be fully opened before the arrival of the foal, but can be closed again by the same operation after its birth and many mares which were barren fluters are able to produce foal after foal because of Caslick's operation.

Coital exanthema Coital exanthema is a disease that is spread from horse to horse during mating. The infection is due to a herpes virus that causes water blisters to appear on the penis or vulva and occasionally on the buttocks and under the tail. The blisters change to pustules which rupture to become large ulcers and finally scabs and these eventually fall off. The only treatment necessary is to dress the affected parts with mild antiseptic lotion or antibiotic ointments to deal with any bacteria that may infect the ulcers.

The course of the disease from the first signs of infection to healing is less than three weeks. If cases do occur it is advisable to stop mating activities for six weeks, after which normal stud work can be resumed. Six weeks is suggested because it seems likely that some animals may not show signs of the disease for more than a month after being infected.

Some animals become carriers. These recover from coital exanthema and show no further signs of it but carry the infection and can pass it on to other horses. Carriers are the means by which this disease may re-appear in subsequent breeding seasons. If a carrier is identified there is no way of eliminating the disease in that animal. Every care should be taken that carriers are not allowed to mate. Stallion carriers should be gelded.

Dourine Dourine, also called maladie du coit, is caused by a trypanosome, equiperdum. The disease occurs in tropical and sub-tropical countries and sometimes reaches into temperate zones. Dourine is spread from one horse to another during the sexual act. It is recognized by the appearance of swollen genital organs, flat swellings under the skin, known as 'dollar spots', and by intermittent increases in temperature. The signs of the disease rise and fall often for months or years, ending in recovery or death in mares but always in death in male animals. Worsening cases develop paralysis, blindness, anaemia and emaciation. Diagnosis is by the signs mentioned and by finding trypanosomes in discharges from the vulva or in the fluid taken from the dollar spots, but the most definite confirmation is by a laboratory examination of a blood sample. Treatment is possible by using trypanocides but in most countries slaughter of known cases is compulsory.

Diseased ovaries (nymphomania) Mares' ovaries may grow very large because of tumour formation by granulomas or teratomas.

The effect is that the mare is constantly in-season and willing or anxious to be mated, a condition of nymphomania. They do not conceive a foal and the only treatment is to remove the enlarged ovary by surgery. The other ovary is not likely to be affected and the mare can resume normal breeding activity when the diseased ovary has been removed.

Pregnancy

Diagnosis Diagnosing pregnancy as early as possible is important, so that mares that have not conceived may be served again before the mating season is over. If the mare comes into oestrus two or three weeks after being mated it may be assumed that she is not pregnant. However, it is not quite so certain that the mare is in foal if she does not come in-season at that time. At this stage manual examination of the uterus through the wall of the rectum by a veterinary surgeon is the only method of detection. At three weeks after conception, the developing embryo – although it is less than half an inch long – causes with its surrounding fluid and membranes a small but definite bulge in one of the horns of the uterus which is confirmation of pregnancy. Although the foal drops forward into the mare's belly as it develops and is out of reach after a few months, manual examination by the expert can always confirm pregnancy. Laboratory tests can diagnose pregnancy from blood samples from the mare between 45 and 90 days after being mated or from urine samples at any time after 150 days. These later confirmations that the mare is in-foal may be needed to allay any suspicion that she has lost her foal in the earlier stages of its development; or for insurance purposes, or in connection with the sale of the mare. When there is an arrangement that the fee for the stallion's service is only payable if the mare becomes pregnant (known as 'no-foal, no fee') settlement is frequently agreed to be due on 1st October so that confirmation of pregnancy at that date is required.

Embryo to foetus Pregnancy usually proceeds uneventfully. At six weeks the embryo has grown to 5 cm (2 in) in length from its face to its rump and weighs over 14 g ($\frac{1}{2}$ oz). Its eyes, limbs and feet are distinguishable as those of a horse, which qualifies it at this age to be promoted from the status of embryo – only recognizable as a developing creature – to rank as a foetus, a foetal horse. At birth, 11 months after conception, the foal weighs about one tenth the weight of its mother – 40 kg (90 lb) for a foal from a 15.5 hand riding horse, having been 13 g ($\frac{1}{2}$ oz) at 6 weeks; 1 kg (2 lb)

The foetus at 10 weeks

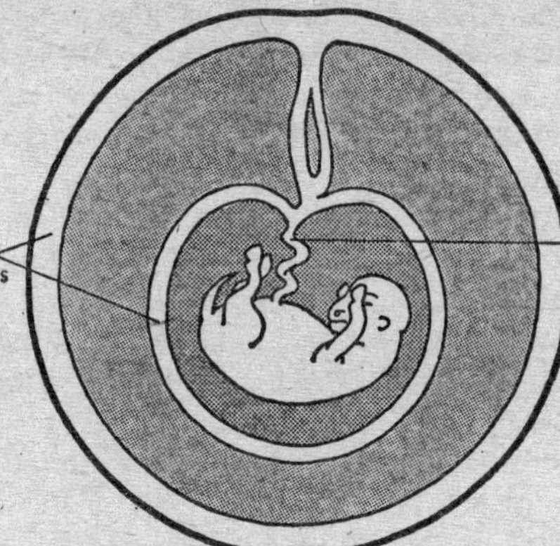

at 4 months; 4.5 kg (10 lb) at 6 months; 13.5 kg (30 lb) at 8 months; and trebling in weight during the last three months to 40 kg (90 lb), adding 27 kg (60 lb) in 90 days.

Loss of the foetus

The most serious mishap that can arise during pregnancy is the loss of the foetus. This can occur in three ways: by resorption, abortion or mummification.

Foetal resorption Resorption is the death of the embryo or very young foetus, up to 8 or 10 weeks after conception, and its disappearance by being re-absorbed inside the womb. There are no outward signs of this occurrence and it is most disappointing, if the mare has been confirmed as pregnant by a veterinary manual examination, to find later that she is empty. The mare which has lost her foal in this way may come into season again after a gap of 2 or 3 months, which is likely to be too late for another mating in that year. The cause of resorption is not known. One suggestion is that an alteration in the embryo's blood supply which occurs one month after conception has failed to adjust correctly and led to its death; another, that lack of suitable nourishment for the mare is responsible, but this is certainly not the usual cause as resorption happens to mares on very well managed stud farms.

Infectious abortion Various infections of the womb or of the membranes enclosing the foetus are a cause of abortion. These cases usually occur singly though they may spread to other mares if isolation of affected animals and good hygienic measures are not observed. Bacteria, viruses or fungi may be responsible. Bacterial infection may be caused by one of the coli group during the first half of pregnancy or by a streptococcus in the second half. The rhino-pneumonitis virus which is present in most studs and stables and is a common cause of coughing, occasionally appears in a form that brings about abortion late in pregnancy. Several fungi may also cause late abortion. These and other infections gain access to the womb through the vulva. Mares in good health manage to keep most infections at bay by their defences of white blood corpuscles and antibodies. Old and debilitated mares are most likely to succumb to infection because of lowered resistance and damage to their organs during previous foalings. One of the main causes of womb infection is the alteration in the alignment of the vulva which changes with advancing age from vertical to nearly horizontal. The lips of the vulva also slacken. As a result, faeces are aspirated into the vagina carrying filth and infection with them. This problem can often be dealt with satisfactorily by Caslick's operation for reducing the size of the vulval orifice.

Outbreaks of infectious abortion are not common and seldom affect more than a few mares and while this state of affairs continues the wide use of preventive vaccination is not recommended.

When an abortion occurs the foetus and the membranes should be collected in a plastic sack for veterinary inspection and a laboratory investigation into the cause. The contaminated area of ground should be scraped and disinfected, and other horses kept away from it. One problem is that a small foetus may not be found and even larger ones may be carried away by foxes so that it may not be discovered that an abortion has occurred. The mares either present no sign of the mishap or a varying amount of discharge from the vulva. In some types of virus-induced abortion, not at present seen in the British Isles, the mares run a high temperature and suffer from circulatory troubles causing swellings on the body and limbs.

Mares that have aborted should be treated with suitable antibiotics given by injection and by syringe into the womb, and oxytocin may be used to help the uterus to contract in size and rid itself of any remnants of the foal's membranes.

Twins and abortion The commonest cause of foal loss by abortion is the conception of twins. It seems likely that twins are present in 2% or 3% of all pregnancies. Many twins develop together for some months, competing against each other for accommodation. One usually manages to occupy an unfair share of the uterus and the other dies of starvation. The dead foal is rejected by the womb with the result that the living foal is also aborted.Some mares carry twins to full term producing one small foal and one of normal size. The small foal seldom survives for more than a few hours and of the larger ones 3 out of 4 are unlikely to survive. It does occur from time to time that a mare produces two healthy foals of equal size that thrive but they do not reach the size of their parents when they mature.

Twins are usually developed from two distinct egg cells but there are times when one egg cell alone produces twins. Such twinning can be detected 3 or 4 weeks after mating and abortion can be induced by dilating the passage from the vagina to the uterus.

Twins may be anticipated if a manual examination of the ovaries before mating detects two follicles that are likely to ovulate at about the same time. The veterinary surgeon may find it possible to puncture one follicle and allow the other to mature in due course; alternatively he may advise missing service by the stallion until a later oestrus when only one follicle appears to be developing. If it seems likely that a mare has been mated when two follicles have matured together, the pregnancy can be terminated if an injection of fluprostenol is given within four days of the service.

Spontaneous abortion This name is given to the condition when mares abort for no apparent reason. The cause may be lack of progesterone, a hormone which is essential to the continuity of a pregnancy. Mares that repeatedly lose their foals may be given additional progesterone by a series of injections or by a long acting implant: or their own progesterone production may be stimulated by injecting gonadotrophin.

Spontaneous abortion may be caused by twins but not recognized as such because only one aborted foetus has been found. It can also be due to some infection and all cases of abortion should be dealt with as though they were infectious as a precaution against the possible spread of disease.

Induced abortion Abortion can be brought about up to four days after mating by injecting the mare with fluprostenol. This may be found of use if she has been mated by accident or it seems likely that she has conceived twins. Later abortions can be effected by dilating the passage from the vagina to the uterus.

Mummification A dead foal in the uterus is usually aborted. Rarely, a foetus may die and be retained in the womb indefinitely as a leathery mummified object varying in size according to its age at death. The mare usually gives no sign of its presence which is only discovered when an examination is made of her genital organs to discover why she is not coming into season. The mare is unlikely to breed again. The dried-up foetus, if small, may be left undisturbed or may possibly be delivered whole or in pieces through the vagina. Larger mummies can only be removed by an abdominal operation.

Premature foals Foals that are born ten months or more after conception but before they are at the full term of eleven months are classed as premature foals and not as abortions. Unless serious disease has been responsible for their early arrival they have a good chance of survival.

Birth

The eleven months of a mare's pregnancy may continue uneventfully until labour actually commences. While older mares bulge visibly, young mares may retain their figures to such an extent that even knowledgeable horsemen may fail to observe that a mare they have bought is pregnant until they find her early one morning suckling her foal.

Most mares show an enlarging udder during the last month of pregnancy and a few days before the foal is due there is often a discharge of sticky milk on the teats that looks like wax. The mare is said to have 'waxed-up'. Sometimes milk runs from the udder at this time. The muscles on either side of the tail slacken and the vulva becomes longer. These are the premonitory signs of foaling but let those who dare forecast when the foal will arrive. Most foals are born in the early hours of the morning, so it is necessary to sit up all night – possibly several nights – to be sure of being present at the birth. Mares prefer to foal alone. When running free they separate themselves from the herd and find a secluded spot. If stabled they have no choice of location but they can control the time. So determined is the mare to keep the proceedings private that if she knows anyone is around she will wait until he goes off for that cup of tea at four a.m. and be nuzzling her offspring when he slips back half an hour later. While it is praiseworthy to know what is going on so that expert help can be obtained in case of trouble, causing the mare to delay foaling may be harmful to both the mare and the foal and the utmost care should be taken to ensure that she is not disturbed. On stud farms where the staff needs to be available in case of difficulties, foaling boxes are arranged around a sitting-up room with small windows through which the attendants can keep an eye on the mares, or closed-circuit television may help one groom to monitor a number of foaling boxes.

Normal birth The time taken from the first pains, the contractions of the womb that are to drive the foal out into the world to complete separation of mother and foal, varies from thirty minutes to one hour. When the contractions begin to get stronger the mare shows colicky signs, looks round at her flanks, crouches down, swishes her tail, and sometimes breaks out into a sweat behind the elbows and on her flanks. The pains may stop for a period then come on again with renewed strength. A bladder appears after a while in the vulval opening. This is the outer wall of the placenta, enclosing the water-bath in which the foal has grown. The placental membrane ruptures and a variable quantity of fluid, sometimes many litres, is discharged. Straining continues and in a few minutes another, white-skinned bladder appears. This is the inner placental membrane which closely surrounds the foal and, before long – if all is well – a front foot will be detectable, blanketed by the placenta. By this time the mare is usually lying down, changing her position frequently and occasionally standing up, to lie down again more comfortably. If anybody is present the mare may foal standing up with more risk of accidental bleeding.

Meanwhile another front foot and the foal's nose bulge in the opening; the inner membrane ruptures discharging a small quantity of fluid, and the forelegs and head are thrust clear. After a pause, very strong expulsive efforts drive the foal's chest through the vulva; there is usually another pause in the onset of pains until some less strenuous contractions deliver the hips and the hind legs. The mare rests exhausted and the foal lies struggling a little, taking gasping breaths into its unaccustomed lungs. The mare and foal are not yet completely separated. The umbilical cord is joining them and for a while there is an invisible delivery of blood to the foal from the placenta. This supply of blood is important and because of it separation of the mare and foal should not be hurried. Complete rest for 10 to 20 minutes is desirable. As long as the foal's nostrils are not covered by membranes (which would cause it to suffocate, and should be pushed to one side) the mare and foal should be left alone, until the mare or the foal gets up and the umbilical cord tears at its natural weak point a short distance from the foal's navel.

The afterbirth The mare usually discharges the placenta, or afterbirth, within an hour or two of delivering the foal. The placenta, purple in colour and spongy in texture, may cling to the inner wall of the womb. When it has been shed by the mare, the afterbirth should be taken out of the stable and inspected to ensure that it has all come away, in which case it will lie out as a large capital 'Y'. If it is obvious that one branch of the Y has been torn off and retained, veterinary advice and help may be needed to prevent infection developing in the womb.

The hippomane Among the membranes may be found a brown oval object, up to 15 cm by 7 cm and 1 cm thick (6 in by 3 in by ½ in), fleshy to the touch. This is known as the 'false tongue' or hippomane. It consists of debris accumulated in the fluid enclosed by the placenta. The hippomane has no significance, but at one time was highly prized as having magical properties associated with fertility.

Induced foaling Mares can be induced to foal by injecting fluprostenol into the neck muscles. This will effectively set in motion the normal processes and the foal is likely to be born in less than four hours. The method should only be used if the mare has carried the foal for at least eleven months and her udder shows that she is ready to foal. The udder should be distended, with bulging teats from which colostrum (see page 340) can easily be drawn with the thumb and finger. This is a sticky yellow-white milk. A brown or straw coloured liquid indicates that the mare is not ready to produce her foal.

Since the majority of mares foal without trouble, induced foaling is not normally required, but there are times, for example, if a mare has been pregnant for over eleven months and is spurting milk, when it would be advantageous to both mare and foal for the birth to take place. If the foaling is to be supervised there are considerable benefits from being able to arrange the foaling at a convenient time.

A number of apparently normal pregnancies end in disastrous foalings. There is no reason to suppose that induction with fluprostenol increases their number, but any mishap that does occur is likely to be attributed, instead of to natural causes, directly to the unnatural induction and this responsibility should be considered before this method of foaling is applied.

Mishaps at foaling

Torsion of the womb As a preparation for birth, the foal – which has been lying curled up on its back for eleven months – is re-aligned. By some remarkable activity of the mare and foal jointly, which can only be described as lurching and pitching, the foal is turned over so that it now lies spine up and belly down, with its front legs stretched out towards the mare's vulva and its head resting on its knees. Japanese research workers have shown that this re-adjustment is not a gradual process but may take as little time as a quarter of a minute. If the strong muscular activities con-

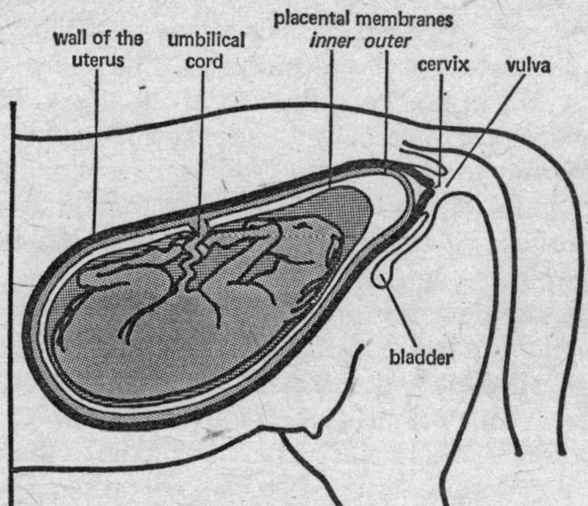

Foetus, fully developed, lying within placental membranes

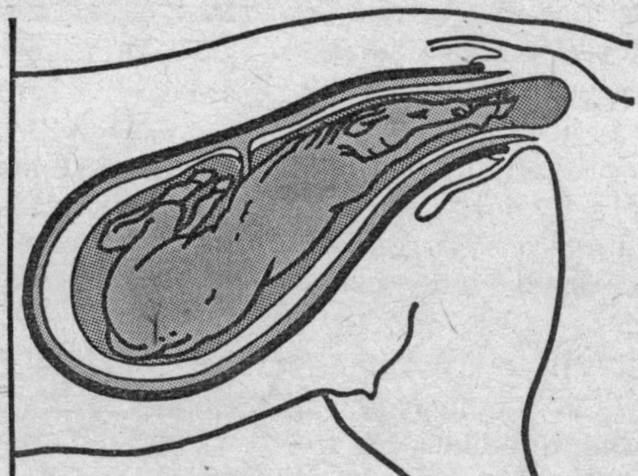
Foetus, self-adjusted in preparation for birth

cerned in this process are not exactly balanced the whole uterus may be turned over instead of just the foal. This puts a spiral twist on the neck of the womb, completely closing it as a passage for the foal's delivery, and no amount of straining by the mare can unwind the twist. Without help the mare will continue to strain and the uterus will be ruptured. A veterinary surgeon may be able to straighten out the twisted uterus by manipulation – or it may be necessary to anaesthetize the mare and, when she is on the ground, roll her over bodily in such a way that the weight of the foal unwinds the neck of the womb. If such adjustments are not possible the foal may have to be delivered by a caesarian operation.

Faulty alignment of the foal The passage of the foal through the mare's bony pelvic girdle resembles a Chinese puzzle whose parts only move on an exact alignment. If the foal is correctly placed for birth, lying on its belly facing the mare's vulva, with its forelegs straight out in front and its chin on its knees, it is thrust through the mare's pelvic girdle without damage to itself or to the mare. If any part of the foal is out of line its progress is impossible and the misalignment must be corrected.

The commonest deviation from the correct presentation is that one of the forelegs is laid back alongside the body. This increases the girth of what is already the thickest part of the foal, the shoulder and chest area. Another fault is when the head is turned on one side or is right back on the full bend of the neck to lie in the foal's flank. Occasionally the foal arrives hind feet first, which causes no trouble; but when it is presented backwards with the hind legs forwards, in what might be described as a sitting position and the parts that can be touched are the buttocks and tail, there are real problems. With all these faulty alignments the mare strains to no avail and the foal makes no progress.

The external indications of this trouble are that, although the mare has burst the waterbed and discharged quantities of fluid from her vulva, the foal's forefeet and nose are not visible and straining continues. The vet's job is to determine how the foal is lying and to make the necessary corrections.

Correcting faulty alignment of the foal The veterinary surgeon can ease the mare's distress and prevent continuous straining by using tranquillizers or other injections. With his own hands, and ropes and instruments designed for the purpose he may be able to draw the forelegs up from the foal's side, or straighten the head and neck so that the foal is normally aligned for delivery. The foal coming backwards in the sitting position may be treated by drawing the hind legs back and pulling it out hind feet first. These manipulations can be very complicated to carry out in the confined space of the genital passage without damage to the mare. The possibility of such adjustments depends a great deal on the relative sizes of the mare and foal. If these manoeuvres prove to be impossible the choice lies between delivering the foal by caesarian operation or carrying out embryotomy.

The delivery of twins Twins do not often cause trouble at birth as they are usually undersized. They sometimes attempt to get out together and consequently jam in the passage. It can be somewhat surprising to find four feet sticking out of the mare's vulva and some ingenuity is required to find out whether they are front feet or hind feet or a few of each and to allocate them correctly. The usual solution to this traffic block is, after tranquillizing the mare, to repel one foal back into the uterus to make room for its brother or sister to be born, after which the second foal should present no problem.

The caesarian operation It is only in the latter half of the 20th century that abdominal surgery has become established in horses. The increased number of large animal-hospitals with full surgical facilities has been a major factor in bringing this change about but new methods of anaesthesia, new surgical techniques and the use of antibiotics have reduced the risks to such an extent that abdominal surgery on horses can now be reasonably attempted in emergencies even when hospital facilities are not available.

The caesarian operation (named after the Roman Emperor Julius Caesar, who came into the world in this way) consists of removing the offspring from its mother through the wall of the abdomen. It is applied to mares when some obstruction, deformity or faulty alignment of the foal prevents its birth in the usual way. The mare is given a general anaesthetic and the foal is delivered through an operation site in the left flank.

Embryotomy If some obstruction, deformity or faulty alignment of a foal prevents its birth in the normal way, an alternative to the caesarian operation is embryotomy which consists of removing a dead foal piece by piece through the vulva. This has the advantage that the mare does not require to be given a general anaesthetic or be subjected to the stress of a major abdominal operation. There are various instruments devised for simplifying the embryotomy operation and for enabling it to be carried out without damage to the mare.

If the foal is alive but cannot be delivered normally the caesarian operation should be chosen. The risks of the death of the mare or the foal or both are considerable in either of these operations because in many cases both have been injured to some extent before the necessity for surgical interference has been appreciated.

Suffocation The foal takes its first gasp of air as soon as its head is clear of the mare's vulva. Care should be taken that the membranes are not preventing air reaching the nostrils. If necessary the membranes can be cut or torn to ensure this; otherwise the foal may suffocate. This can also happen if the mare foals quickly and easily dropping the foal in its surrounding membranes which may not have separated to allow the head and forelegs through. The membranes should be opened at once over the face and nostrils to give the foal air.

Some foals have been partially suffocated during foaling by pressure on the blood vessels in the umbilical cord interfering with the delivery of oxygen to the foal by that route. Premature foals may also have difficulty in commencing to breathe.

All these cases may be helped by oxygen from an oxygen cylinder or their lungs may be stirred into activity by the kiss of life.

Monsters (defective foals) One of the causes of delay or difficulty in foaling may be the faulty development of the foal. During the rapid growth of the foetus mistakes do occasionally occur so that a foal may reach full term with some vital part missing altogether or spectacularly duplicated. Some of the digestive organs may be absent or the foal may have two heads or five or six legs. These pathetic oddities are named with the peculiar beasts of imaginative story-telling as 'monsters' and, if not already dead, they are painlessly destroyed.

Rib injuries to the foal The bulkiest part of the foal to squeeze through the mare's pelvic bones is the girth, including the shoulders and that part of the chest which accommodates the heart. In a deep-chested foal, even when it is perfectly aligned, the pressure required to drive the foal through the pelvis may be so great that the young ribs crack or break low in the chest. If these rib injuries are not severe the foal may be none the worse but more extensive damage can force the fractured bones against the heart with fatal results to that organ. The pain from this injury may interfere with the establishment of breathing immediately after birth and the administration of oxygen may be of some assistance.

Wounds and tears in the mare When the foal's limbs are even slightly out of alignment, the mare's thrusts during delivery may force a foot into her soft tissues, tearing deep wounds in the wall of the vagina or even through the vaginal wall into the rectum – an injury that requires considerable veterinary skill to repair. Wounds and tears of the mare's vulva may be caused by the expansion necessary to accommodate a large foal's shoulder girdle. These must be carefully repaired to avoid scars that might distort the vulva and allow dirt and infectious organisms to reach the vagina and the uterus leading to disease and causing abortion or sterility.

Rupture of the womb The mare's straining to deliver her foal is a combination of muscular activity in the wall of the uterus helped by the mare holding her breath and contracting her chest and belly muscles. If this enormous pressure is resisted by an immovable foal, the womb may rupture and the large waterbed empties itself into the mare's abdomen. The only indication of this serious accident, which is likely to be fatal, is that the mare stops straining because, with the womb emptied of a large quantity of fluid, the pressure has disappeared. The mare usually bleeds to death rapidly from blood vessels damaged in the torn uterus. If skilled help was immediately available the foal's life, and possibly the mare's as well, might be saved by a caesarian operation.

Bone injuries to the mare The process of foaling is often distressing for a mare, especially if she has not previously produced a foal. In the preliminary restless phase and during the occurrence of her pains she may lie down and get up again frequently. A generous amount of bedding is required and this should be redistributed from time to time as the mare's restless movement may pile it up in one place and leave other areas clear. There is a danger that she may throw herself down so violently that she breaks a leg or fractures her pelvis if she lands on a solid floor. If this happens she either cannot get up again or, if she does, she will be very lame. Such accidents are usually fatal but some of these injuries, where the broken bones are not seriously displaced, can be repaired.

Bleeding at foaling The injuries that are liable to occur during the delivery of an exceptionally large foal or one that has been mis-aligned usually cause some bleeding which is not serious unless a large blood vessel is ruptured. If that does happen, blood streams from the vulva or it may accumulate in the uterus and be thrown out periodically in clotted masses. Such blood loss is dangerous, and professional help should be called. In the meantime, it is reasonable to try to suppress the flow by inserting clean towels in the vagina. These may help by compressing the damaged vessels and encouraging the blood to clot, which is part of the natural process of staunching blood loss from a vein or artery. The clotting mechanism is attempting to form a clot in the blood vessels to stop the bleeding, while blood pressure from the beating heart is driving blood out of the broken vessel. The more blood that is lost the lower the blood pressure becomes and the more chance there is that the blood will clot and the bleeding stop. If the mare lies down or collapses on to the floor, she should not be disturbed as movement interferes with clotting.

A torn vessel may bleed into the mare's abdomen without any blood discharging from the vulva. This internal bleeding may be quite unnoticed until the mare shows signs of severe blood loss by unsteadiness, collapsing on to the ground and change of colour of the membranes of the lips and gums from a clear pink to pale primrose or white. Both internal and external bleeding are very difficult to control and are likely to lead to the death of the mare.

If the bleeding does stop, the mare can make a rapid recovery even from such a severe loss of blood that she is unable to stand. Standing or lying she should be disturbed as little as possible. The foal should be left with her because taking it away would rouse the mare's maternal instinct to be with her foal come what may. If she is standing the foal will suckle as it requires. If the mare remains lying down some of her milk should be drawn off at hourly intervals and fed to the foal from a bottle at blood heat. The mare should be offered cold water to drink every half hour. Even when the blood loss has been enormous, horses that survive recover their normal behaviour within a few hours. Their activity must be restricted because the increase in blood pressure from movement might cause further haemorrhage. The quantity of blood lost is soon made up by water taken into the blood stream. The quality of blood will obviously be weakened by this dilution but the blood-forming organs can replace all the deficiencies in a few days.

Complete eversion of the womb (uterine prolapse) Prolapse of the womb is the most spectacular mishap that can occur at a foaling. After the foal and the afterbirth have been delivered the mare's womb turns itself inside out and hangs from the vulva down to the ground if she is standing up or stretches out behind her if she is lying down. The womb is an enormous bag-like organ capable of accommodating a foal of 36 to 45 kg (80 to 100 lb) and many litres of fluid. The uterus has turned itself inside-out because, during the recent foaling process, some part of the membranes have stayed attached to the inside wall at the tip of the uterus and pulled it down just like the end of a glove finger being inverted. The inverted end of the uterine horn forms a thickening or a lump that the walls of the uterus resent and they contract to drive the lump out after the foal. The further the walls of the uterus drive the in-turned tip the more of the walls have to follow it until the tip is driven through the vulva and all the rest of the womb follows after it.

Turned out of the mare, the womb inside-out is exposed as a soft, dark-red mass with a spongy surface that tears and bleeds easily. The worst thing that can happen at this stage is that the mare should get up, take fright at the object hanging behind her and plunge away, either tearing the womb or putting a foot through it, which is likely to be fatal. She should be tranquillized, and a plastic sheet laid under the uterus. Any dirt or straw is then washed off with quantities of tepid salt water; 25 g (1 oz) of salt to every 4½ litres (1 gal). The uterus is then to be wrapped in a clean cloth or bed-sheet. Gravity is helpful in the process of returning the uterus to its proper place. If the mare is on the ground the womb can be lifted in the plastic sheet. If she is standing up the same thing applies, but some ingenuity and kitchen chairs may be needed for the helpers to raise the uterus above the level of the vulva. There is a natural tendency for the uterus to reduce in size after it has ejected the foal and this is encouraged by raising it so that blood may drain out of it back to the mare's body. If the womb is left hanging the blood accumulates and it swells even larger. Dusting a pound or two of domestic sugar over the womb helps it to shrink, and obviously the smaller it becomes the easier it will be to return it. By its own weight and by pressure to constrict it at the entrance to the vulva the organ will gradually disappear back into the mare. Attempts to invert it from its extremity are fruitless as the same contracting muscles that drove the uterus out come into play again and thrust against the inversion. The replacement, slow at first, gradually gains momentum until the whole organ disappears. The veterinary surgeon, to prevent a repetition of the event, must ensure that inversion is complete, usually by filling the uterus with a warm and mild antiseptic solution which the mare will rapidly eject if all is in order. A re-occurrence is unusual in mares and any risk diminishes rapidly as the uterus quickly continues its shrinking process, helped by injections of oxytocin. Stitching across the vulva is not advised. If the womb did prolapse again the stitches would be torn away causing extensive wounds.

After-treatment is by antibiotics to protect the mare against the dangers of infection. It is remarkable that this major calamity may often be overcome without any permanent harm to the mare or any likelihood that such a mishap will recur at subsequent foalings.

New-born foals

Adjustments at birth The foal, having been born and become a separate individual, needs to make a lot of adjustments. The mare has supplied food and oxygen through the blood vessels in the placenta. Now the foal has to acquire oxygen and food for itself. As soon as its head has appeared through the membranes at the mare's vulva its lungs have gasped for air. There is a new job for the heart too, because it has to switch its blood circulation from the placenta to the lungs. This is brought about quite simply by the closure of a large gap in the wall between the two sides of the heart. At birth, using a stethoscope, the blood can be heard gushing through the gap. Within forty-eight hours the gushing sound fades away because the gap has closed. Another alteration takes place in the bladder. The foal's urine has emptied into the main waterbed in the placenta through an opening known as the urachus, at the forward end of the bladder. That route closes at birth and the bladder has to empty at the other end through the penis or the vulva. The digestive tract suddenly becomes important and a healthy foal's first motivation is soon seen to be based on suckling.

Standing up Within an hour of birth foals are making valiant attempts to stand up. Their legs are extremely long and the muscles are quite unaccustomed to controlling them – as is seen by the foal's early struggling and tumbling about; but a state of balance is rapidly acquired and the objective is the mare's udder. Within 2 or 3 hours of birth the foal should be having his first drink. This is no ordinary milk but colostrum.

Colostrum Each mare during the course of her life has been in contact with a number of diseases and infections and has become resistant to them. This resistance is carried in the blood in the form of minute particles known as antibodies, and it would be helpful to the foetus if the mare could pass her resistance on to it; but the mare's blood and the foetal blood are quite separate and the antibodies are physically unable to filter across the placenta to the foetus. However, antibodies can be secreted in the milk. The mare's milk for the first day or two is colostrum, which means that it is full of antibodies. It is vitally important that a new-born foal should be suckling well for the first day of its life to gain protection against the diseases that are likely to attack it – most particularly because after that period of twenty-four hours the foal's digestive tract alters and cannot absorb any more antibodies. The mare's milk changes to an ordinary nutritious food, but the foal's blood now carries a supply of antibodies which lasts effectively for several weeks. The foal is by then capable of producing its own antibodies against infections and diseases.

The bond between mare and foal Foals should never be out of their mother's sight until they are weaned. The importance of being within sight and touch of each other is a tremendously strong bond from birth, and if the mare and foal are separated they will both ignore all obstacles to get to each other again. Terrible damage can occur if a foal happens to stray to the wrong side of a barbed-wire fence. Even though they are in the same box the mare becomes very upset and difficult to handle if she loses sight of the foal only for a moment, though its reply to her whinnying eases her distress. When anything has to be done to the mare it is as well to have a second person in the box to keep the foal in her view and to allow her to touch it with her nose for mutual re-assurance from time to time. The bond between mare and foal weakens a little as the months go by and the foal frisks with others at some distance. Nevertheless there are still whinnyings and cantering about in search of the foal if it does go out of sight, and there is always some upset when the foal is weaned at 6 months however carefully this is planned. This is reduced to a minimum if the foals can be separated from the mares for a few days by a simple post and rail fence. The mares and foals can contact each other but the foals cannot suckle. This arrangement is further helped if a barren nurse mare can be left running with the weaned foals for a while.

Handling foals New-born foals weighing 45 kg (90 lb) or so are not easily handled. They may have to be picked up to move them to a more convenient part of the box or to help them suckle the mare, or it may be decided to lay them down to rest if they are unwilling to lie down themselves. A foal standing up can be held with one hand grasping the up-turned tail near its root and the other hand round the front of the neck. Pressure on the neck should be as light as possible as the windpipe is easily compressed, suffocating the foal or cracking the rings of cartilage that form the tube. The foal can be moved about with the same hold, using the tail for propulsion and the neck for steerage. To lay a foal down, start with the same hold, stand very close to the foal's body, slide the hand at the front of the foal down and round to the far elbow and the hand at the tail down and round the far buttock. Shuffle forward and lift the foal. The weight of the foal's body will tip its back away as it slides on its side down to the ground. The reverse procedure needs two people to lift the foal. One stands close to the foal's belly with a hand round below the neck to the lower elbow and the other round the lower buttock. If this person lifts unaided the foal will just turn on its back. The second person should stand at the foal's spine and, as lifting starts, help to lever the foal into a standing position, holding the tail in one hand and balancing the head with the other.

To control a recumbent foal conveniently for bottle feeding, giving medicine by mouth or taking its temperature, the helper should sit near the wall so that he can rest his back against it. The foal should lie to his left with its back parallel to the wall and its head resting in his lap. To take the foal's temperature a second helper should slip a dampened thermometer into the foal's anus to a depth of 8 cm (3 in) and hold the projecting tip for the required time – sensibly as long as two minutes. The normal temperature of a foal should be 37.8° to 38.1 °C (100° to 100.5°F).

Feeding A new-born foal should be suckling within 2 or 3 hours after its birth. If after 4 hours it has not managed to suckle. the mare should be held while another helper guides the foal to the udder and draws some milk with finger and thumb which may interest the foal enough to begin suckling on its own. If the foal is not suckling because it cannot stand up, being premature or sick, it should have milk from its mother as an urgent matter because of the antibodies in the colostrum. Milk should be drawn from both the mare's teats into a warm (blood heat) jug. The milk is drawn by gripping the base of the teat gently between the ball of the thumb and the side of the first finger and sliding them with slight pressure towards the tip of the teat. About 0.25 litres (½ pint) makes a reasonable feed for a foal.

Even if the mare is flush with milk and lets it flow readily, not more than this quantity should be drawn off for each feed because the more milk is taken the more the mare will produce. If there is difficulty in drawing milk, less will do for the first feed, but 0.25 litres (½ pint) should be taken if possible after an hour. The milk should be transferred to a baby's feeding bottle with the hole enlarged sufficiently to allow a pin-head through easily. Foals suckle by instinct and usually take milk from a bottle teat without hesitation. If the milk does not flow the hole in the teat should be enlarged further. If the foal will not suckle from the bottle, which probably means that it is really ill, the milk may be dribbled into its mouth through a big hole in the teat. Feeding 0.25 litre (½ pint) at hourly intervals will suffice; but a strong foal may be given larger feeds at wider intervals, though strong foals usually draw their own milk supply. Weakly foals should be fed hourly for a week, after which the interval and quantities may be increased if the foal's progress is satisfactory. Milk should never be poured into a foal's mouth. When a foal sucks at a mare or a bottle teat it sucks and swallows in a gentle rhythm. A large quantity of milk causes it to gulp and some of the milk is likely to enter the windpipe, run down into the lungs and cause pneumonia.

Medicines Most veterinary treatments of foals are given by hypodermic syringe, but if a medicine is to be given by mouth it should be out of a baby's feeding bottle to avoid these same risks of pneumonia.

Infectious conditions A great number of bacteria affect newborn foals. They acquire the infections from their mothers, sometimes while still in the womb, or from unclean stables, especially those that have already been used for mares to produce their foals. The foal's resistance to infection is lowered by being premature, having the umbilical cord torn and tied, and by lack of colostrum if the mare has run milk before foaling.

Rossdale and Ricketts, Newmarket veterinary surgeons, have suggested in *The Practice of Equine Stud Medicine* (Baillière Tindall, London, 1974) that foal infections should be grouped under the heading of septicaemic diseases – since they all show the characteristics of a high temperature, lethargy and an accelerating reduction in the inclination to suckle from the mare. These notes are largely derived from their writings on this subject.

The onset and course of foal infections is rapid: so rapid in some cases that sudden death is the only intimation of disease.

Usually in illness a slight dullness appears on the second day after birth; then a reduction in the amount of milk taken so that the mare's udder is distended and drips milk. Soon the temperature, pulse rate and breathing rate all rise significantly, the foal stands drooped and shows no inclination to suckle the mare: the skin loses its elasticity and the eyes sink back into the head. Various systems may be particularly affected, giving rise to convulsions, diarrhoea, colic, lameness, swollen joints, or pneumonia. In a day or two untreated cases collapse, the temperature falls, and death supervenes. These generalized infections have been named according to the particular signs presented: sleepy foal disease, meningitis, joint-ill, navel-ill, scours, enteritis, pneumonia, hepatitis, and nephritis.

Treatment of isolated cases should consist of a broad-spectrum antibiotic three times a day, continued for two days after the signs of disease have subsided. For rapid and effective action the antibiotic should be injected into the spinal canal if the nervous system is involved, into the joints if they are swollen, or given by mouth in cases seriously affecting the bowels. Transfusions of whole blood or plasma from the mare may be needed if signs of anaemia appear. In outbreaks of foal diseases or when a number of cases occur in an area, sensitivity tests will indicate which antibiotic or combination of antibiotics is most likely to counter the particular infection. Careful nursing is of the first importance in saving these foals from an early death.

Maladjusted new-born foals Foals suffer from a number of conditions causing distress and disturbed behaviour that are not due to bacterial infections. Rossdale and Ricketts have again simplified a confused picture by suggesting that barkers, wanderers, dummies and convulsive foals, which are all suffering from failure to adjust to the requirements of an independent existence, should be considered maladjusted foals. The main causes of maladjustment are thought to be bleeding into the brain brought about by excessive pressures during the process of birth, or damage to the brain from an insufficient supply of oxygen. The common signs of these conditions are an increased rate of breathing, complete loss of the ability to follow the mare or to suckle even if led to the teat, and apparent blindness. The barker foals breathe so sharply that they produce a noise like a yapping terrier; the wanderers drift aimlessly around, falling over or pressing their heads against any obstruction; the dummies stand or lie unresponsive to all efforts to help them, and the foals lying in convulsions strain, twist and jump as their muscles contract in violent spasms. The temperature of maladjusted new-born foals is usually normal or sub-normal, though it may rise considerably during periods of excitement or in convulsions.

Treatment is to give phenytoin by injection or by mouth in all the conditions, to encourage sleep, and to control the nervous signs. Feeding from a bottle is needed at regular intervals. If the foal cannot suck from the bottle the feed may have to be given by stomach tube. Oxygen can be helpful and intravenous sodium bicarbonate or normal saline may be necessary to correct acidity and dehydration. Some foals affected in this way chew at quantities of straw, and this should be prevented by muzzling them between feeds. Unremitting care is worthwhile as many of these cases recover over a period of days or weeks and if recovery does occur it is complete.

The use of oxygen The foal's life depends on a constant supply of oxygen to the lungs. In pneumonia the lungs are inflamed, usually by some infection, and because the lungs – being partially blocked by catarrhal discharges – have a reduced capacity to absorb oxygen the breathing is speeded up in an attempt to improve the supply. If the placenta is separated too soon foals may be seriously deprived of oxygen before they have had time to acquire it through the lungs by establishing a proper breathing rhythm. During the process of birth some foals are starved of oxygen from the placenta by a twist in the umbilical cord, or they may be prevented from breathing by membranes lying across their nostrils. These foals may have suffered brain injury from oxygen deficiency and they are greatly helped by supplies from an oxygen cylinder. The tube from the cylinder should be attached to a plastic funnel large enough to accommodate a foal's muzzle without fitting tightly. Oxygen should be released at the rate of 4.5 litres (1 gal) a minute for just one minute while the plastic funnel is held loosely over the muzzle. Turn on and off at intervals of a minute for a quarter of an hour. By that time one should be able to judge if the treatment is helping the foal, and the effects of an increase in time and quantity may be tried and continued for another quarter of an hour. If the foal appears to have benefited one may repeat the half hour's treatment after a rest of one hour. If the foal becomes worse during that hour, further oxygen may be given immediately. Some foals may settle to comfortably established breathing after only a few minutes of oxygen supply. Others, especially pneumonia cases, may benefit from a number of half hour periods through the day and night for several days.

Persistent urachus (leaking umbilicus) While in the mare's womb the foetus produces an amount of urine, most of which passes out of the opening at the front of the bladder and empties into the main waterbed in the placenta. This opening from the bladder is the urachus. Ordinarily the urachus closes at birth, the bladder emptying itself from then on through the penis or the vulva. Occasionally the urachus fails to close completely and leaks urine through or around the stump of the umbilical cord causing raw areas of wet skin. There is usually some infection present. Treatment consists of antibiotics to counter the infection and dusting the umbilical area with a wound powder, or applying an antiseptic dressing held in place with a strip of crêpe bandage tied over the foal's back. The urachus, properly cared for, usually closes up satisfactorily in a few days.

Penis retention in foals Newly-born colt foals, soon after they have suckled for the first time, may sometimes be seen to straddle their hind legs into the staling position, but are in some distress as they can neither protrude the penis nor pass any urine. The untried penis may be found folded back in the sheath and is readily straightened by the fingers to effect a complete cure.

Meconium Within a few hours of birth foals begin to pass their first droppings. These are an accumulation, not of food, but of debris collected up in the bowels during the later stages of development as a foetus. This debris, known as meconium, is projected from the rectum for half a metre ($1\frac{3}{4}$ ft) or more and varies in consistency from moist firm segments to small hard pellets and in colour from grey to brown. It is a matter of considerable satisfaction to the stud groom to observe the foal ridding itself of the meconium, because some foals have great difficulty in passing it and show signs of colic by strenuous efforts to rid themselves of it, and sometimes by rolling on the ground or by lying on their backs with all four legs in the air. The hard lumps of meconium can be felt by passing a lubricated finger into the foal's rectum.

Treatment consists of giving enemas of soapy water from an ordinary enema syringe or inserting glycerine suppositories. A pint of equal parts of medicinal liquid paraffin and glycerine may be given by the stomach tube. This should be followed by half doses at twelve-hour intervals and treatment may have to be continued for 2 or 3 days. Success is recognized by the arrival of orange-yellow droppings which are the first sign of digested milk. Very hard knobs of meconium may be helped through the rectum with the large, smooth-headed forceps sometimes used to help a bitch when she has difficulty in delivering her puppies. It is not understood why some foals develop this trouble while the majority of foals rid themselves easily of their meconium. No satisfactory means of preventing these cases is known.

Ruptured bladder (water belly) The pressure imposed on the foal during its delivery may cause its bladder to rupture with the result that the urine leaks into its abdomen. There are no signs of this accident until, after two or three days, the accumulating urine begins to distend the foal's belly. The foal lies down more than usual, frequently attempts to pass urine without success and shows signs of abdominal pain. If the foal's belly is handled, the urine can be felt flooding from side to side, and from this the name water belly arises. An abdominal operation is required to drain off the urine and stitch up the tear in the bladder which is usually on the middle line of its upper surface. The chances of complete recovery are good.

Scrotal hernia At birth, colt foals sometimes appear to have a scrotal hernia, noticed as a very large scrotum containing the testicles and a considerable quantity of small intestines which have descended from the abdomen. This state of affairs would be serious but for the fact that within forty-eight hours the bulge has disappeared and the scrotum is normal in size. There do not appear to be any records of scrotal hernia in young foals causing any trouble at the time or later in life.

Umbilical hernia A few days or weeks after foaling, a hernia may appear at the foal's umbilicus. On examination, a gap in the wall of the abdomen can be felt through the skin, large enough to accommodate two or three fingers. Most of these umbilical hernias disappear by the time the foal is three months old. Some of them persist as an unsightly bulge, and the larger ones may contain abdominal fat that has forced its way through the tear and lies under the skin. These persisting ruptures require stitching up, an operation usually carried out when the foal is 4 or 5 months old. Occasionally some of the small intestine is pinched in the hernia giving rise to a very severe bowel injury which needs immediate surgery.

Contracted tendons Foals are sometimes born with what appear to be unusually short tendons at the back of the front legs below the knee so that they cannot put their feet flat on the ground. They try to walk on their toes but may knuckle over and end up walking on the front of the fetlock joints. If the fault is only slight the muscles accommodate themselves after a few days and the foal walks normally. More severe cases may be helped back to normal by putting each foreleg in a well padded plaster-cast below the knee while the foot is pulled as far forward as it will go. A fresh cast is applied every few days, gaining a little on the shortened tendon each time. Badly bent limbs may need the tendons to be cut through before the foot is extended and the cast applied. The severed tendons eventually re-unite, but the process is tedious and involves so much work that only valuable foals warrant this treatment. If a mild case has not been treated as a foal it may be helped later by shoeing with a toe extension which encourages the young horse to put its heel down to the ground.

Bent legs When new-born foals stand up for the first time and wobble their way to the mare's udder it may sometimes be noticed that the hind legs are both bent the same way at the hocks – so that, seen from behind, the feet are both well to the left or well to the right. Fortunately this is only due to immaturity and slackness of the ligaments and, in almost every case, the condition corrects itself in the next forty-eight hours.

Overshot and undershot jaws The foal is born with two upper and two lower incisor teeth. The upper and lower teeth should meet each other precisely. Sometimes the lower jaw is a little shorter or a little longer than it should be. This is not important if it only makes one of the rows of teeth overlap the other slightly; but if the teeth do not meet at all the growing animal will have difficulty in grazing and as the molar teeth are also likely to overlap, this can lead to more serious feeding problems. (See Dentistry.) Foals which are overshot or undershot by more than about 1 cm ($\frac{1}{2}$ in) may not be worth raising. There is no treatment for this condition, which is thought by some people to be hereditary though there does not appear to be any evidence for this.

Inturned eyelids (entropion) Young foals sometimes develop an eye injury due to the lower eyelid turning in – a condition known as entropion, in which the eyelashes rub on the eye's surface. This causes the surface of the eye to inflame, showing a spreading area turning white. Entropion is more likely to occur in sickly foals than in robust ones because the sick foal's eyes are inclined to sink back in their sockets encouraging the lids to turn in.

Treatment is simply to insert a few 1 cm ($\frac{1}{2}$ in) stitches into the skin of the eyelid, at right angles to the long axis of the eye, so that when the stitches are tied they draw the edge of the eyelid back from the eye's surface. The application of an eye ointment is needed for a few days, after which the stitches may be removed. The condition is not likely to recur.

Jaundice Jaundice in foals is a result of the mare and foal having antagonistic blood groups. The disease develops quite simply. In spite of the fact that the mare's blood and the blood of the foetus do not come into direct contact with each other, some of the blood cells from the foetus do leak through the placenta to the mare. Because the blood groups are incompatible, the mare treats these blood cells as though they were infectious bacteria and develops antibodies against them. These antibodies accumulate with others in the mare's first milk, the colostrum; and when the new-born foal suckles the colostrum it receives a massive dose of antibodies against its own blood cells. The antibodies break down the blood so rapidly that the foal becomes anaemic. The pigment from the damaged blood corpuscles causes jaundice so that after a day or two the foal's mouth and eyes and skin take on a golden-yellow colour. Unless the foal can be given a fresh supply of blood cells from another horse, which is a major operation that can only be undertaken at a fully equipped equine hospital, the foal will die. The disease can be prevented if the foal is not allowed to suck from its mother for twenty-four hours, because after that time the foal's bowel cannot absorb antibodies (which are the cause of the trouble) from the mare's milk. The difficulty is to know that the mare is producing a foal with an antagonistic blood group. A suspect mare can be checked by a weekly laboratory blood test during the last month of pregnancy. A mare that has produced a jaundiced foal is likely to do so again, so her foals should always be prevented from suckling for the first twenty-four hours. They must be fed with artificial food or, if possible, colostrum from another mare or from a colostrum bank, kept at some equine hospitals.

Foals in intensive care Premature and weak foals have a good chance of growing into normal horses if they are carefully nursed for some days to make up for their early arrival and to protect them from infection. The foals concerned are those which are unable to stand up and suckle within two hours of birth. With a little help and encouragement some foals rapidly gain strength and only need supervising and periodic aid, but there are those which need intensive care for several days or even a week or two before they have built up the required strength to manage on their own.

The room or box temperature in which the foal lies should be at 21 to 23°C (70 to 74°F) with through-ventilation using an extrac-or fan to keep the air moving if necessary, and infra-red lamps to keep the temperature up. The foal should be dressed in an insulated nylon foal-rug, and laid on a clean rug on a straw bed with a simple plastic tent over it with adequate air intake and outlet and a supplementary oxygen supply. The primary purpose of the tent is to enable the air to be boosted by oxygen tubed into the tent at about 10 litres (2 gal) a minute from an oxygen cylinder. It also helps to keep the foal in an atmospheric temperature of 22°C (72°F). The tent should be removed when the foal is to be turned or dealt with in other ways, and it and the oxygen supply can be discarded when the foal's breathing is less than 40 respirations each minute and the heart beat below 100 per minute.

The foal should be fed at hourly intervals for the first 12 hours with colostrum from the mare, about 250 to 300 ml (½ pint) at each feed: then rather larger feeds at 2-hourly intervals. After the first 24 hours this may be continued at intervals of 2 hours during the day and 3 hours at night up to 4 days, and then spaced to 3 hours by day and 4 hours at night – the milk being taken from the mare if she is able to be milked. If that source dries up the foal should be fed as suggested below for orphan foals.

The foal should never be allowed to lie for more than an hour on one side. When turned over it should be gently massaged by hand rubbing and given an opportunity to use its legs in attempts to stand up. If the first bowel evacuation, the meconium, is not passed within twelve hours of birth a gentle enema of warm soapy water should be given and repeated at six-hourly intervals until the meconium has come away and is followed by yellowish soft faeces.

It is extremely important that a weak or premature foal should receive a daily injection of an antibiotic drug for the first five days of its life.

Pneumonia in suckling foals A serious and usually fatal pneumonia may occur in foals at 3 or 4 months of age due to a bacterial infection by *Corynebacterium equi*. The signs of this disease are deceptive. The foal does not appear to be ill, just not thriving. There is some watery or gummy discharge from the nose and an inclination to follow slowly behind the mare instead of the galloping about and playing with the other foals that is usual at this age. The temperature is raised to 39°C (102°F) or a little more. It is very difficult to appreciate that the foal is really ill until, using a stethoscope, the rattling and crackling sounds in the lungs make it obvious that the foal has pneumonia. This particular infection causes the formation of large abscesses and cavities in the lungs and once these are established there is very little chance of preventing the foal's death.

The infectious organism, *Corynebacterium equi* lives in soil and once it has occurred on land used for horse breeding it is essential to move the horses to other accommodation, otherwise fatal cases will occur year after year. If affected ground is cultivated and cropped for two years it may then be safe for horses.

It seems likely that the foals take up the infection by mouth from soil in the pastures, and that some of the bacteria enter the blood stream and settle in the lungs which have been previously damaged by worm larvae migrating through the lung tissues.

This disease is not a common one but outbreaks and isolated cases occur from time to time in all parts of the world where horses are raised.

If those in charge of young foals have been alerted to this risk by previous cases or by noticing that a foal is unusually listless, a course of antibiotic treatment may restore the foal to health before the *Corynebacterium equi* has become sufficiently established to break up the lung tissue. Careful worm treatment of all horses and foals is a further safeguard that may avoid this disease.

Orphan foals

Some mares die foaling; others suffer injuries or illnesses that prevent them from producing milk; while a few refuse to have anything to do with their new-born foals. In all these cases the owner is left with a foal to rear by hand or by fostering on to some other recently foaled mare.

It should not be forgotten that a number of foals die at birth and that every year there are more mares that have lost their foals than foals that have lost their mothers. Fostering a foal on to a mare has so many advantages over hand-rearing that every effort should be made to find a bereaved mare.

The most urgent requirement for a new-born foal is colostrum. This must be provided within the first twelve hours of life because, about that time, or shortly after, the foal's intestines become unable to absorb the antibodies from the mare's colostrum which protect them from disease. If the mare is still alive but unable or unwilling to allow the foal to suckle, milk should be drawn from her udder every hour and fed to the foal from a bottle and teat. If the mare is dead it may be possible to obtain a supply of colostrum from an equine veterinary hospital, a friendly stud farm or in Great Britain from the National Foaling Bank at Newport in Salop, where colostrum is kept in deep freeze.

Antibiotic drugs are also useful as a protection against infection, and should be given daily by injecting them for the first five days.

For the next month the foal needs warmth, frequent feeds of milk, a little hay, grass and water, company and exercise; and for the next three months less milk, more hay, grass and water, small quantities of foal pellets, and exercise in company.

The ambition to hand-rear an orphan foal may be irresistible, but compared with fostering there are many drawbacks. Hand-rearing requires devoted attention for many hours a day and, in the early stages, at night as well: food has to be freshly and frequently prepared, as cow's milk is not the best substitute; and there are problems associated with exercise and grazing because foals do not know how to graze until they have it demonstrated to them! The company of another foal or at least some close association with other horses is necessary to prevent the foal becoming so orientated to humans that, in later life, it neither mixes normally with other horses nor accepts from people the disciplines of proper behaviour. Finally, the fact must be faced that hand-reared foals seldom thrive or grow as well as fostered ones.

With fostering the main problem is to persuade the mare to accept a foal that is not her own. Unfortunately, a mare with her own foal alive will never accept another foal, so the fostering must be by a mare that has lost her foal. When the foal is accepted the mare provides the necessary warmth, suitable food at the right times and at the right temperature, and teaches the foal a great many things it ought to know – by supervision, control and example. Weak or sickly foals that have been in intensive care for more than a day or two lose the instinct to suckle, and so cannot be adopted by a foster mother.

There is a third choice, that of raising foals on an automatic calf-feeding machine which mixes milk powder and warm water and delivers it by pipeline to a series of teats from which the foals can draw their meals.

Fostering

The first need when fostering orphan foals is to find a suitable foster mother. It is nearly always an urgent problem because it is unexpected. As more foals than mares die at foaling there should always be a mare available somewhere. One's own horse contacts, equine veterinary hospitals and stud farms may know of an available mare. In Great Britain the National Foaling Bank at Newport in Salop deals with about 500 foals a year and may be able to give help or advice.

Having discovered a bereaved mare, the next obstacle – the major one – is to persuade her to adopt the foal. The rapport between a mare and her foal is extremely strong and, as far as the mare is concerned, depends very largely on her acute sense of smell. To persuade her to adopt a strange foal it should be made to smell like her own foal or else her sense of smell must be confused. The dead foal's skin with the feet still attached may be draped over the orphan before it is introduced to the mare. The orphan's feet can be slipped through slits in the skin to hold it in place. If the foal's skin is not available, the afterbirth may be used instead. Otherwise, a strong smelling ointment should be smeared around the mare's nostrils and over the foal. The mare may be given a tranquillizer to make her less aware of what is going on and she should be held while the foal is allowed to suckle.

The foal is not usually as particular as the mare. It should not have been fed for several hours before the introduction and, being hungry, will be only too pleased to suckle, especially if it has already learnt the art of suckling from its own mother. If it has been bottle-fed before attempting to foster it on to a mare, it may be reluctant to suckle but in such a case care should be taken to ensure that it is really hungry. When the foal has had a little milk it should be taken away for a few minutes in the hope of rousing some maternal instinct in the mare so that she will call for the foal and be more likely to accept it on its return. Attendants to hold the mare and help the foal should wait for some time to see what progress is made with the adoption, because some mares appear to accept the foal while she is held, but will turn on it, kicking and biting, when they are left alone. In such a case the foal should be taken away for half an hour before trying again. Some more resentful mares take to a strange foal after several attempts and then turn out to be extremely possessive foster mothers. Once the mare has accepted the foal there is nothing further to do other than to treat them as a normal mare and foal.

Hand-rearing Various milk powder preparations which are specially compounded for feeding foals, are obtainable from animal foodstuff suppliers or chemists. They have the essential ingredients of a complete ration and the packages carry printed instructions about strength and quantity.

The foal should be given a drink of colostrum hourly for the first twelve hours and, after that, at intervals of two hours. If colostrum cannot be obtained the foal will manage on the milk substitute with the protection of an injection of antibiotic drugs each day for the first five days against infection.

After the first day the foal requires bottle feeding with the milk substitute every two hours through the day and at three-hourly intervals at night until the fourth day when the interval can be extended to three hours by day and four hours at night. The quantity given should be increased according to the foal's willingness to accept it, and the intervals between feeds are widened to six feeds per twenty-four hours at a fortnight, five feeds at a month, four feeds at six weeks, three feeds at two months, and one feed in the morning and one in the evening at three months of age. The foal should be persuaded to drink its milk from a bucket soon after the first month.

Orphan foals are usually independent of milk feeding soon after four months, though a daily 0.5 litres (1 pint) of cow's milk until five or six months is nourishing and simple to provide. The foals are weaned on to hay, grass, foal-nuts and water. This introduction to food should be a gradual process starting when the foals are two weeks old with very small quantities placed in front of them and frequently changed to ensure that the food is fresh. The foals will play with the food without eating much for a week or two but they will be accustomed to it by the time they find themselves hungry enough to want to eat. Water should be limited in the early weeks because, if it is always available, the foals may not clear up their full milk ration. They should be eating about 0.5 kg (1 lb) of dry food each day by the time they are eight weeks old, and as much again a month later. From then on they will not require increased rations for some time because they will be grazing freely until late autumn.

Foals require company. A foal raised in isolation for several months, except for human companionship, never establishes a comfortable relationship with other horses. It is frightened of them at first and shuns them as far as possible thereafter. This is partially obviated by raising two foals together, but an adult should be involved if possible. A quiet mare or gelding or a donkey may be stabled alongside the foal or foals so that some contact is established, and after a month or so they can share a box with advantage. Foals need the example of an adult. Turned into a field without an older animal they have no idea of grazing but just wait anxiously at the gate to be brought in for their next feed. They also need exercise from very early life and will soon learn to be led in a halter; but, from three to four weeks, if the weather is suitable, they will take a lot of exercise in company in a paddock, with intervals of sound and healthy sleep in the open air.

The first two or three months of a foal's life are not likely to be uneventful: digestive upsets and coughs and colds may cause setbacks, and it requires a fund of determination and optimism to continue ministering to a dejected foal that appears to be losing condition day after day. They have remarkable powers of recovery, and it may all have been worth while but rearing foals by hand can lead to terrible disappointments and fostering has many advantages.

Automatic foal feeders Automatic milk dispensers are frequently used for raising groups of calves. The system is directly applicable to foals especially if several orphan foals are to be raised. The machine mixes a given quantity of milk powder and warm water and delivers it to a small tank and then by pipeline to a number of teats set in the walls of the foals' boxes or, later, to inverted funnels from which the older foals can drink. When the mixture in the tank falls to a certain level the machine produces a further supply. Foals need company, and single foals do not thrive on this system, nor is it suitable for very small numbers of foals because the machine needs a fair amount of attention and maintenance is not worth while unless several foals are benefiting.

The advantages are that a foster mother does not have to be found for each foal; the foals do not need a great deal of individual attention; and they do not develop a fixation for the person supplying them with food, because they get that from a teat in the wall or a plastic funnel for which they are not likely to develop a lifelong attachment. Their milk consumption may reach as high as

25 litres ($5\frac{1}{2}$ gal) a day at three months of age.

Two foals in a box are company for each other for six weeks or so. Thorough ventilation in the boxes is essential to avoid coughs and colds. As they get older and more active, the foals are better in more roomy accommodation which a group can share with the tutor pony or donkey so essential to the foals' outdoor training.

Foals raised in this way may tend to become obese and constipated. This should be corrected by adding laxatives to the feed and increasing their exercise.

Foals requiring intensive care can be raised on this system. If they cannot suckle from the wall teat they must be fed from a bottle with a teat that will dribble the milk, or from a bowl. When they have learnt to drink from a bowl they can take their meals from the plastic funnel.

Foals and yearlings

Care of the feet Foal's feet at birth are soft and rubbery. They harden to some extent as they come into use, but considerable flexibility remains until the true and harder horn has grown down from the coronet reaching the bottom of the hoof wall at about five months.

Foals at pasture seldom require any attention to their feet. Those running on exceptionally soft ground may suffer from lack of wear so that the overgrown feet spread and break at the edges, allowing gravel to work into the white line. On unusually hard ground foals may wear their feet away too fast, especially at the toe, and develop high heels and contracted feet. A look round once a month by a farrier is a wise precaution to ensure that the feet are kept in good order. An added advantage is that this accustoms the young animals to having their feet held and trimmed, so that a battle with the farrier is avoided when regular shoeing begins.

Some foals are born with bent fetlock joints or with feet that turn in or out. Others develop one or other of these stances as they grow. These defects of conformation do not correct themselves: they steadily increase and throw the joints off-balance as far as the knee, causing the rapidly developing bones to grow out of alignment. Corrective shoeing in later life may be too late. Correction by rasping the feet can begin at the age of one month to guide foot growth and to keep the joints level. When the hoof wall is hard enough at six months of age to hold the shoeing nails, light tips or half-shoes can be used if correction is still needed; but the most important adjustments are made by the early use of the rasp.

Upright pasterns Some foals at the age of from three to five months quite suddenly develop a stilted action with a re-alignment of the fore feet so that the heels do not reach the ground and the foot appears blocky, its front line approaching the vertical. The fetlock joints are often swollen. This condition occurs most frequently at stud farms where the mares and foals are carefully tended and stabled at night. Such horses are generously fed in the stable and, on wet and cold days, are often kept in or only turned out for a few hours. The bad action and the stumpy feet result from a combination of over-feeding with excessively rich milk and unlimited supplies of manger food, and from lack of exercise at a time when the foal's limbs are growing fast. It is an interesting aspect of bio-mechanics that tendon lengthening cannot keep up with the speed of growth of the cannon bones and the stronger flexor tendons at the back of the limb pull harder than the extensor tendons in front and cause the fetlock joint to become upright.

Treatment of the condition is rapidly effective if the mare and foal are left out in the field both day and night with little or no supplementary feeding. This should cause no hardship as there is likely to be an adequate supply of summer grazing, and both mare and foal soon accustom themselves to the vagaries of the weather.

Prevention of the disease on farms where it has occurred consists of altering the management of the mares and foals so that the foals do not grow too fast for their own healthy development. This is most easily accomplished by turning them out with their mothers and leaving them out except in the worst weather conditions.

Upright fetlocks Yearlings may suddenly become upright in their fetlock joints, usually in the summer months when they are at pasture. The fetlock area thickens and there may be lameness. One or both forelegs may be affected.

The cause is over-feeding in the same way that foals suddenly develop upright feet. Because the condition appears in the summer months it is often attributed to the hard ground; but the basic cause is the very high nutritive value of summer grazing, which is probably being supplemented with generous grain feeding to improve the animals' condition at a time when they are becoming a saleable commodity.

Treatment and prevention of this condition are both related to food intake. Supplementary feeding should be stopped and the yearlings should be pastured on poorer land if that is available, or grazed over paddocks that have had the flush of grass eaten off by other stock. This treatment does not stunt their growth, it only delays it – a great advantage, since horses grow soft bone fast or hard bone slowly and soft-boned animals have short working careers.

Colts and stallions

Colts are uncastrated young male horses. They start off as colt foals; the following year they are yearling colts; the next, two-year-old colts, and so on. If they are castrated they become geldings. Colts that are used for breeding are spoken of as stallions when they start their stud duties. Those that are neither gelded nor used at stud may continue to be called colts indefinitely, though in some breeds they are known as 'entire' horses, or just as 'horses' from the age of four.

Well nourished colts can mate successfully while they are yearlings: that is, during the summer of the year after their birth. Such matings are avoided as far as possible in horses under control because more dependable matings by older horses are usually desired. These precocious activities are unlikely to occur in groups of horses running free, because food shortages limit the development of the colts and they are exposed to the authority and rivalry of older horses. Two-year-old colts may sire a number of mares and a reasonable fertility rate is likely. But it is more usual to use 3- or 4-year-olds, by which time the horse will be well developed and, at 4, capable of mating a full complement of mares (which may be forty or more). This can continue until over the age of 20, when a natural decline is likely to reduce the stallion's vigour and fertility.

Colts running free with mares or fillies have little or no difficulty in mating with them when they come in season. It is the colts that have been broken and disciplined for riding or driving and are suddenly presented with a mare ready for service that are likely to be shy and difficult. They have not had the opportunity of prenuptial play that leads naturally to the physical and mental developments that are desirable for the sexual act and, furthermore, they are confused by the presence of men to whom they have learned to be subservient. Even the shyest young horse will gradually overcome his inhibitions if he is treated with patience and given time to become adjusted to his new role. There is no reason why such a horse should not continue with other activities for which he has been trained.

In many establishments the stallion is set aside to be used for stud purposes only. This may keep him fully occupied during the mating season with little time or vigour for other activities; but if, for the remaining 6 or 7 months of the year, he is stabled away from other horses and given no work to do, he is likely to become sour in temperament and put on fat. This leads to his acquiring a reputation for being dangerous and, in consequence, he is liable to become more isolated and his exercise more limited so that he develops a fatty heart leading to decreasing vigour and early death. Stallions do far better if they are regularly ridden or driven – not just for exercise, but given actual work to do. They then remain disciplined and amenable, keep much fitter and retain their vigour for stud duties for years longer than they would if they were treated as something too precious or too dangerous to put to work.

Male infertility The purpose of keeping a colt or stallion is that he shall be able to reproduce his kind. His reputation depends on his fertility record. Infertility may be due to some disease on the part of the mare, but that only means one foal the fewer. A sterile stallion may mean no foals at all, while one of poor fertility may result in only a small proportion of the mares becoming pregnant.

Stallion infertility is not a common complaint, though it may occur in horses that are too young or too old, or in animals that are in poor health from improper feeding, or from neglect – and it may be associated with such diseases as dourine and brucellosis. Stallions that have become savage from being shut away and inadequately worked are sometimes underfed to reduce their tendency to be aggressive, and these may well be infertile in consequence. Horses which have been pushed in early life for maximum development and performance by the use of corticosteroid preparations are often infertile and cause great disappointment if, after a successful career, they are put to stud and produce no offspring. Nearly all these cases of stallion sterility not traceable to a particular disease will recover with proper feeding and exercise, but one or more crops of foals may have been lost and the horse's reputation degraded.

Castration Male horses are usually castrated, by complete removal of the testicles and associated ducts, if they are not likely to be required for breeding purposes. This is because colts and stallions become difficult to manage as they get older and they need to be kept away from fillies and mares during the breeding season, which creates huge difficulties over paddock fencing. Also, if they are highly fed for strenuous or competitive activities, they are likely, in the presence of mares, to fail to give proper attention to the work in hand. The view that castration is unnecessary is sometimes expressed and is supported by seeing stallions and mares in some countries working steadily together throughout the year. These are cold-blooded draught horses which are naturally amenable and are not comparable to the lighter, more active breeds used in sporting and competitive activities. Nevertheless, colts and stallions are used by some horsemen for riding and driving in competitive events, and it is beneficial that stallions at stud should be involved in such activities out of the breeding season; but these horses need to be in the hands of fully experienced people who have firm control of their animals.

Castration is usually carried out when the colt is two years old. Some breeders have colt foals operated on at the age of three months, as being less disturbing to a suckling foal than to a horse later in life. This may be true, but there is a rather higher risk of scrotal hernia following the operation in foals and it is probably to their advantage to have the benefit of male hormones derived from the sexual organs during their early growth period. Other breeders carry this last point further and maintain that the colt should be allowed to grow to full masculine stature before being castrated. This would postpone the operation to five years of age and defeat the main purpose of gelding the animals, which is to prevent troublesome behaviour. In the spring about two years after their birth remains the time at which most colts are castrated.

Colts are usually castrated under a general anaesthetic given by hypodermic injection which causes them to fall unconscious to the ground. This complete control, even though the horse is unaware of it except during the recovery period, appears to have the effect of permanently subduing the animal, helping in the process of accustoming it to discipline. This effect of complete control was known to the great horse-breakers of the 19th century, such as Galvayne and Hayes, who depended on casting horses to the ground with ropes and manpower as the basis of their subjugation of vicious horses. Some racehorse trainers do not wish their colts to have their sense of freedom and independence reduced in this way and they prefer to have their animals castrated under local anaesthesia. The operation is the same but the animal remains standing, controlled by the bridle and a twitch. The standing operation is able to be performed without pain or distress on horses that have already been well handled and are accustomed to grooming and head harness.

Rigs Rigs are colts in which one or both testicles have failed to migrate from the abdomen into the scrotum during the development of the foetus. Testicles retained in the abdomen do not produce fertile sperm. If neither testicle has descended the animal appears to be a gelding but behaves like a colt. It is more usual that only one testicle is retained in the abdomen while the other is present in the scrotum. If this one is removed by a castrator and the other left in the abdomen, again the animal resembles a gelding but retains coltish behaviour and will mate with mares. Rigs are objectionable in that the condition is hereditary and likely to occur in their male offspring; their fertility rate is low, and their behaviour is more coltish than colts. Rigs should be castrated and this usually involves an abdominal operation.

Some geldings show signs of sexual interest in mares. This is due to the production of male hormones from other tissue than the removed testicles. Such horses are sometimes known as 'rough-cut' – implying that the castrator has not removed the usual amount of extra tissues associated with the testicles. This is not often the case though some lose their masculinity if more tissue is removed from the scrotum. Rough-cut geldings are considered by some horsemen to have extra competitive spirit. Such geldings are seldom capable of mating with mares, and certainly cannot get them in foal. They usually lose their sexual interest as they become older and more fully involved in other activities.

There are sometimes difficulties in determining if an animal is a rather masculine gelding or an actual rig. This question can be settled with a high degree of accuracy by a laboratory test for the concentration of male hormones in blood samples.

Masturbation Two-year-old colts in racing stables on the routine of concentrated feeding and long hours of idleness may develop the habit of masturbating by rubbing the erected penis against the belly. Ivory or plastic rings about 35 mm ($1\frac{1}{2}$ in) in diameter, known as 'pollution rings', may be slipped on to the penis to lie in the groove just behind its terminal cap to discourage them by causing pain when the penis becomes distended. A natural wax accumulates on these rings and they need cleaning from time to time. They can be dangerous, causing pain and swelling if forgotten about, or if the colt is transferred to another stable which is not informed of the ring. If there is difficulty in removing the rings they should be cut or broken. Many trainers ignore masturbation as the colts usually discontinue the practice as their work increases.

Symptoms chart

Appearance and behaviour as indications of health, injury or disease

Symptom	Cause
The whole horse	
Unable to move (standing)	broken limb, acute laminitis, azoturia, tetanus, injured back
Unable to move (lying)	lack of oxygen, winded, broken back, cast, heart trouble, embolism
Throwing itself down	acute colic, stubborn temper
Swaying or reeling action	exhaustion, spinal or pelvic injury, wobbler, failing heart
Rolling, at grass or in stable	relaxation
Getting up and down and rolling repeatedly	colic pains
Lying on back or in other awkward positions	colic pains, cast
Marked changes in temperament	excitement, fright, rabies
Not feeding	mouth injury or tooth trouble or disease, pain, general infection, unsuitable food
Loss of general alertness	general infection, pain, heart trouble
Easily tired	unfit, fat, pregnant, old age, heart trouble, general infection
Swellings	abscess, haemotoma, gas gangrene, purpura haemorrhagica, failing heart
The skin	
Short hair, shiny coat with supple skin	natural in summer
Long hair, matted greasy coat with supple skin	natural in horse not worked in winter
Dull, dry coat with skin difficult to pick up	starvation, worms, indigestion, tooth problems
Spots and pimples	acne, urticaria, ringworm, filarial worms, warbles, glanders (farcy), ulcerative lymphangitis, epizootic lymphangitis

Symptom	Cause
Sores	galls, sit-fast, wounds, warbles, sweet-itch, photo-sensitization, rain-scald, bursati, sporotrichosis
Lumps and growths	warts, abscesses, haemotoma, sebaceous cysts, bursitis, actinomycosis, actinobacillosis
Tense or soft swellings	abscess, haemotoma, gas gangrene, purpura haemorrhagica, failing heart
White hair marks	result of galls from saddle, rug, rope or girth injury, insect bites
White patches of skin near lips or eyes	leucoderma
Loss of hair: diffuse or patchy	natural in spring
Loss of hair: patchy and scaly	mange
Loss of hair: on mane and tail	lice, sweet-itch
Loss of hair: on tail	tail rubbing, pin worms
Pale insect eggs on hair	bots
The limbs	
One whole leg swollen: fore leg to elbow or hind leg to stifle	lymphangitis
Short pace with any limb	lame that leg
Tripping, stumbling	foot too long, pain in foot, arthritis, blindness
Limbs advanced, weight back on the heels	acute laminitis
Fore foot resting on toe	lame that leg
Hind foot resting on toe:	
occasionally	natural
continuously	pain that leg
One fore foot placed in advance of other	navicular disease
Fore foot dragged	shoulder injury, dropped elbow
Hind foot dragged	hip injury
Hind foot extended back and fixed	slipped stifle
Hind legs paralysed	pelvic or spinal injury, thrombosis, azoturia, wobbler
Striking with fore feet	offence or defence
Scraping with fore feet	pain, excitement
Kicking the box walls	loneliness, boredom
Head nodding as fore foot meets the ground	lame other limb

Symptom	Cause
Hock points covering different range of action	lame in leg having less range of action
Kicking at belly	colic pains
Foreleg stilted action (young stock)	upright pasterns
The feet	
Long foot	overgrown
Short foot	slow growth
Mis-shapen foot	chronic laminitis, blocky foot
The sole:	
Pain on pressure	thin, corn, bruise, burn, puncture, abscess
Convex sole	dropped sole, chronic laminitis
The frog:	
Pain on pressure	thrush, foreign body
Wet discharge	thrush, canker
The wall:	
Pain on pressure	acute laminitis, gravel abscess, nail bind, prick, arthritis, fracture, keratoma
Ridges on wall	grass rings, chronic laminitis
Concave front of wall	chronic laminitis
Front wall separating from the toe	seedy toe
Wall bulged in front	keratoma
The Coronet:	
Pain on pressure	tread, ringbone, quittor, sandcrack, thorn
Discharging coronet	tread wound, quittor, foot abscess
Coronet prominent in front	ringbone, subluxation
Coronet prominent at sides	sidebones
The hoof heels:	
High narrow heels	contracted foot, thrush
The foreleg and the pastern	
Heels:	
Sore and inflamed heels	cracked heels, mud-fever, rope gall
Moist discharging heels	mud-fever, horse pox
Thick ridged skin in heels	grease
Sensitive knob each side of back tendon	un-nerving neuroma
Bony enlargement on the pastern front or sides	ringbone
Tender mid-line of pastern	split pastern, thorn
The fetlock joint:	
Wounds or scars inner side	brushing

Symptom	Cause
Wounds or scars on front of joint	knuckling over
Wounds or scars at back of joint	over-reach
Swollen fetlock joint	joint-ill, bursitis
Small lateral swellings	wind-galls
Diffuse swelling over and behind joint	poor circulation
Vertical line of swelling over front of joint	bruised extensor tendon sheath
Bony enlargements at the sides of the joint	periostitis, rickets, ankle bones
Thickened joint	jarred joint, strained joint ligament
Upright joint	strained tendons, upright pasterns in young stock
Joint in advance of hoof	knuckled over, old age, pain in foot, strained tendons, subluxation
Pain on flexion of fetlock joint	sesamoiditis, ringbone
Sensitive knob each side of back tendon	un-nerving neuroma
The cannon bone:	
Tender mid-line front of cannon bone	crack, fracture, thorn, bruised extensor tendon
Diffuse tenderness in front	sore shins
Insensitive bulging front	bucked shins
Bony swelling on splint bone	splint, fractured splint bone
The back tendons:	
Diffuse swelling	filled leg, poor circulation
Swelling confined to tendon area	inflamed tendon sheath
Swollen tendons; soft and painful	recent tendon strain or injury
Swollen tendons; hard and painless	old tendon strain or injury
Tender between tendons and cannon bones	strained suspensory ligament
The knee	
Knee painful when flexed	arthritis, fracture
Vertical line of swelling over front of knee	bruised extensor tendon sheath
Front of knee tender	bruise, thorn
Small fluid swellings	popped knee, synovitis
Acute pain back of the knee	fractured accessory carpal bone
Scaly skin back of the knee	eczema

Symptom	Cause
The elbow:	
Elbow joint held low, leg dragged	dropped elbow, shoulder paralysis
Swollen point of elbow	capped elbow
Point of elbow painful and movable	fractured bone
Flexion of elbow joint painful	arthritis
The shoulder:	
Bony bulge at shoulder joint	dislocated joint
Pain and swelling above the shoulder joint	fractured shoulder blade
Pain and swelling below the shoulder joint	torn muscles or fractured humerus
Wasted muscles above the shoulder joint	muscle injury, nerve damage
Pain on drawing shoulder mass away from body	damaged pectoral muscles
Pain at point of shoulder	fractured shoulder blade point, arthritis
The hind leg	
The foot to the hock:	
As fore limb except:	no navicular disease, wear of shoe at toe indicates spavin
The hock:	
Bony swelling low on the inner front of the hock	spavin
Soft swelling low on the inner front of the hock	bog spavin
Soft bulging swelling in front of the point of the hock	thoroughpin
Hard thickening (sometimes soft bulge) low on back line of hock	curb
Swelling on the point of the hock	capped hock
Tendon usually riding over cap of the hock diverted to run outside the hock joint	slipped flexor tendon
The stifle:	
Swelling over the stifle	bursitis
The hip:	
Point of the hip flattened	hip down, minor pelvic fracture
The buttock:	
Point of the buttock flattened	minor pelvic fracture

Symptom	Cause
The head	
Swelling on poll	bursitis, poll-evil
Swellings on face	tooth root infection, sinusitis, osteomalacia, osteodystrophy, urticaria, purpura haemorrhagica, African horse sickness
Pink skinned and white haired areas inflamed	photosensitization, blue-nose
Head shaking, head tossing	painful bit, ear irritation, head pain, tooth trouble
Head pressing against wall	brain injury or disease, colic pain
Turning head to flanks	colic pains
Ears laid back	temper
Ears excessively active	blindness
Raising head and turning upper lip back	assessment of a smell
Tucking chin in and swallowing air	wind sucking, crib-biting
The eyes	
Eye kept closed	injury, irritation, foreign body, periodic ophthalmia
Tears running on face	irritation, entropion, blocked tear duct
Eye white filmed	injury, ulcer, entropion
White mark on eye	scar from previous injury
Growth on eye	dermoid cyst
Protrusion from eye	punctured eyeball
Sunken eye	punctured eyeball
Both eyes sunken	emaciation, dehydration
3rd eyelid seen	emaciation, dehydration, tetanus
Permanently distended pupil	blindness, brain damage
Slightly triangular upper lid	periodic ophthalmia
Opaque area in lens	cataract
The mouth	
Mouth and eye membranes, pink	healthy
pale to white	anaemia, shock, internal haemorrhage
primrose to yellow	jaundice
orange to dark red	infection, toxaemia
blood flecked	virus infection
Saliva dripping	irritant, ulcer, loose tooth crown or other foreign body
Blood in saliva	ulcer, mouth wound from teeth or foreign body

Symptom	Cause
Food rejected from mouth	ulcer, wound, sharp teeth
Inflamed gums	new teeth erupting, peridontal disease
Angled wear on front teeth	crib-biting
Sour smell from mouth	lodged food, ulcer, indigestion
Food rejected from nostrils	oesophageal obstruction, choke pharyngitis
Food bolted	hunger, excitement, tooth trouble or bad habit
Eating earth, twigs, bark, planking	natural source of minerals, vitamins, savoury tit-bits
Eating droppings	indigestion, worms
The lower jaw	
Lump on jaw bone	halter damage
Swellings under jaw bones	infected tooth roots or sockets
Scabby swellings between jaw bones	glands infected from mouth or throat
Fluid swelling	poor circulation
Limited movement	tetanus, strangles
The nose and throat	
Throat swellings	strangles, guttural pouch infection, purpura haemorrhagica, anthrax, African horse sickness, haemorrhagic septicaemia
Swelling on side of larynx	enlarged thyroid gland
Coughing	any respiratory infection, dry food in throat, lung worms
Nasal catarrh, watery	irritant, virus infection
Nasal catarrh, thick	any respiratory infection, tooth root infection
Blood from nostril	broken wind, guttural pouch ulcer, ethmoid haemangioma
Food or water from nostril	oesophageal obstruction, choke pharyngitis
Stinking breath	diseased tooth root, ulcer
Breathing	
Rapid breathing assisted by abdominal muscles	exertion, respiratory infection, general infection
Rapid breathing assisted by double action of abdominal muscles	broken wind

Symptom	Cause
Snorting, at rest or at various paces	natural expression of fear, exhibitionism or habit
Noisy inhalation	roaring or whistling
Groaning while sleeping	contentment
Grunting when shocked or threatened with stick	roaring, whistling, pleurisy
Short grunt when jumping	back pain, arthritis
Choking up when galloping	soft palate disease
Whinnying	communication, loneliness
The neck	
Blood pulsing in jugular groove	jugular pulse
Painful turning	arthritis, fracture, muscular strain
The back	
Tender withers	saddle gall, rug gall
Swollen withers	bursitis, fistulous withers, fractures
Small mid-line swellings	bursitis
Mid-line scab	setfast
Pain over loins	setfast, azoturia
Grunting or hollowing back when girthed or mounted	spinal arthritis
Bucking	spinal arthritis, high spirits
Not lowering spine under fingernail pressure	spinal arthritis, muscle injury
Stiff back, turning like a ship	spinal arthritis, muscle injury
Discomfort in backing or turning in tight circle	back injury, arthritis
Unequal outline to quarters	muscle wasting, fractured point of hip, displaced pelvis
Tail trembling when backed	shivering
Tail and croup muscles slack	croup paralysis
Erratic gait, hindquarters	spinal or pelvic injury, jinked back, wobbler, exhaustion, failing heart
Paralysed hindquarters	iliac thrombosis, embolism, back injury
The belly	
Painful signs	colic, mare in-foal, impending foaling, foals – retained meconium
Distended belly	excess fat, wind from indigestion or colic, mares – in-foal, foals – ruptured bladder
Small belly with poor condition	starvation, indigestion, chronic disease
Small belly with good condition	extreme fitness
Umbilical swelling	hernia, foals – joint-ill, persistent urachus

Symptom	Cause
The anus	
Grey scum around anus	pin worms
Black growths around anus	melanoma
Pink fleshy mass protruding from anus	anal prolapse
Droppings	
Lemon-sized boluses that break on falling	normal
Small hard droppings	indigestion, fever
Soft watery droppings	diarrhoea, worms
Droppings streaked with mucus	indigestion
Blood in droppings	bowel infection, colitis-X, intussusception
Whole grains of corn in droppings	tooth trouble, indigestion
Foul smelling droppings	indigestion, bowel infection
Stubby maggots in droppings	bots
Large white worms or small red worms in droppings	worms
Occasionally passing wind with or without droppings	normal
Passing excessive amounts of wind repeatedly	indigestion
Urine	
Urine turbid, primrose-yellow to light brown	normal
Urine in excessive quantity and pale	kidney irritation or infection
Urine colour of black coffee	azoturia
Horse straddling to urinate but passing no urine	colic, bladder inflammation
The penis	
Penis not protruded to pass urine	smegma accumulation in sheath
Ulcers on penis	coital exanthema
The scrotum	
One testicle slightly larger than the other	normal
Testicles enlarged and tender	infection
Only one testicle in scrotum	rig
No testicles in scrotum	gelding or rig

Symptom	Cause
The vulva	
Vulval lips opening and shutting a few times after urinating	normal
Squealing and kicking, opening and shutting lips of vulva and emitting small squirts of urine especially if touched on the quarters	in season
Persisting in season as above for weeks	nymphomania
Discharge from vulva	womb infection, abortion
Ulcers on vulva	coital exanthema
Aspirating air through vulva	wind sucking, fluter
Hind legs apart and croup lowered	normal urinating position
Urinating position and straining	impending foaling
Urinating position, straining and white bladder showing from vulva	foaling in progress
Straining for half an hour and no bladder showing	foaling obstruction
Purple membranes protruding from vulva after foaling	placental membranes being shed naturally
Large red bladder protruding from vulva after foaling	prolapsed womb
The udder	
Mare NOT in-foal, udder tense and painful	infection
Mare in-foal, enlarging udder	approaching foaling
Thin straw-coloured fluid from udder	approaching foaling
Wax on teats	impending foaling
Sticky thick yellowish milk secreted from udder a day or two before and a day or two after foaling	colostrum
Thin fluid milk from a day or two after foaling	normal milk
Udder tense and painful a day or two after foaling	foal not sucking, infection

Symptom	Cause
Foals	
New-born foals (up to 3 or 4 days old) weak, sleepy, dull, diarrhoea, distressed breathing, lameness, swollen umbilicus, swollen joints, collapse, cold and clammy, unable to stand, no interest in sucking	infection of new-born foals
New-born foals (up to 3 or 4 days old) wandering, headpressing, blindness, convulsions, spasmodic breathing, no interest in sucking	maladjusted new-born foal
Unsuccessful attempts to pass droppings	retained meconium, colic
Damp umbilicus	persisting urachus
Unsuccessful attempts to urinate	penis folded in sheath, retained meconium, colic, ruptured bladder
Swollen belly	ruptured bladder
Older foals	
Eating other horses' droppings	normal diet adjustment
Coughing	worms, foal pneumonia
Stilted gait	upright pasterns

Index

Frank Manolson
C is for Cat £1

The comprehensive guide to every aspect of cats and their care. This handbook covers everything that cat owners need to know about the habits, personality and problems of their pets.

'An encyclopedia worth its weight in gold' DAILY TELEGRAPH

D is for Dog £1

The comprehensive guide to the care, training and upbringing of all well-known breeds of dog. This invaluable handbook covers everything from choosing a breed to exercising and grooming.

Dick Moller and Jeffrey Feinman
21 days to a trained dog £1·25

A new, effective and humane approach to training your puppy or full-grown dog. In only 21 days, your dog will sit, heel, stand, stay, lie down and come when called – not out of fear, but out of delight in pleasing you. Basing their technique on natural behaviour patterns, the authors show how to raise a happy, obedient dog, how to break bad habits and control the dog on crowded streets, and how to teach advanced commands, with a complete section on housetraining puppies. Fully illustrated, with an introduction by Stanley Dangerfield.

John Slater

Just Off the Motorway £1·95

The new and enlarged edition of a sensational bestseller. Introduction by Russell Harty.

Here's the new, bang-up-to-date edition of the handbook everyone needs. Detailed research, careful sampling, and more than 150 maps show where you can find any service you require – cheaper and better – by turning off at a junction and driving no more than three miles off the Motorway – eating, drinking, overnight stops, breakdown services, petrol, visits.

'Worth a detour to buy it' DAILY MAIL

Cyril A. Reilly and Renee Travis Reilly

An Irish Blessing £2·25

The traditional blessing of old Ireland draws its imagery from the soft green landscape, the sparkling waters and the warm-hearted folk of Erin's isle. Each line of the time-honoured verse is brought to life in this interpretation, in superb colour photographs that will transport you to the blue lakes of Killarney, to the misty headlands of Connemara, and to the sea roads of Donegal.

David Taylor

Zoovet 75p

The drowning Hippo ... the arthritic Giraffe ... the Killer Whale with ulcers ... all just part of a day's work for the flying animal-doctor whose missions of mercy take him to Loch Ness, Arabia and Red China, as he answers cables from zoos, circuses and wildlife parks across the globe.

'Good humour and abounding energy on every page' WASHINGTON POST

'Wildly funny' SUNDAY MIRROR

John Holgate
Make a Cow Laugh 85p

To give up commuter life for the daily grind of a Welsh border farm takes something special. You might need imagination, dedication or just sheer lunacy ... but you do need a sense of humour!

'Packed with humorous incidents ... if his farming is as good as his writing he should have left London years ago' WESTERN MAIL

On a Pig's Back 85p

John Holgate and Family, suburbanites turned farmers, have not only survived their first year on the land ... they even seem to be getting good at it! Their increasing confidence, however, is not always justified by results as they tackle the muck-spreading and cow-chasing, haymaking and harvest ... all to the wry amusement of the locals round the bar of The Forge.

'Hilarious' SUNDAY EXPRESS

Rob Buckman
Out of Practice 95p

Do you need a course of yellow fever injections to enter a Chinese restaurant? Did your father ever strip naked, do handsprings against the bathroom door while shrieking out French irregular verbs? No? Between the covers of this book lurk the innermost thoughts and crazy experiences of a practising medic – the only man to invent a cure for which there is no known disease. Illustrated by Bill Tidy, this hilarious book's author is still a practising registrar in a London hospital.

'The funniest thing to come out of a hospital since Richard Gordon' SHERIDAN MORLEY

Edward Vernon

Practice Makes Perfect 85p

Out in the waiting room lurk a confused old lady, a timid vet, a puzzled diabetic, a lonely housewife, a hypochondriac athlete, a tipster with an ulcer, a nun with dandruff, and a persistent young lady with abundant charms and perfect health!

Inside the surgery there is the general practitioner, filling out countless forms, outwitting the pill-freaks, destroying indestructible plastic syringes, watching pharmaceutical salesmen fill his office with gimmickry, and dreading the small hours phone call from a patient with a hangover!

'An entertaining and often hilarious look behind the surgery door... make a bedside book of it' DAILY TELEGRAPH

Practise What You Preach 95p

More medical misadventures with the harrassed Dr Vernon, who takes over a new practice in the Midlands... There's the embarrassed vicar with a guilty secret, a private patient who pays him to keep her ill, a beautiful young creature who insists on being examined in the bath, a marble-swallower (aged six), and other trials to keep a GP practising.

The hilarious sequel to *Practice Makes Perfect.*